T0321449

Vitamins and Cancer

Experimental Biology and Medicine

Vitamins and Cancer

**Human Cancer Prevention by
Vitamins and Micronutrients**

Edited by

**Frank L. Meyskens, Jr.
and Kedar N. Prasad**

Humana Press • Clifton, New Jersey

Library of Congress Cataloging-in-Publication Data
Main entry under title:

Vitamins and cancer.

(Experimental biology and medicine)
"The Second International Conference on the Modulation and Mediation
of Cancer by Vitamins was held in Tuscon, Arizona, from February 10-13,
1985"--
Pref.
   Includes index.
   1. Vitamin therapy--Congresses. 2. Cancer--Prevention--Congresses.
3. Vitamins in human nutrition--Congresses. I. Meyskens, F.L. (Frank L.)
II. Prasad, Kedar N. III. International Conference on the Modulation and
Mediation of Cancer by Vitamins (2nd : 1985 : Tucson, Ariz.) IV.
Series: Experimental biology and medicine (Clifton, N..) [DNLM: 1.
Neoplasms--drug therapy--congresses. 2. Neoplasms--prevention &
control--congresses. 3. Vitamins--therapeutic use--congresses. QZ
267 V8365 1985]
RC271.V58V58 1986   616.99'4'0654   85-27134
ISBN 0-89603-094-6

© 1986 The Humana Press Inc.
Crescent Manor
PO Box 2148
Clifton, NJ 07015

Printed in the United States of America

PREFACE

In the past five years, a surprising and intense resurgence in interest in vitamins and other micronutrients and their role in health and disease has occurred. The recognition has emerged that vitamins not only are essential for life in that severe nutritional deficiencies occur in their absence, but that these compounds may also serve as natural inhibitors of cancer. Synthetic alterations of the basic vitamin A molecule have also resulted in the production of compounds that are more potent as anticancer agents than the natural substance and may have substantial therapeutic activity as well. Whether other vitamins can be changed or altered to produce a better anticancer effect than the native compound has been little explored to date, but should be a fruitful pursuit for future study.

In our concluding remarks to the First International Conference in 1982, we speculated that rapid advances in our understanding of vitamins would occur in the next few years and that large-scale intervention trials of vitamins as preventive agents in defined human populations would be started. This anticipated generation of data on vitamins and their interactions has proceeded rapidly and the importance of interactions between vitamins and other micronutrients in the prevention setting has become better appreciated. Currently, more than 25 intervention trials with a variety of target populations using vitamins and other micronutrients have been started, but it remains too early for meaningful analysis of the results to date. A number of major methodological issues concerning prevention trials in humans have been identified, and difficult areas of experimental design, choice and administration of agents, and compliance have been extensively addressed. The proper execution of these trials clearly requires very careful experimental design and input to varying degrees from epidemiologists, nutritionists, pharmacologists, and basic scientists to assure their success.

A large group of investigators from the sciences of cell biology, biochemistry, nutrition, oncology, epidemiology, and public health have contributed to our new knowledge of vitamins. The positive interactions between individuals in these diverse disciplines during and following our First International Conference suggested that a second conference would be productive. The Second International Conference on the Modulation and Mediation of Cancer by Vitamins was held in Tucson, Arizona, from February 10–13, 1985. The series of papers in these proceedings indicate the excitement and breadth of science that human prevention trials must encompass to be successful.

Frank L. Meyskens, Jr.
Kedar N. Prasad

INTRODUCTION AND
FUTURE PERSPECTIVES

Kedar N. Prasad and Frank L. Meyskens, Jr.

Animal data have convincingly established that optimal intake of certain supplemental nutrients reduces the risk of cancer induced by a
wide range of tumor initiators and promoters, whereas a decreased
intake of some nutrients enhances cancer risk. Examples of protective
nutrients include vitamins A, C, and E, as well as folic acid and selenium. The effects of these nutrients are both site- and tumor-specific.

A standard approach to test the relationship between vitamin intake and the risk of cancer in human beings has been to perform epidemiological investigations. However, the results have not always
been consistent. Frequently this may be because they have measured
only one or two biological parameters of the many that are involved
in human carcinogenesis.

Human cancers are the result of extracellular and cellular events,
as well as host-mediated events; therefore, in any epidemiological
study the crucial parameters of all relevant events should probably be
measured in order to generate consistent data. For example, extracellular events include the formation of nitrosamine in the stomach from
nitrate and biogenic amines and the formation of fecal mutagens
from a variety of food substances, especially meat. These extracellular events may be more important for some tumors than others. Both
vitamin C and alpha-tocopherol may block the formation of nitrosamines and also reduce the level of fecal mutagens. The combined effects of vitamin C and alpha-tocopherol would be expected to be
greater than the individual vitamins in reducing the levels of fecal
mutagens and a single agent trial may not produce significant results.
Therefore, in order to evaluate the role of vitamins A, C, and E and
other nutrients in human carcinogenesis through an epidemiological
approach, one should optimally measure the following:

(a) Amounts of vitamin intake based on extensive dietary records
(b) Levels of vitamins
(c) Levels of fecal mutagens

Unfortunately, in previous human studies only one of these parameters has been measured in any given study, and indeed most of the prior studies on cancer risk are based on dietary intake of vitamins or a "vitamin index."

Cellular events include at least tumor initiation and promotion, which lead to transformation, and certain other intracellular events that become responsible for maintaining the transformed phenotype in an irreversible state. Vitamins A, C, and E and selenium may influence the cellular events of carcinogenesis in more than one way. For example, the vitamins may block the action of tumor promoters and initiators or induce cell differentiation in newly transformed or established tumor cells. In general, vitamin A and its synthetic and natural derivatives preferentially induce cell differentiation in established cancer cells of epithelial origin, although potent effects on certain stages of hematopoiesis are also evident. Vitamin C can reverse newly transformed cells to normal phenotype in vitro. However, after time the transformed phenotype becomes irreversibly fixed. Vitamins E and D may also cause cell differentiation in some established tumor cells (at least in culture), as well as permanently inhibit their growth.

If one considers these mechanisms of action by vitamins on cells, it becomes evident that the measurement of plasma levels alone for vitamins and other nutrients in target tissues (normal, dysplastic, and neoplastic) will be important. Unfortunately, the tissue levels of vitamins have not been determined in any previous epidemiological study. In order to influence the cellular events of carcinogenesis, knowledge of the tissue level of nutrients may be more crucial than the plasma level in estimating the cancer risk of the target tissue.

Even in plasma, measurements are usually very limited. For vitamin A, one must measure not only the levels of retinol and retinoic acid, but also the levels of all relevant carotinoids. Similarly, for vitamin E, one should measure its types. Although the biological activity of gamma-tocopherol is only one-tenth that of alpha-tocopherol, its level in our diet is twice that of alpha-tocopherol. Therefore, the level of gamma-tocopherol could contribute significantly to the plasma level of tocopherol. The plasma level of vitamin C fluctuates markedly as a function of dietary intake; therefore, the levels of plasma vitamin C in any epidemiological study would be difficult to interpret with respect to cancer risk. The leukocyte level of vitamin C appears to be a reasonable indicator of tissue level of vitamin C; however, there are no substantive data to support this contention.

In addition to extracellular and cellular events of carcinogenesis, the cancer risk is also influenced by host-mediated events. These include at least competency of the immune system and detoxification and metabolic activation of chemical carcinogens. Vitamins seem to stimulate cellular immunity, accelerate the detoxification of some carcinogens, and in some cases block the metabolic activation of chemical carcinogens.

Thus, in order to obtain meaningful data, we must estimate the levels of nutrients based on dietary intake, determine the actual levels of nutrients in plasma and tissues (normal, preneoplastic, and neoplastic), and monitor host-mediated events. Such a comprehensive epidemiological study will be critical to evaluating the role of vitamins and other nutrients in human carcinogenesis.

Conclusive results regarding the role of nutrients will come from intervention studies in which the effect of one or more nutrients on the incidence of cancer among a high-risk population is evaluated. However, we have not yet performed experiments in humans analogous to the animal studies. Such experiments can only be accomplished using carefully controlled intervention studies among populations at high risk of developing cancer. Some of these studies are in progress, but it will be at least five years and possibly longer before conclusive data will be available.

Nevertheless, intervention trials in humans are not as simple as they might appear because of great variations in dietary habits and in life style and attitudes toward the proposed studies. We have made considerable progress in the last few years in defining the methodological issues that may reduce the impact of the above confounding factors on the interpretation of results. In the design of human intervention studies, we have found that the appropriate methodologies and experimental design may be more important than the particular nutrients used in the chemoprevention. It is important to estimate the intake of nutrients based on dietary intake, determine the actual levels of nutrients in plasma and tissues (normal, preneoplastic, neoplastic), and monitor the immune competency of the host closely. In the absence of such a comprehensive effort, the results of human intervention studies may well be difficult to interpret.

Laboratory experiments have given us sufficient biological rationale for using combinations of nutrients in human cancer prevention studies. For example, the fact that vitamin E (alpha-tocopherol) in combination with selenium (sodium selenite) is more effective than the individual agents suggests the possibility that vitamins may interact with other nutrients, as well as with other molecules in the body. It has recently been reported that d-alpha-tocopheryl succinate, which is the most effective form of vitamin E, enhances the level of morphological differentiation of murine neuroblastoma (NBP_2) in culture induced by a cAMP-stimulating agent, prostaglandin A_2. This suggests that vitamin E succinate may regulate at least some effects of cAMP on mammalian cells in culture. Further studies on the interaction of vitamins with other nutrients and other anticancer agents normally present in the body (cAMP, butyric acid, protease inhibitors) must be performed in order to define the role of nutrients in carcinogenesis.

It appears that an excessive intake of fat increases the risk of cancer. The exact mechanisms of this effect are unknown. It has been proposed that the excessive consumption of fat increases the production of prostaglandin E_2, which is known to suppress immune response. The involvement of cholesterol in the etiology of colon cancer has been suggested. More studies are needed to substantiate the precise role of fats and fat-related substances in human carcinogenesis.

The studies on the role of vitamins in the treatment of cancer remain at an early stage. Biological features must be considered when developing a treatment protocol. These considerations include the forms of vitamins, dose and dose schedules, route of administration, and tumor tissue accumulations. It should be stressed that any biological modifier, including vitamins, may need to be used differently from chemotherapeutic agents. Therefore, in any protocol, the use of vitamins must be made on a firm biological rationale with a prolonged treatment time until the compound is limited by toxicity of the vitamin and/or rapid growth of tumor. The studies on the value of retinoids in the treatment of some tumors appear very encouraging, and more basic studies are needed to improve the effectiveness of retinoids in the treatment of human neoplasms. The clinical studies with vitamin E are very limited. More preclinical studies on the value of vitamin E succinate in human neoplasms are needed. In addition, more preclinical studies are essential to confirm positive studies of the role of vitamins (A, C, and E) in favorably modifying the effects of currently used therapeutic agents (chemical, radiation, and hyperthermia).

We are very much encouraged by the new mechanistic data on the effect of nutrients on animal and human carcinogenesis from numerous laboratories around the world. We believe that in the very near future modification of old concepts will be made and new ones developed. From animal studies it appears that for the first time we have in our hands molecules that, when properly used, may reduce the incidence of human cancer. There is no doubt that we have a long way to go before our goals of reducing cancer incidence and achieving more effective cancer prevention (and treatment) are reached—but we believe that an excellent beginning has been made.

CONTENTS

CHEMOPREVENTION (HUMAN)

Methodological Issues

CONTRIBUTORS

J. ABRAHM • *Philadelphia Veterans Administration Medical Center, Philadelphia, PA*

D. S. ALBERTS • *Sections of Hematology/Oncology, Pharmacology, and Cancer Center, Arizona Health Sciences Center, University of Arizona, Tucson, AZ*

L. ANDREONI • *C. Golgi Institute of General Pathology, Centro Tumori, University of Pavia, Pavia, Italy*

A. ARNABOLDI • *C. Golgi Institute of General Pathology, Centro Tumori, University of Pavia, Pavia, Italy*

P. BERMOND • *Centre Hospitalier, Reims, France*

E. C. BESA • *Department of Medicine, Section of Hematology-Oncology of Medical College of Pennsylvania, Philadelphia, PA*

A. BIANCHI • *Institute of Pharmacology II, University of Pavia, Pavia, Italy*

L. BIANCHI • *C. Golgi Institute of General Pathology, Centro Tumori, University of Pavia, Pavia, Italy*

C. W. BOONE • *National Cancer Institute, Bethesda, MD*

C. BOREK • *Departments of Pathology and Radiology, Columbia University, College of Physicians and Surgeons, New York, NY*

S. A. BROITMAN • *Boston University School of Medicine, Boston, MA*

M. P. CARPENTER • *Biomembrane Research Program, Oklahoma Medical Research Foundation and Department of Biochemistry and Molecular Biology, University of Oklahoma Health Sciences Center, Oklahoma City, OK*

M. W. CONNER • *Massachusetts Institute of Technology, Cambridge, MA*

F. L. CRANE • *Department of Biological Sciences, Purdue University, West Lafayette, IN*

T. P. DAVIS • *Department of Phamacology, University of Arizona, Tucson, AZ*

J. J. DeCOSSE • *Memorial Sloan-Kettering Cancer Center, New York, NY*

R. M. DETSCH • *Center for Vitamins and Cancer Research Department of Radiology, University of Colorado Health Sciences Center, Denver, CO*

W. D. DEWYS • *National Cancer Institute, Bethesda, MD*

L. EDWARDS • *Section of Dermatology, Arizona Health Sciences Center, University of Arizona, Tuscon, AZ*

P. FEIGL • *Swedish Hospital Tumor Institute, Fred Hutchinson Cancer Research Center, University of Washington, Seattle, WA*

L. S. FREEDMAN • *Memorial Sloan-Kettering Cancer Center, New York, NY*

G. E. GOODMAN • *Swedish Hospital Tumor Institute, Fred Hutchinson Cancer Research Center, University of Washington, Seattle, WA*

L. S. GOTTLIEB • *Boston University School of Medicine, Boston, MA*

P. GREENWALD • *Division of Cancer Prevention and Control, National Cancer Institute, Bethesda, MD*

S. GROSHEN • *Memorial Sloan-Kettering Cancer Center, New York, NY*

A. HANCK • *Department of Clinical Research, Hoffman-La Roche, Basel, Switzerland*

M. M. HENDERSON • *Swedish Hospital Tumor Institute, Fred Hutchinson Cancer Research Center, University of Washington, Seattle, WA*

C. H. HENNEKENS • *Departments of Medicine, and Preventive Medicine and Clinical Epidemiology, Harvard Medical School and Brigham and Women's Hospital, Brookline, MA*

M. HYZINSKI • *Philadelphia Veterans Administration Medical Center, Philadelphia, PA*

G. J. KELLOFF • *National Center Institute, Bethesda, MD*

M. KELLY • *Department of Anatomy and Cell Biology, University of Cincinnati College of Medicine, Cincinnati, OH*

A. R. KENNEDY • *Department of Cancer Biology, Harvard School of Public Health, Boston, MA*

G. D. KLEINMAN • *Swedish Hospital Tumor Institute, Fred Hutchinson Cancer Research Center, University of Washington, Seattle, WA*

H. KUPCHIK • *Boston University School of Medicine, Boston, MA*

H. A. LADNER • *University of Freiburg, Freiburg, West Germany*

C. M. LAZARO • *New York University Medical Center, New York, NY*

M. J. LEE • *Department of Biochemistry, UMDNJ-New Jersey Medical School, Newark, NJ*

J. Y. LI • *Department of Epidemiology, Cancer Institute, Chinese Academy of Medical Sciences, People's Republic of China*

R. LOTAN • *Department of Tumor Biology, The University of Texas, M. D. Anderson Hospital and Tumor Institute, Houston, TX*

B. LUND • *Swedish Hospital Tumor Institute, Fred Hutchinson Cancer Research Center, University of Washington, Seattle, WA*

W. F. MALONE • *National Cancer Institute, Bethesda, MD*

S. MAYRENT • *Departments of Medicine, and Preventive Medicine and Clinial Epidemiology, Harvard Medical School and Brigham and Women's Hospital, Brookline, MA*

D. L. MCCORMICK • *ITT Research Institute, Chicago, IL*

R. G. MEHTA • *ITT Research Institute, Chicago, IL*

C. METTLIN • *Roswell Park Memorial Institute, Buffalo, NY*

F. L. MEYSKENS, Jr. • *Section of Hematology/Oncology, Cancer Center, Arizona Health Sciences Center, Tucson, AZ*

H. H. MILLER • *Memorial Sloan-Kettering Cancer Center, New York, NY*

K. W. MILLER • *Department of Biochemistry, UMDNJ-New Jersey Medical School, Newark, NJ*

R. C. MOON • *ITT Research Institute, Chicago, IL*

T. E. MOON • *Biometry, Computing and Epidemiology, Arizona Cancer Center, University of Arizona, Tucson, AZ*

F. MORISHIGE • *Fukuoka Nakamura Memorial Hospital, Fukuoka, Japan*

N. MORISHIGE • *Fukuoka Nakamura Memorial Hospital, Fukuoka, Japan*

D. J. MORRÉ • *Department of Medicinal Chemistry and Pharmacognosy, Purdue University, West Lafayette, IN*

M. MOSESON • *New York University Medical Center, New York, NY*

N. NAKAMURA • *Fukuoka Nakamura Memorial Hospital, Fukuoka, Japan*

T. NAKAMURA • *Fukuoka Nakamura Memorial Hospital, Fukuoka, Japan*

P. M. NEWBERNE • *Massachusetts Institute of Technology, Cambridge, MA*

P. NOWELL • *Department of Pathology and Laboratory Medicine of the University of Pennsylvania School of Medicine, Philadelphia, PA*

G. S. OMENN • *Swedish Hospital Tumor Institute, Fred Hutchinson Cancer Research Center, University of Washington, Seattle, WA*

Y. M. PENG • *Department of Internal Medicine, Arizona Cancer Center University of Arizona, Tucson, AZ*

R. PIZZALA • *C. Golgi Institute of General Pathology, Centro Tumori, University of Pavia, Pavia, Italy*

K. PRASAD • *Center of Vitamins and Cancer Research Department of Radiology, University of Colorado Health Sciences Center, Denver, CO*

R. PRENTICE • *Swedish Hospital Tumor Institute, Fred Hutchinson Cancer Research Center, University of Washington, Seattle, WA*

B. N. RAMA • *Center for Vitamins and Cancer Research Department of Radiology, University of Colorado Health Sciences Center, Denver, CO*

C. RAVETTO • *C. Golgi Institute of General Pathology, Centro Tumori, University of Pavia, Pavia, Italy*

S. RODNEY • *Biometry, Computing and Epidemiology, Arizona Cancer Center, University of Arizona, Tucson, AZ*

R. M. SALKELD • *University of Freiburg, Freiburg, West Germany*

G. SANTAGATI • *Institute of Pharmacology II, University of Pavia, Pavia, Italy*

L. SANTAMARIA • *C. Golgi Institute of General Pathology, Centro Tumori, University of Pavia, Pavia, Italy*

J. SCHINDLER • *Department of Anatomy and Cell Biology, University of Cincinnati College of Medicine, Cincinnati, OH*

T. F. SCHRAGER • *Massachusetts Institute of Technology, Cambridge, MA*

R. SEROKMAN • *Arizona Cancer Center, University of Arizona, Tucson, AZ*

M. A. SESTILI • *National Cancer Institute, Bethesda, MD*

R. E. SHORE • *New York University Medical Center, New York, NY*

I. SUN • *Cancer Center, Purdue University, West Lafayette, IN*

D. D. THOMAS • *Swedish Hospital Tumor Institute, Fred Hutchinson Cancer Research Center, University of Washington, Seattle, WA*

A. K. VERMA • *Department of Human Oncology, Wisconsin Clinical Cancer Center, University of Wisconsin, Center for Health Sciences, Madison, WI*

Y. M. WANG • *Department of Experimental Pediatrics, University of Texas, M.D. Anderson Hospital and Tumor Institute, Houston, TX*

R. R. WATSON • *Department of Family and Community Medicine, Cancer Center, University of Arizona, Tucson, AZ*

C. S. YANG • *Department of Biochemistry, UMDNJ-New Jersey Medical School, Newark, NJ*

BASIC EXPERIMENTAL APPROACHES

STUDIES ON THE MECHANISM OF THE

ANTIPROLIFERATIVE ACTION OF RETINOIDS USING

RETINOID-RESISTANT MELANOMA CELL MUTANTS

Reuben Lotan

Department of Tumor Biology, The University of

Texas - M.D. Anderson Hospital and Tumor Institute

at Houston, TX.   77030

INTRODUCTION

An increasing number of reports, over the past few years, on the ability of retinoids (vitamin A analogs) to modulate cell transformation, proliferation, and differentiation has highlighted the importance of this group of compounds for prevention and suppression of malignancy (1-3). Although the mechanism(s) by which retinoids modify such fundamental processes is not clear, there are strong indications that these compounds can alter gene expression (1-7) and cell membrane glycoprotein synthesis and structure (1,3,8-14). Consequently, the two most likely cellular targets for retinoid action are the nucleus and the plasma membrane.

The involvement of retinoids in the maintenance, regulation or induction of differentiation of a variety of cell types, including embryonal carcinoma cells, in vivo and in vitro strongly implied that retinoids influence gene expression (1,4-7). It has been suggested that specific cellular retinoid-binding proteins recognizing either retinol (CRBP) or retinoic acid (CRABP) mediate this action by transporting the lipophilic retinoids via the hydrophilic cytoplasm to

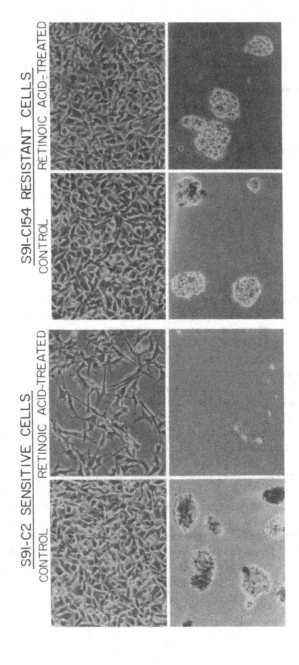

Fig. 1. Photomicrographs of S91-C2 and S91-Cl54 melanoma cells grown on plastic for 5 days (upper panels) or in 0.5% agarose for 10 days (lower panels) in the absence or presence of 10 μM retinoic acid phase contrast. x85.

the nucleus (1,4,5,15). However, little is known about the mechanism by which retinoids alter gene expression or whether the binding proteins are essential for retinoid action in all cells.

Various studies with cells or isolated membranes have demonstrated that retinol can be phosphorylated and that the retinylphosphate formed can be glycosylated (8,14). These derivatives were able to transfer monosaccharides, in particular mannose, to endogenous membrane components (8,14). Other reports described retinoid-enhanced activity of galactosyltransferase in several cell types (16-20). Thus, a role for retinoids in the glycosylation of membrane glycoproteins has been proposed (8,20). At present it is not clear whether changes in the glycosylation of cell membrane components may lead to altered growth and/or differentiation.

Studies with a considerable number of cultured tumor cells of human and rodent origin have demonstrated that retinoids can suppress the expression of different properties associated with the transformed phenotype (1-3). Our laboratory has been interested in the mechanism of this effect of retinoids and, in particular, in the mechanism by which retinoids inhibit cell proliferation. We have employed murine melanoma cell line S91-C2 (clone C2) as a model system for studies on the mechanism of the growth inhibitory action of a representative retinoid-β-all-trans retinoic acid (RA). We believe that such studies are not only important for the understanding of how this group of vitamin A analogs modulate cell behavior, but also for unraveling basic cellular regulatory mechanisms through which the transformed phenotype can be manipulated and suppressed.

EFFECTS OF RETINOIDS ON S91-C2 MELANOMA CELLS

The treatment of cultured S91-C2 cells with RA at concentrations ranging from 1 nM to 10 μM resulted, within 48-72 hr, in marked alterations in growth and morphology (21, 22). The rate of cell proliferation was reduced in a dose-dependent and a time-dependent fashion, and the cells assumed a more elongated and dendritic appearance (Figs. 1 and 2). Furthermore, the expression of properties characteristic of transformed cells was suppressed by RA. Thus, the abilities of the S91-C2 cells to synthesize DNA while suspended in a

liquid medium above a non-adhesive plastic substrate
coated with polyhydroxyethyl methacrylate (23) or to
form multicellular colonies by multiplication of single
cells suspended in a semisolid medium (22) were
dramatically suppressed by RA treatment (Figs. 1 and
2). These effects were not the result of cytotoxicity
of RA but rather were due to cytostatic, reversible
restoration of "normal" growth control to the malignant
cells.

Attempts at unraveling the mode of retinoid action
on the S91-C2 cells were focused on both nuclear
expression and membrane modification. The putative
"shuttle" for RA transport to the cell nucleus—CRABP—
was found in the cell cytoplasm (Fig. 3A) and a good

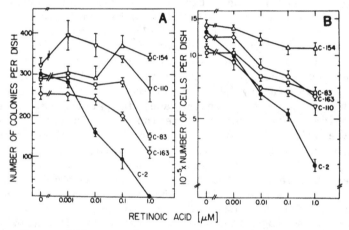

Fig. 2. Effect of retinoic acid on anchorage-
independent growth (A) and on anchorage-dependent growth
(B) of S91-C2 melanoma cells and retinoic acid-resistant
clones.
(A) The cells were suspended in medium containing 0.5%
agarose and either dimethysulfoxide (DMSO) or the
indicated concentrations of retinoic acid and plated at
$2x10^3$ cells/3.5-cm dish on top of a precast layer of 1%
agarose. The number of colonies was counted after 10
days.
(B) Cells grown on plastic dishes for 24 hours were
refed liquid medium containing either DMSO or the
indicated concentrations of retinoic acid at $1x10^4$
cells/3.5-cm dish and counted after 6 days. All
cultures were refed every 72 hours.

correlation was established between the ability of RA analogs possessing a free carboxyl group at carbon 15 to bind to CRABP and their ability to inhibit the proliferation of the S91-C2 cells (24). These findings indicated that CRABP may be involved in RA action. An obvious next question was what effects does RA have on gene expression in the S91-C2 cells. Analyses of [^{35}S] methionine-labeled proteins separated by two-dimensional polyacrylamide gel electrophoresis (PAGE) failed to reveal reproducible qualitative or quantitative changes following treatment of the cell with RA (Fig. 4, upper panels). Isolation of poly (A^{+}) RNA and translation in vitro also failed to demonstrate specific changes induced by RA (25).

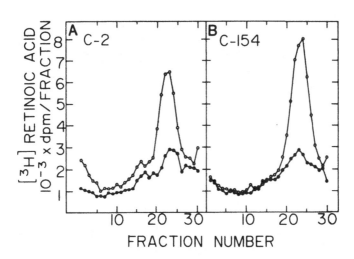

Fig. 3. Sucrose gradient sedimentation profiles of radioactivity obtained after incubation of cell extracts (2 mg protein in 0.2 ml of 50 mM Tris-HCl, pH 7.5: 2 mM dithiotreitol) with 30 pmol (403,000 dpm) of [11,12-^{3}H]retinoic acid for 8 hours at 4°C in the dark in the absence (0) or presence (●) of a 200-fold excess of unlabeled RA. After adsorption of unbound radioactivity on charcoal dextran, the samples were placed on top of 5 to 20% sucrose gradients and centrifuged at 189,000 x g for 16 hours. Fractions were then collected from the bottom of the tubes and the radioactivity was counted (26).

In contrast, a comparison of glycoprotein synthesis and cell surface membrane glycoprotein structure in untreated and in RA-treated cells was more rewarding (10). We found that RA increased the incorporation of radiolabeled monosaccharides, including mannose, fucose, and glucosamine into a single glycoprotein (gp160) exhibiting an apparent M_r of 160,000 on sodium dodecyl sulfate (SDS):PAGE (Fig. 5, lanes A and B). Analyses of cell surface glycoproteins by methods that radiolabel specifically either sialic acid or galactose (or galactosamine) residues exposed on intact cells demonstrated that gp160 is a constituent of the cell

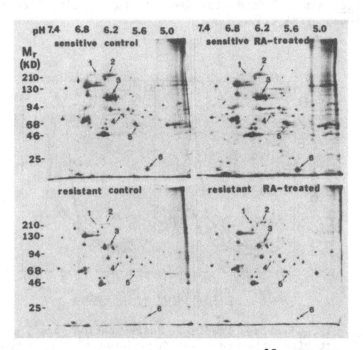

Fig. 4. Two-dimensional patterns of [^{35}S]methionine-labeled proteins from retinoic acid-sensitive (S91-C2) or resistant S91-C154 cells grown for 5 days without or with 10 µM retinoic acid. The first dimension (isoelectric focusing) was from left to right and the second dimension SDS:PAGE was from top to bottom. Conditions for labeling and electrophoresis were as described elsewhere (25). The arrows point to proteins that are labeled differently in sensitive and resistant cells.

surface membrane and that it contains more sialic acid and more galactose than the gp160 counterpart molecule of untreated cells (Fig. 5, lanes E and F, I and J). The increased glycosylation of gp160 in RA-treated cells correlated well with our observation that RA-induced augmentation of the activity of galactosyltransferase

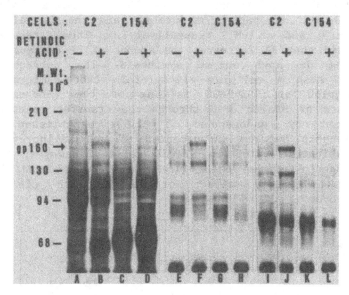

Fig. 5. Effect of retinoic acid on the glycosylation of cellular and cell surface glycoproteins of sensitive (S91-C2) and resistant (S91-C154) cells. (A-D) Cells were grown for 3 days without or with 10 µM retinoic acid and were then labeled for 48 hours with [³H]glucosamine. The cells were then solubilized and the labeled glycoproteins were separated by PAGE in the presence of SDS and identified by fluorography, as described earlier (10). (E-H) Cells were grown in the absence and in the presence of 10µM retinoic acid for 5 days and then the sialoglycoproteins that were exposed on the cell surface were labeled by oxidation with NaIO₄ followed by reduction with tritiated borohydride. (I-L) Cells grown as the latter were labeled by treatment with neuraminidase followed by oxidation of galactoproteins with galactose-oxidase and reduction with tritiated borohydride. The labeled cells were then solubilized and the glycoproteins were analyzed as above. For further details see Lotan et al. (27).

(20) and sialyltransferase (11), which are the enzymes involved in the covalent attachment of monosaccharides to the oligosaccharide side chain of glycoproteins.

The increase that RA caused in sialyltransferase (ST) activity was time dependent and was detectable by 24 hours of treatment (Fig. 6). The Vmax values calculated for ST in untreated and in RA-treated cells were 90 and 285 pmol/hr/mg protein and the Km values were 2.9 and 3.1µM, respectively. These results suggested that RA increases the amount of ST perhaps by inducing de novo enzyme synthesis. The subsequent finding that a cellular glycoprotein that comigrates with gp160 on SDS:PAGE is one of the endogenous acceptors of sialic acid through the transfer reaction catalyzed by endogenous ST (11) established a relationship between RA-augmented ST and RA-increased sialylation of gp160 in S91-C2 cells. However, the relationship between these biochemical changes and the growth inhibitory effect of RA is not clearly understood.

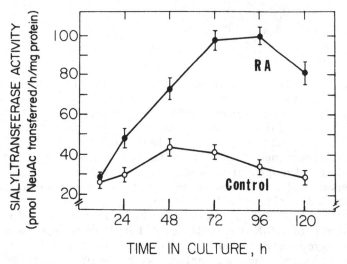

Fig. 6. Effect of retinoic acid on sialyltransferase activity in S91-C2 melanoma cells. Cells were grown in the absence and in the presence of 10µM retinoic acid for the indicated time and then assayed for enzymatic activity using asialofetuin as an exogenous acceptor of [^{14}C]sialic acid (NeuAc) from CMP-[^{14}C]sialic acid, as described elsewhere (11).

ISOLATION AND ANALYSIS OF MELANOMA CELL MUTANTS
RESISTANT TO THE ANTIPROLIFERATIVE ACTIONS OF RETINOIDS

Because retinoids exert pleiotropic effects on
cells, it is possible that some changes induced by RA
may be unrelated to the growth inhibitory effects, and
others may be the indirect result of the decrease in the
rate of cell proliferation. Since we were interested in
identifying specific biochemical changes induced by RA
that cause changes in growth, we developed RA-resistant
mutants from the sensitive S91-C2 cells (26). These
mutants, we hoped, would provide a powerful tool for
determining the relevance of the different effects of RA
for growth inhibition.

Our approach to the isolation of RA-resistant
mutant melanoma cells was based on the complete
suppression of growth of the parental cells in semisolid
medium in the presence of 1µM RA (Figs. 1 and 2). Thus,
only resistant mutants should be able to form colonies
in agarose in the presence of RA. Such colonies were
indeed obtained after mutagenesis of S91-C2 cells with
ethylmethane sulfonate. These colonies were isolated
and the cells were propagated on plastic tissue culture
dishes to expand the population. After recloning and
initial analyses of stability of the resistant phenotype
and the ability of the cells to take up [^{3}H]retinoic
acid from the medium, we identified stable mutants that
were not defective in RA uptake (26). The four mutants
that were studied extensively exhibited varying degrees
of resistance to inhibition of anchorage-independent and
of anchorage-dependent growth (Fig. 2). CRABP was found
in the cytosol of most of the mutants (26), and the
level of this putative mediator of RA action in the most
resistant mutant, S91-C154, was significantly higher
than in the sensitive parental S91-C2 cells (Fig. 3).
These findings demonstrated that the presence of CRABP
is not sufficient to confer sensitivity to the growth
inhibitory effects of RA. Since we have not studied the
function of CRABP in the mutant cells (e.g. whether it
can transport RA to the nucleus) it is not possible to
exclude the possibility that CRABP plays a role in
inhibition of growth by RA.

A preliminary comparison of the [^{35}S]methionine-
labeled proteins produced by RA-sensitive S91-C2 and RA-
resistant S91-C154 revealed several (at least six)
quantitative changes (Fig. 4). However, there were no

such differences between other resistant clones and the
parental S91-C2 cells. Thus, there are at present no
indications for specific changes in protein synthesis
that are associated either with the resistant phenotype
or with the sensitive phenotype.

Since the most striking effects that RA exerted on
the sensitive S91-C2 cells were the increases in ST and
in gp160 glycosylation, we used the RA-resistant clones
to explore whether cell surface modulation by RA is
related to growth inhibition. We have isolated several
subclones of S91-C2 cells, not treated with mutagen,
after recloning in agarose in the absence of RA. All
these subclones were susceptible to the growth-
inhibitory effect of RA, and their exposure to RA also
resulted in a several-fold increase in ST activity
(Table 1) and in an increased glycosylation of gp160
(27). In contrast, RA-treatment of the four RA-
resistant mutant clones failed to increase either ST
(Table 1) or the glycosylation of gp160 (Fig. 5) (27).

Since the synthesis of certain macromolecules may
fluctuate during the cell cycle and considering the fact
that RA increases the proportion of cells in the G_1
phase of the cell cycle as a result of growth inhibition
(22), the question arose as to whether the changes
induced by RA in ST and in gp160 are secondary to growth
inhibition. Having previously observed that the tumor
promotor 12-0-tetradecanoyl-phorbol-13-acetate (TPA) can
inhibit the growth of S91-C2 cells similarly to RA, we
used this compound in an attempt to resolve the above
question. TPA inhibited the growth of both S91-C2 and
the RA-resistant S91-C154 clone without increasing ST in
any of these cells (Table 2). Likewise, TPA failed to
increase the glycosylation of gp160 (27). These
findings indicate that inhibition of growth of S91-C2
cells is not sufficient to alter ST and gp160.
Consequently, we propose that RA-induced changes in
glycoprotein glycosylation may be the cause rather than
the outcome of growth inhibition.

Although the function of gp160 and how this
function may be altered by RA-induced changes in gp160
glycosylation are not known, we have preliminary
indications that gp160 is involved in growth control.
This assumption is based on the ability of anti-gp160
polyclonal antibodies (prepared in rabbits against gp160
that is shed by S91-C2 cells) to inhibit the anchorage-
independent and the anchorage-dependent growth of S91-C2

TABLE 1. EFFECT OF RETINOIC ACID ON SIALYLTRANSFERASE (ST) ACTIVITY OF SENSITIVE S91-C2 CELLS AND SUBCLONES AND RESISTANT MUTANT CLONES

Clone	Relative resistance to RA[a]	ST activity (pmol NeuAC/hr/ mg protein)[b]	
		Control	RA-treated
S91-C2	1.0	14.9 ± 1.0	48.9 ± 0.4
S91-C2-A1	1.1	15.4 ± 1.1	32.2 ± 2.1
S91-C2-A2	0.7	13.8 ± 0.9	57.4 ± 1.7
S91-C2-A3	1.2	13.1 ± 0.3	40.3 ± 0.8
S91-C2-A4	1.3	18.4 ± 0.6	46.5 ± 0.9
S91-C83	170	11.3 ± 0.8	15.1 ± 1.1
S91-C110	500	17.5 ± 0.2	18.7 ± 0.4
S91-C154	2500	12.9 ± 0.1	13.1 ± 0.4
S91-C163	275	18.7 ± 1.0	16.2 ± 0.1

[a]The numbers are the -fold increase in RA concentration required for 50% inhibition of cell proliferation.
[b]Cells were grown in the absence or presence of 10 μM RA for 5 days before ST analysis. The values are mean ± S.E

TABLE 2. COMPARISON OF THE EFFECTS OF RA AND TPA ON THE GROWTH AND SIALYLTRANSFERASE ACTIVITY OF SENSITIVE AND RESISTANT CELLS

Clone	Treatment	% of growth inhibition	ST activity (pmol NeuAc/hr/ mg protein)
S91-C2	None	0	14.7 ± 1.1
	RA, 10μM	85.5 ± 2.4	61.5 ± 1.2
	TPA, 0.5μM	80.2 ± 3.5	16.3 ± 0.3
S91-C154	None	0	16.1 ± 1.4
	RA, 10μM	16.2 ± 1.1	19.7 ± 0.8
	TPA, 0.5μM	77.8 ± 2.7	12.8 ± 0.9

Cells were grown without or with the indicated agents for 5 days and then counted to determine % inhibition and used for ST analysis.

cells (Deutsch and Lotan, unpublished).

Our hypothesis is that gp160 is a receptor for an
exogenous growth-promoting ligand and that its
modification by increased glycosylation induced by RA or
its "masking" by anti-gp160 antibodies, abrogate ligand
binding, which results in growth inhibition.

Our findings suggest that the initial action of RA
might be on the expression of genes coding for glycosyltransferases. These enzymes then increase the
glycosylation of certain glycoproteins, which may then
exhibit alteration in function. That this mechanism is
not limited to the melanoma cells is indicated by the
increasing number of reports from different laboratories
(16-19), as well as our own (11,20), documenting that RA
increases the activities of various glycosyltransferases
and modifies the glycosylation of specific membrane
glycoproteins (10-12).

REFERENCES

1. Lotan, R. Effects of vitamin A and its analogs
    (retinoids) on normal and neoplastic cells.
    Biochim. Biophys. Acta, 605: 33-91, **1980.**

2. Lotan, R., Thein, R. and Lotan, D. Suppression of
    the transformed cell phenotype expression by
    retinoids. In: "Modulation and Mediation of
    Cancer by Vitamins" (F.L. Meyskens and K. N.
    Prasad, eds.) pp. 211-221, S. Karger AG. Basel,
    1983.

3. Roberts, A.B. and Sporn, M.B. Cellular Biology and
    Biochemistry of the Retinoids. In: "The
    Retinoids" (M.B. Sporn, A.B. Roberts and D.S.
    Goodman, eds.) Vol. 2, pp. 210-286. Academic
    Press, Florida, **1984.**

4. Omori, M. and Chytil, F. Mechanism of vitamin A
    action. Gene expression in retinol-deficient
    rats. J. Biol. Chem., 257: 14370-14374, **1982.**

5. Chytil, F., Omori, M., Liau, G. and Ong, D.E.
    Retinoids, Cellular Retinoid Binding Proteins,
    Nucleus and Cancer. In: "Diet and Cancer" (D.
    Roe, ed.) pp. 117-123 A.R. Liss, New York, **1983.**

6. Fuchs, E. and Green, H. Regulation of terminal differentiaiton of cultured human keratinocytes by vitamin A. Cell. 25: 617-625, 1981.

7. Strickland, S. and Sawey, M.J. Studies on the effect of retinoids on the differentiation of teratocarcinoma cells in vitro and in vivo. Dev. Biol., 78: 76-85, 1980.

8. DeLuca, L.M. The direct involvement of vitamin A in glycosyl transfer reactions of mamalian membranes. Vitam. Horm., 35: 1-57, 1977.

9. Sasak, W., DeLuca, L.M., Dion, L.D. and Silverman-Jones, C.S. Effect of retinoic acid on cell surface glycopeptides of cultured spontaneously-transformed muse fibroblasts (Balb/c 3T12-3 cells). Cancer Res., 40: 1944-1949, 1980.

10. Lotan, R., Neumann, G. and Deutsch, V. Identification and characterization of specific changes induced by retinoic acid in cell surface glycoconjugates of S91 murine melanoma cells. Cancer Res., 43: 303-312, 1983.

11. Deutsch, V. and Lotan, R. Stimulation of sialyltransferase activity of melanoma cells by retinoic acid. Exp. Cell Res., 149: 237-245, 1983.

12. Meromsky, L. and Lotan, R. Modulation by retinoic acid of cellular, surface-exposed and secreted glycoconjugates in cultured human sarcoma cells. JNCI 72: 203-215, 1984.

13. Adamo, S., DeLuca, L.M., Silverman-Jones, C.S. and Yuspa, S.H. Mode of action of retinol. Involvement in glycosylation reactions of cultured mouse epidermal cells. J. Biol. Chem. 254: 3279-3287, 1979.

14. Shidoji, Y., Sasak, W., Silverman-Jones, C.S. and DeLuca, L.M. Recent studies on the involvement of retinyl phosphate as a carrier of mannose in biological membranes. Ann. N.Y. Acad. Sci., 395: 345-357, 1981.

15. Chytil, F. and Ong, D.E. Cellular retinol and
     retinoic acid binding protein. In: "Advances in
     Nutritional Research" (H.H. Draper, ed.) pp. 13-
     29, Plenum Publishing Corp. New York, **1983.**

16. Moskal, J.R., Lockney, M.W., Marvel, G.C., Mason,
     P.A., Sweeley, C.C., Warren, S.T. and Trosko,
     J.E. Regulation of glycoconjugate metabolism in
     normal and transformed cells. In: "Cell Surface
     Glycolipids" (C.C. Sweeley, ed.) Vol. 128, pp.
     241-260, ACS Symposium Series, Washington D.C.
     1980.

17. Plotkin, G.M. and Wolf, G. Vitamin A and
     galactosyltransferase of tracheal epithelium.
     Biochem. Biophys. Acta, 615: 94-102, **1980.**

18. Creek, K.E. and Morr'e , D.J. Effects of retinol
     and retinol palmitate on glycolipid and
     glycoprotein galactosyltransferase activities of
     rat liver plasma membranes. Biochem. Biophys. Res.
     Commun. 95: 1775-1780, **1980.**

19. Durham, J.P., Ruppert, M. and Fontana, J.A.
     Glycosyltransferase activities and the
     differentiation of human promyelocytic (HL-60)
     cells by retinoic acid and a phorbol ester.
     Biochem. Biophys. Res. Commun., 110: 348-355,
     1983.

20. Lotan, R., Deutsch, V. and Meromsky, L. Modulation
     of tumor cell membrane glycoconjugates by Vitamin A
     acid. In: "Membranes in Tumor Growth". (T.
     Galeotti, A. Cittadini, G. Neri, and S. Papa, eds.)
     pp. 121-126. Elsevier Biomedical Press, Amsterdam,
     1982.

21. Lotan, R. Giotta, G., Nork, E. and Nicolson, G.L.
     Characterization of the inhibitory effects of
     retinoids on the in vitro growth of two malignant
     murine melanomas. JNCI, 60: 1035-1041, **1978.**

22. Lotan, R., Neumann, G. and Lotan, D.
     Characterization of retinoic acid-induced
     alterations in the proliferation and
     differentiation of a murine and a human melanoma

cell line in culture. Ann. N.Y. Acad. Sci., <u>359</u>: 150-170, **1981.**

23. Lotan, R., Stolarsky, T., Lotan, D. and Ben-Ze'ev, A. Retinoic acids restores shape-dependent growth control in neoplastic cells cultured on poly (2-hydroxyethyl methacrylate)-coated substrate. Int. J. Cancer, <u>33</u>: 115-121, **1984.**

24. Lotan, R. Neumann, G. and Lotan, D. Relationships among retinoid structure, inhibition of growth, and cellular retinoic acid-binding protein in cultured S91 melanoma cells. Cancer Res., <u>40:</u> 1097-1102 **1980.**

25. Lotan, R., Fischer, I., Meromsky, L. and Moldave, K. Effects of retinoic acid on protein synthesis in cultured melanoma cells. J. Cell Physiol., <u>113</u>: 47-55, **1982.**

26. Lotan, R., Stolarsky, T. and Lotan, D. Isolation and analysis of melanoma cell mutants resistant to the antiproliferative action of retinoic acid. Cancer Res. <u>43</u>: 2868-2875, **1983.**

27. Lotan, R., Lotan, D. and Meromsky, L. Correlation of retinoic acid-enhanced sialytransferase activity and glycosylation of specific cell surface sialo-glycoproteins with growth inhibition in a murine melanoma cell system. Cancer Res. 44: 5805-5812, **1984**

RETINOIDS, POLYAMINES AND

TERATOCARCINOMA DIFFERENTIATION

JOEL SCHINDLER AND MICHAEL KELLY

DEPARTMENT OF ANATOMY AND CELL BIOLOGY,
UNIVERSITY OF CINCINNATI COLLEGE OF MEDICINE,
CINCINNATI, OHIO 45267

Teratocarcinomas are tumors of gonadal tissue origin which contain an array of differentiated cell phenotypes derived from a population of undifferentiated stem cells known as embryonal carcinoma (EC) cells. These undifferentiated EC cells are the primary malignant cells of such tumors, while their differentiated derivatives are benign.

Murine embryonal carcinoma cells have proven to be a useful model system for the study of mammalian development (1). A large number of EC cell lines have been established and maintained in vitro (2,3). Cells from such cell lines differ in their ability to differentiate in response to a variety of inductive stimuli including high density growth (3,4,5), aggregate formation (2,3), and certain biochemicals (6-11; see Table 1 and below). Additionally, microinjection of individual EC cells from either tumors (12) or cell lines (13) into a mouse blastocyst can contribute to chimeric mouse formation, indicating that EC cells can contribute to normal development when introduced to an appropriate microenvironment. Thus, murine EC cells represent an excellent model system for studies related to malignancy, cytodifferentiation and mammalian embryogenesis.

TABLE 1

INDUCTION OF DIFFERENTIATION BY VARIOUS STIMULI IN
SEVERAL EC CELL LINES

MEANS OF INDUCTION OF DIFFERENTIATION	CELL LINES		
	PCC4aza1R	Dif(RA)$^{-}$1	Nulli-SCC1
High density growth[a]	-	-	-
Aggregation[a]	++	-	-
Retinoic acid[a]	+++	-	+++
α-Difluoromethyl-ornithine[b,c]	+++	+++	-

Cells from the various cell lines were induced to
differentiate by the means indicated. (-) denoted no
response; (++) denotes >60% of the cells responded;
(+++) denotes >90% of the cells responded. The data is a
compoite of previously reported observations: a - Sherman
et al., 1981 (14); b - Schindler et al., 1983 (9);
c - Schindler et al., 1985 (10).

POLYAMINES AND DIFFERENTIATION

A growing number of studies indicate that polyamines
play an important role in various developmental processes.
The use of highly specific inhibitors of certain polyamine
biosynthetic enzymes, in particular α-difluoromethyl-
ornithine (DFMO), an enzyme activated irreversible
inhibitor of ornithine decarboxylase (ODCase) (15) has
facilitated such investigations.

In vivo studies have shown that abnormal levels of
polyamines can impair the normal development of polycheates
(16), sea urchins (17), chickens (18), and several
mammalian species (19,20). Extensive in vitro studies on a
variety of different cell phenotypes have demonstrated that
the exact nature of polyamine involvement in cellular
differentiation is complex. While elevated levels of
polyamines seem to be necessary for bone (21), chondrocyte

(22) or adipocyte differentiation (23), reduction in the
level of polyamines is necessary for neuroblastoma cells
(24), HL-60 cells (25) and murine embryonal carcinoma cells
(9-11) to differentiate. Thus, polyamines have the ability
to influence the differentiative state of a variety of
different cell phenotypes - a characteristic shared by
another class of molecules, the retinoids.

RETINOIDS, POLYAMINES AND CANCER

If cancer is considered a developmental disease (26),
it is reasonable to suggest that inducing undifferentiated
malignant stem cells of a tumor to differentiate could
result in a population of differentiated cells expressing
a benign phenotype. Retinoids do influence the state of
cellular differentiation (27), and a series of studies have
shown that retinoids can influence the malignant phenotype,
perhaps by modulating levels of polyamines. For example,
observations with HL-60 cells, a human promyelocytic
leukemia cell line, indicate that retinoid induced
differentiation of these cells involves a large increase in
intracellular levels of polyamines (28) and complete
depletion of intracellular spermidine blocks this retinoid
effect (25). Also, murine neuroblastoma cells treated with
retinol show lowered levels of ODCase activity (29), and
treatment with DFMO induces differentiation (30).

Perhaps the most compelling argument for the possible
role of retinoid-polyamine interactions in cancer stems
from observations made on the induction of mouse epidermal
tumors involving a two-step initiation promotion protocol
for carcinogenesis (31). One of the earliest events in
phorbol ester induced tumor promotion is the induction of
ODCase activity (32). Compounds which block the induction
of ODCase also block tumor formation (33). Among the most
potent of such compounds are retinoids (34). Thus, the
ability of retinoids to prevent phorbol ester-induced tumor
formation is likely to be the direct result of retinoid
mediated inhibition of both ODCase induction and putrescine
accumulation.

POLYAMINES AND EC CELL DIFFERENTIATION

One of the most effective inducers of EC cell differentiation is retinoic acid (RA) (6,7). Since RA can induce extensive differentiation of EC cells, and can directly influence polyamine levels in several biological systems, we reasoned that RA-induced differentiation of EC cells could be mediated through alterations in polyamine metabolism. Therefore, if we could interfere with polyamine metabolism by some alternative means, we should be able to mimic RA-induced differentiation.

Effect of DFMO on EC Cell Behavior

To investigate the role of polyamines during EC cell differentiation, the effect of DFMO on cells from several EC cell lines was tested. The results are shown in Table 2. Whereas cells from two of the cell lines studied (PCC4aza1R and Dif(RA)$^-$1) respond very well to DFMO, cells from cell line Nulli-SCC1 fail to differentiate. These cells do, however, exhibit altered growth characteristics, indicating that DFMO did have an effect on these cells, and that the induction of differentiation in the responsive cells was not simply a result of altered growth rates.

If polyamines are related to the actual induction of differentiation, it is likely that changes in their levels would occur shortly after exposure to any inducers. Therefore, the level of ODCase activity, as well as the actual levels of polyamines, were determined within hours of exposure to DFMO. These results are shown in Table 3. All cells treated with DFMO (even Nulli-SCC1 cells, which fail to differentiate) show markedly reduced levels of enzyme activity and polyamines, as compared to untreated controls. These results suggest that changes in the levels of polyamines may represent an early event in the different- iation of EC cells.

Effect of RA on EC Cell Polyamine Metabolism

As stated above, our studies on the role of polyamines during EC cell differentiation stem from our interest in understanding the mechanism of action of retinoids on the induction of EC cell differentiation. If RA does modulate

TABLE 2

THE EFFECT OF DFMO ON EC CELL BEHAVIOR IN VITRO

CELL LINE	TREATMENT	% MORPHOLOGICAL DIFFERENTIATION	% SSEA-1	% CELLULAR ACTIN	DOUBLING TIME (Hr)	FINAL DENSITY (x 10^6)
PCC4aza1R	untreated	0	98.5	9	10	5.6
	2.1 mM DFMO	100	3.5	87	19	0.8
Dif(RA)$^{-1}$	untreated	0	98	20	10	8.0
	2.1 mM DFMO	100	2.2	97	18	0.8
Nulli-SCC1	untreated	0	99	26	11	4.5
	21 mM DFMO	0	99	26	48	0.57

Cells from the EC cell lines listed were plated at 10^5 cells/60 mm dish. Twenty-four hours after inoculation, DFMO was added to the concentration indicated. Samples were counted every 24 hr. Doubling times were taken from the steepest portion of the growth curves. The percent of morphological differentiation was determined 96 hr after the addition of DFMO. These results are taken from previously published observations (9,10).

TABLE 3

ALTERATIONS IN LEVELS OF ODCase ACTIVITY AND POLYAMINES
FOLLOWING 8 HR EXPOSURE TO EITHER DFMO OR RA

CELL LINE & TREATMENT	% LEVEL OF UNTREATED CONTROL			
	ODCase activity	Putrescine	Spermidine	Spermine
PCC4aza1R + DFMO	33	6	5	120
" + RA	37	8	18	80
Dif(RA)¯1 + DFMO	8	7	30	110
" + RA	95	92	98	90
Nulli-SCC1 + DFMO	12	12	80	133
" + RA	96	87	120	106

Cells from the EC cell lines listed were grown as indicated
in the legend to Table 2. Following 8 hr. of incubation in
either 2.1 mM DFMO or 10^{-6} M RA, cells were harvested and
assayed for either ODCase or levels of polyamines. The
results are a compoite of data previously reported (35).

intracellular levels of polyamines, and this modulation is
related to the induction process (i.e. is an early event),
alterations on the levels of polyamines should be detected
shortly after exposure to RA. The results of studies
intended to address this question are shown in Table 3. In
the case of cells from cell line PCC4aza1R, RA treatment
leads to a reduction in both the activity of ODCase and the
levels of polyamines. The extent of this reduction is
virtually identical to that seen in DFMO treated cells.
Dif(RA)¯1 cells fail to show any effect of RA on either
ODCase activity or polyamine levels. Since these cells are
refractory to RA induced differentiation (36), it is not
unexpected that RA fails to influence these parameters.
Nulli-SCC1 cells present an intriguing dilemma. Whereas
DFMO fails to induce these cells to differentiate, levels of
ODCase and putrescine are significantly reduced. RA, which
does induce Nulli-SCC1 differentiation, has little effect on

ODCase or putrescine levels. These observations suggest
that while polyamine levels are important in determining
the state of EC cell differentiation, reduction in these
levels alone is not sufficient to induce EC cell differentiation in all cell lines.

Possible Retinoid-Polyamine Interactions During Embryonal
             Carcinoma Cell Differentiation

     Several observations indicate that a direct inter-
action between RA and ODCase, similar to that in the TPA-
induced tumor promotion system, is unlikely for explaining
the influence of RA on polyamine metabolism. First, as
discussed above, Nulli-SCC1 cells respond to RA but not
DFMO, despite no effect on ODCase activity by the former,
but by the later. Second, exogenous polyamines fail to
prevent RA-induced EC cell differentiation, while they do
block DFMO-induced differentiation. Third, studies
utilizing other inhibitiors of polyamine biosynthetic
enzymes (methylglyoxal bis (guanylhydrazone) (MGBG), which
inhibits S-adenosylmethionine decarboxylase (37) and
dicyclohexylammonium sulfate (DCHA), which inhibits
spermidine synthase (38) - refer to Figure 1) fail to
effect cells from EC cell line PCC4azalR. Together,
these observations suggest that putrescine, not spermidine
or spermine, is the polyamine most important in
influencing EC cell behavior. The influence of RA on
putrescine levels is not, however, the result of direct
interaction with ODCase. Therefore, the ability of
retinoids to interact with polyamine metabolism and induce
EC cell differentiation might involve alterations at other
polyamine biosynthetic sites. Such possible sites are
identified in Figure 1.

     If the mechanism of action of RA induced EC cell
differentiation does share common elements with polyamines,
it is likely that suboptimal levels of both RA and DFMO
together could stimulate a cellular response. In order to
test this possibility, Nulli-SCC1 cells were treated with
DFMO, which fails to induce differentiation, and a level
of RA which fails to stimulate a cellular response. The
results are shown in Table 4. It is clear that neither
DFMO nor RA (at 10^{-10}M) can alone successfully induce
Nulli-SCC1 cellular differentiation, but the two together,
added to the cell cultures in either order, can induce

FIGURE 1

POLYAMINE BIOSYNTHETIC PATHWAYS

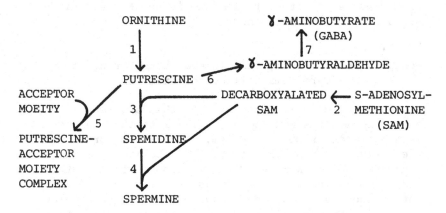

Enzymes involved in aspects of polyamine metabolism:
1) ornithine decarboxylase;   2) S-adenosylamethionine
decarboxylase;   3) spermidine synthase;   4) spermine
synthase;   5) transglutaminase;   6) diamine oxidase;
7) aldehyde dehydrogenase

successful differentiation, as determined by both
morphological and biochemical criteria. This observation
suggests that retinoids and polyamines do share a common
pathway for the induction of EC cell differentiation.

A possible site of such an interaction could be a
transglutaminase (TGase) reaction. As shown in Figure 1,
the transglutasminase reaction utilizes putrescine as a
substrate, and covalently binds this molecule to the
glutamine residue of another acceptor protein. In the
case of EC cell differentiation, levels of this putative
putrescine-acceptor moiety complex may be related to EC
cell differentiation, with changes in the level of this
compound directly influencing the differentiative state
of the cells. Alterations in the level of this putative
putrescine-acceptor moiety complex could result from changes
in putrescine levels (as demonstrated by DFMO treatment),
changes in enzyme activity (there is precedent for retinoid
mediated changes in TGase activity-39,40), or changes in
the endogenous acceptor moiety, preventing its normal
participation in the putrescine reaction.

TABLE 4

THE EFFECT OF RA + DFMO ON EC CELL BEHAVIOR

Treatment	% Morphological Differentiation	% Cellular Actin	% SSEA-1
Untreated	0	7	96
RA (10^{-6} M)	70	68	4
RA (10^{-10} M)	0	6	98
DFMO (2.1 mM)	0	8	97
RA (10^{-10} M) + DFMO (2.1 mM)	80	72	7
DFMO (2.1 mM) + RA (10^{-10} M)	80	74	5

Cells from EC cell line Nulli-SCC1 were plated 10^5 cells/ 60 mm dish. Twenty four hours after innoculation, inducers were added. If two inducers were used, the second inducer was added 48 hrs. after the first. The extent of differentiation was determined 96 hrs. after the full set of inducers was added.

Since TGase could be involved in regulating EC cell differentiation, initial attempts to monitor activity in EC cells were made. Cells from both cell lines PCC4azalR and Nulli-SCC1 were exposed to RA for short periods of time, and the levels of TGase determined. The results are shown in Table 5. In the case of both cell lines, treatment with RA, at levels that normally induce differentiation, causes increases in TGase activity. PCC4azalR cells exhibit an early (1 hr) increase in TGase activity which decreases with time. Nulli-SCC1 cells show a less pronounced early increase in enzyme activity, but exhibit substantially elevated levels after 6 hr of exposure to RA. These preliminary observations indicate that TGase activity can be modulated by retinoids and suggest a series of possible experiments to explore the role of transglutaminase activity in regulating EC cell differentiation.

TABLE 5

TRANSGLUTAMINASE ACTIVITY IN EC CELLS

Sample		Time	Cpm/mg Protein
PCC4aza1R	Control	1 hr.	4904
	+ RA (10^{-6}M)	1 hr.	7626
	Control	6 hr.	5733
	+ RA (10^{-6}M)	6 hr.	6816
Nulli-SCC1	Control	1 hr.	3912
	+ RA(10^{-6}M)	1 hr.	4740
	Control	6 hr.	1866
	+ RA (10^{-6}M)	6 hr.	3744

Cells were harvested in trypsin and sonicated. Cellular
debris was removed by centrifugation and enzyme activity
was measured by determining the amount of radioactive
putrescine incorporated into TCA precipitable material,
using casein as an exogenous acceptor protein.

OVERVIEW

     A role for retinoids in influencing cellular behavior
in well established (27), yet no firm mechanism of action
has been determined. Several possibilities have been
suggested, including: 1) glycosylation reactions (41),
2) specific intracellular retinoid binding proteins (42),
or 3) modulation of protein kinase activities (43). In
addition, our studies on the differentiation of murine
embryonal carcinoma cells suggest that retinoids may
function by interacting with intracellular polyamines.

     The ubiquitous nature of polyamines, and the
complexity of their regulation, preclude a single role in
the cell for this family of molecules. Retinoids, as a
class of molecules, exhibit pleiotropic effects on cell
behavior similar to those of polyamines. The mechanisms
mentioned above for retinoid action do not rule out a
direct interaction with polyamines. If transglutaminase
activity is related to the mode of action of retinoids,

it could be mediated via a binding protein, a protein kinase or a glycosylation reaction. Our observations with murine embryonal carcinoma cells provide some intriguing evidence regarding the interaction of retinoids and polyamines and offer a useful experimental system to further investigate the exact nature of that interaction.

REFERENCES

1. Graham, C. Teratocacrinoma cells and normal mouse embryogenesis. In: M.I. Sherman (ed.), Concepts in Mammalian Embryogenesis, pp. 315-362. Cambridge, Mass: M.I.T. Press, 1977.
2. Sherman, M.I. Differentiation of teratoma cell line PCC4aza1 in vitro. In: M.I. Sherman and D. Solter (eds.), Teratomas and Differentiation, pp. 189-196. New York: Academic Press, 1975.
3. Martin, G.R., and Evans, M.J. Differentiation of clonal lines of teratocarcinoma cells: Formation of embryoid bodies in vitro. Proc. Natl. Acad. Sci. USA, 72: 1441-1444, 1975.
4. McBurney, M.W. Clonal lines of teratocarcinoma cells in vitro: Differentiation and cytogenetic characteristics. J. Cell Physiol., 89: 441-449, 1976.
5. Sherman, M.I., and Millar, R.A. F9 embryonal carcinoma cells can differentiate into endoderm-like cells. Dev. Biol., 63: 27-33, 1978
6. Jetten, A.M., Jetten, M.E.R., and Sherman, M.I. Stimulation of differentiation of several murine embryonal carcinoma cell lines by retinoic acid. Exp. Cell Res., 124: 281-288, 1979.
7. Strickland, S., and Mahdavi, V. The induction of differentiation in teratocarcinoma stem cells by retinoic acid. Cell, 15: 393-398, 1978.
8. Jakob, H., Dubois, P., Eisen, H., and Jacob, F. Effects de l'hexamethylene-bisacetamide sur la differentiation de cellules de carcinome embryonnaire. C.R. Acad. Sci. Ser. D. 286: 109-114, 1978.
9. Schindler, J., Kelly, M., and McCann, P.P. Inhibition of ornithine decarboxylase induces embryonal carcinoma cell differentiation. Biochem. Biophys. Res. Commun., 114: 410-414, 1983.
10. Schindler, J., Kelly, M., and McCann, P.P. The response of several murine embryonal carcinoma cell

lines to stimulation of differentiation by α-difluoromethylornithine. J. Cell Physiol, 122: 1-6, 1985.

11. Heby, O., Oredsson, S.M., Olsson, I. and Marton, L.J. A role for the polyamines in mouse embryonal carcinoma (F9 and PCC3) cell differentiation but not in human promyelocytic leukemia (HL-60) cell differentiation. Adv. Polyamine Res., 4: 727-742, 1983.

12. Mintz, B., and Illemensee, K. Normal genetically mosaic mice produced from malignant teratocarcinoma cells. Proc. Natl. Acad. Sci. USA, 72: 3585-3589, 1975.

13. Dewey, M.J., Martin, Jr., D.W., Martin, G.R., and Mintz, B. Mosaic mice with teratocarcinoma-derived mutant cells deficient in hypoxanthine hosphoribosyltransferase. Proc. Natl. Acad. Sci. USA, 74: 5564-5568, 1977.

14. Sherman, M.I., Matthaei, K.I., & Schindler, J. Studies on the mechanism of induction of embryonal carcinoma cell differentiation by retinoic acid. Ann. N.Y. Acad. Sci. 359: 192-199, 1981.

15. Mamont, P.S., Duchesne, M.-C., Grove, J., and Bey, P. Antiproliferative properties of DL-α -difluoromethylornithine in cultured cells. A consequence of the irreversible inhibition of ornithine decarboxylase. Biochem. Biophys. Res. Commun. 81: 58-66, 1978.

16. Heby, O., and Emmanuelsson, H. Role of the polyamines in germ cell differentiation and in early embryonic development. Med. Biol., 59: 417-423, 1981.

17. Brachet, J., Mamont, P., Boloukhère, M., Baltus, É., Hanocq-Quertier, J. Effets d'un inhibiteur de la synthèse des polyamines sur la morphogénèse, chez l'oursin, le chétoptère et l'algue, Acetabularia. C.R. Acad. Sci. [D] (Paris), 287: 1289-1292, 1978.

18. Lowkvist, B., Heby, O., Emanuelsson, H. Essential role of the polyamines in early chick embryo development. J. Embryol. Exp. Morphol., 60: 83-89, 1980.

19. Fozard, J.R., Part, M.-L., Prakash, N.J., Grove, J., Schechter, P.J., Sjoerdsma, A., and Koch-Weser, J. L-ornithine decarboxylase: An essential role in early mammalian embryogenesis. Science, 208: 505-507, 1980.

20. Fozard, J.R., Part, M.-L., Prakash, N.J., and Grove, J. Inhibition of murine embryonic development by

ɑ-difluoromethylornithine, an irreversible inhibitor of ornithine decarboxylase. Eur. J. Pharmacol., 65: 379-385, 1980.

21. Rath, N.C., and Reddi, A.H. Changes in polyamines, RNA synthesis, and cell proliferation during matrix-induced cartilage, bone, and bone marrow development. Dev. Biol. 82: 211-216, 1981.

22. Takano, T., Takigawa, M., and Suzuki, F. Role of polyamines in expression of the differentiated phenotype of chondrocytes in culture. Med. Biol., 59: 423-427, 1981.

23. Bethell, D.R., and Pegg, A.E. Polyamines are needed for the differentiation of 3T3-L1 fibroblasts into adipose cells. Biochem, Biophys. Res. Commun., 102: 272-278, 1983.

24. Chen, K.Y. and Liu, A.Y.-C. Differences in polyamine metabolism of differentiated and undifferentiated neuroblastoma cells. FEBS Lett. 134: 71-74, 1981.

25. Sugiura, M., Shafman, T., Mitchell, T., Griffin, J., and Kufe, D. Involvement of spermidine in proliferation and differentiation of human promyelocytic leukemia cells. Blood (in press).

26. Pierce, G.B., Shikes, R., and Fink, L.M. Cancer - A Problem of Developmental Biology. Prentice Hall, Englewood Cliffs, N.J., 1978.

27. Sporn, M.B., and Roberts, A.B. Role of retinoids in differentiation and carcinogenesis. Cancer Res., 43: 3034-3039, 1983.

28. Huberman, E., Weeks, C., Herrmann, A., Callaham, M., and Slaga, T. Alterations in polyamine levels induced by phorbol diesters and other agents that promote differentiation in human promyelocytic leukemia cells. Proc. Natl. Acad. Sci. USA, 78: 1062-1066, 1981.

29. Chapman, S.K. Antitumor effects of vitamin A and inhibitors of ornithine decarboxylase in cultured neuroblastoma and glioma cells. Life Sciences, 26: 1359-1363, 1980.

30. Chen, K.Y., and Liu, A.Y.-C. The role of polyamines in the differentiation of mouse neuroblastoma cells. Adv. Polyamine Res., 4: 743-750, 1983.

31. Boutwell, R.K. The function and mechanisms of promotors of carcinogenesis. CRC Crit. Rev. Toxicol. 2: 410,437, 1974.

32. O'Brien, T.G. The induction of ornithine decarboxylase as an early, possibly obligatory, event

in mouse skin carcinogenesis. Cancer Res., 36:
2644-2650, 1976.

33. Weekes, R.G., Verma, A.K., and Boutwell, R.K.
    Inhibition by putrescine of the induction of epidermal
    ornithine decarboxylase activity and tumor promotion
    caused by 12-O-tetradecanoylphorbol-13-acetate.
    Cancer Res., 40: 4013-4018, 1980.

34. Verma, A.K., Rice, H.M., Shapas, B.G., and Boutwell,
    R.K. Inhibition of of 12-O-tetradecanoylphorbol-13-
    acetate-induced ornithine decarboxylase activity in
    mouse epidermis by vitamin A analogs (retinoids).
    Cancer Res., 38: 793-797, 1978.

35. Kelly, M., McCann, P.P., & Schindler, J. Alterations
    in polyamine metabolism during embryonal carcinoma
    cell differentiation in vitro. Dev. Biol. in press.

36. Schindler, J., Matthaei, K.I., & Sherman, M.I.
    Isolation and characterization of mouse mutant
    embryonal carcinoma cells which fail to differentiate
    in response to retinoic acid. Proc. Natl. Acad. Sci.
    USA, 78: 1077-1081, 1981.

37. Williams-Ashmann, G.H., and Schenone, A.
    Methylglyoxal bis (Guanylhydrazone) as a potent
    inhibitor of mammalian and yeast S-adenoxylmethionine
    decarboxylase. Biochem. Biophys. Res. Commun.,
    46: 1-14, 1981.

39. Yuspa, S.H., Ben, T., and Steiner, P. Retinoic acid
    induced transglutaminase activity but inhibits
    cornification of cultured epidermal cells. J. Biol.
    Chem., 257: 9906-9912, 1982.

40. Yuspa, S.H., Ben T., and Lichti, U. Regulation of
    epidermal transglutaminase activity and terminal
    differentiation by retinoids and phorbol esters.
    Cancer Res., 43: 5707-5712, 1983.

41. Deluca, L.M. The direct involvement of vitamin A
    in glycosyl transfer reactions of mammalian membranes.
    Vitam. Horm., 35: 1-7, 1977.

42. Chytil, F., and Ong. D. Cellular retinol- and
    retinoic acid-binding proteins in vitamin A action.
    Fed. Proc., 38: 2510-2516, 1979.

43. Plet, A., Evain, D., and Anderson, W.B. Effect of
    retinoic acid treatment of F9 embryonal carcinoma
    cells on the activity and distribution of cyclic
    AMP-dependent protein kinase. J. Biol. Chem.,
    257: 889-893, 1982.

The authors wish to acknowledge support for aspects of this work from a Biomedical Research Support Grant (NIH) and a grant from the Elsa U. Pardee Foundation. The Authors also wish to thank Dr. Peter P. McCann, Merrell Dow Research Institute, Cincinnati, Ohio for kindly providing α-difluoremethylornithine and performing polyamine analyses.

BIOCHEMICAL MECHANISM OF INHIBITION OF PHORBOL ESTER-INDUCED MOUSE EPIDERMAL ORNITHINE DECARBOXYLASE BY RETINOIC ACID

Ajit K. Verma

Department of Human Oncology, Wisconsin
Clinical Cancer Center, University of
Wisconsin, Center for Health Sciences,
Madison, WI 53792 (USA)

INTRODUCTION

Retinoic acid (vitamin A acid), a natural metabolite of retinal or retinyl esters, is required to maintain normal growth and differentiation of epithelial tissues (1-4). Since neoplastic transformation usually results in the loss of cellular differentiation, and vitamin A and its analogs (retinoids) play a role in maintaining the normal differentiation of epithelial cells, it is evident that retinoids may play a potential role in the development of cancer. Excellent reviews are available about the role of retinoids in the prevention and treatment of cancer (5-15). The exact molecular mechanism of action of retinoids remains undefined (16-22).

The two-stage (initiation and promotion) model of mouse skin tumor formation is an excellent quantitative model for the investigation of the mechanism of action of agents, such as retinoids, which modify tumor formation (22-27). Initiation can be accomplished by a single application of a carcinogen (e.g., 7,12-dimethylbenz[a]-anthracene) at a sufficiently small dose that will not lead to the formation of visible tumors during the life span of the animal. However, many tumors develop following repeated and prolonged applications of a tumor promoter to the initiated skin. Application of a tumor promoter alone elicits none or a few tumors; it is only

35

their applications following initiation that elicits many
tumors. 12-0-Tetradecanoylphorbol-13-acetate (TPA), a
component of croton oil, is a potent mouse skin tumor
promoter (27-29). Retinoic acid inhibits skin tumor promotion by interference with the promotion and not with the
initiation stage of carcinogenesis (24). Retinoic acid
inhibition of skin tumor promotion is partially reversible. Our results (22, 24-26) of the effect of retinoic
acid on skin tumor promotion by TPA indicate that the
mechanism of its inhibition of skin tumor promotion is via
its inhibitory effect on ornithine decarboxylase (ODC,
EC 4.1.1.17) induction by TPA, which will be the focus of
this chapter. Data showing that retinoic acid inhibits
TPA-caused ODC synthesis at the transcriptional level will
be summarized.

EXPERIMENTS AND RESULTS

1. <u>ODC induction as an essential component of tumor
promotion by TPA</u>. Application of TPA to mouse skin
elicits numerous biochemical and biological effects which
include primary interactions with plasma membranes, induction of ornithine decarboxylase, induction of dark
keratinocytes and inhibition of metabolic cooperation
(28-33). Although the exact molecular mechanism of tumor
promotion by TPA remains unclear, the available data
indicates that TPA induction of ODC (200-fold above the
control) is an essential component of the mechanism of
tumor promotion by TPA (34-36). ODC, which decarboxylates
ornithine to putrescine, is the first enzyme in the pathway of polyamine biosynthesis and is characterized by its
inducibility and rapid turnover rate ($t \frac{1}{2}$ ~17 min)
(37-39). The nature of the role of polyamines in cell
proliferation, differentiation and malignant transformation is not defined, but polyamines influence the
synthesis of nucleic acids and proteins (37-39). The
availability of α-difluoromethylornithine (DFMO), an
enzyme-activated irreversible inhibitor of ODC (40), has
enabled us to establish an essential role for ODC in skin
tumor promotion by TPA (35). Thus, DFMO, when given in
the drinking water (1%, w/v) inhibited the number of
papillomas per mouse by 90% and the number of mice bearing
papillomas by 56%. DFMO treatment completely inhibited
TPA-induced ODC activity and the accumulation of
putrescine and spermidine (35).

   2.   Inhibition of ODC induction by retinoids.   As
shown in Figure 1, application of 1.7 nmol of retinoic
acid 1 hr before application of 17 nmol of TPA to the
shaved backs of mouse skin, inhibited the induction of ODC
activity.

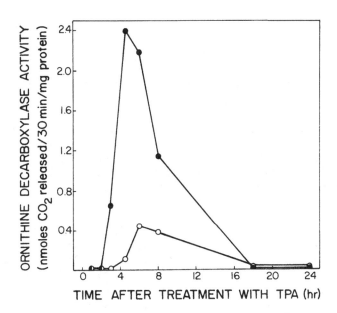

TIME AFTER TREATMENT WITH TPA (hr)

Figure 1.   The effect of pretreatment with retinoic acid
on TPA-induced epidermal ODC activity.   Groups of mice
were treated with 1.7 nmoles of retinoic acid (o) or
acetone (●) 1 hr before treatment with 17 nmoles of TPA.
Mice were killed for enzyme assay at the indicated times
after application of TPA.   Each point in the graph
represents the average of triplicate determinations of
enzyme activity from soluble epidermal extracts prepared
from 4 mice.

Retinoic acid treatment did not inhibit the induction of
S-adenosylmethionine decarboxylase activity by TPA. The
inhibition of the induction of ODC activity by retinoic
acid was dose-dependent. Enzyme induction was suppressed
at a dose above 1.7 pmol; 57% inhibition was observed
after pretreatment with 0.17 nmol of retinoic acid whereas
3.4 nmol completely inhibited the ODC induction by TPA
(24-26, 41). We have also shown that oral administration
of retinoic acid inhibits ODC induction by topically
applied TPA (26).

There was a good correlation between the ability of
retinoids to inhibit the induction of epidermal ODC
activity and skin tumor promotion by TPA. A few examples
will be cited. Application of 1.7 nmol of retinoic acid
1 hr prior to each treatment with TPA inhibited TPA-
induced ODC by 60-80%. In tumor induction experiments,
application of 1.7 and 17 nmol of retinoic acid 1 hr
before each promotion treatment with 17 nmol of TPA
inhibited 57 and 75%, respectively, the number of papillomas per mouse. Application of certain retinoids which
inhibited TPA-induced ODC, inhibited skin tumor promotion
by TPA and conversely the retinoids which did not inhibit
ODC induction failed to inhibit tumor promotion by TPA
(24). The results indicate that the mechanism of inhibition of promotion of tumor formation by retinoids involves
their ability to inhibit TPA-induced epidermal ODC and the
associated elevated putrescine levels (24-26).

We analyzed the mechanism by which retinoic acid
inhibits ODC induction by TPA and found that retinoic acid
inhibits the synthesis of ODC caused by TPA. The results
are shown in Figures 2 and 3. SDS-7.5% polyacrylamide
tube gel electrophoresis of immunoprecipitates of soluble
epidermal extracts indicates that application of acetone
to mouse skin, which did not induce ODC activity, resulted
in neither detectable [^{3}H]DFMO binding nor [^{35}S]methionine
incorporation. In contrast, TPA application, which
resulted in a dramatic induction of ODC activity, elicited
a single peak of [^{3}H]DFMO binding and two peaks of
[^{35}S]methionine incorporation. The total number of dpm
associated with [^{3}H]DFMO and [^{35}S]methionine peaks were
2188, 123 and 277, respectively; a minor peak of
[^{35}S]methionine incorporation copurified with the [^{3}H]DFMO
peak which is the peak of active ODC protein (Figure 2).

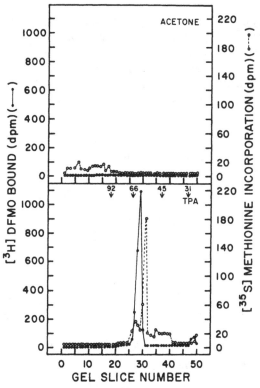

Figure 2.   Effect of TPA on [^{35}S]methionine incorporation
into mouse epidermal ODC.   Acetone or 10 nmol of TPA in
acetone was applied to mouse skin; mice were killed 6 hr
after application.   [^{35}S]Methionine was given intraperitoneally to label ODC protein <u>in vivo</u> 1 hr before
killing.   Epidermis from individual mice was separated by
a brief heat treatment (57° for 20 sec).   The epidermal
preparations from 20-30 mice were pooled, homogenized in
50 mM Tris-HCl (pH 7.5) containing 0.1 mM EDTA, 0.1 mM
pyridoxal phosphate, 1 mM phenylmethylsulfonyl fluoride,
1 mM 2-mercaptoethanol, 0.1% Tween 80, and 0.1 mM dithio-
threitol (Buffer A).   The homogenates were centrifuged at
100,000 x g for 60 min.   The soluble epidermal extract was
fractionated with ammonium sulfate.   The protein precipi-
tating between 35 and 55% ammonium sulfate saturation was
reconstituted in 1 ml volume of buffer A and dialyzed
overnight with two changes against 2 liters of buffer A.
This partially purified epidermal ODC extract was used for
[^{3}H]DFMO binding assays (42).   [^{3}H]DFMO-bound ODC was
immunoprecipitated using monoclonal ODC antibody and, the
second antibody, rabbit anti-mouse IgG (43) and the
immunoprecipitate was subjected to tube gel

electrophoresis (44). The gels were sliced into 2.2 mm
slices. The gel slice was solubilized by heating with
1 ml of 30% H_2O_2 at 50° overnight and the associated
radioactivity in each gel slice was measured using 10 ml
of xylene-based scintillation fluid. ODC activity (nmol
CO_2/30 min/mg protein): acetone, 0.1; TPA, 12.1.

As shown in Figure 3, the application of 17 nmol of
retinoic acid 1 hr before application of 10 nmol of TPA to
mouse skin inhibited the induction of ODC activity and
also the incorporation of [^{35}S]methionine into ODC protein
as detected by the ability to bind [^{3}H]DFMO.

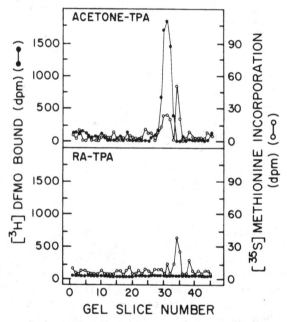

Figure 3. Effect of pretreatment with retinoic acid on
[^{35}S]methionine incorporation into mouse epidermal ODC.
Acetone or 17 nmol of retinoic acid in acetone was applied
1 hr before application of 10 nmol of TPA in acetone to
mouse skin. Mice were killed 5 hr after the second treatment. [^{35}S]Methionine (50 μCi in 0.2 ml saline/mouse) was
injected intraperitoneally 1 hr before killing of mice.
[^{3}H]DFMO binding to [^{35}S]methionine-labeled ODC extract
was determined as described in Figure 2. ODC activity
(nmol CO_2/30 min/mg protein): acetone-TPA, 19.8; retinoic
acid (RA)-TPA, 0.2.

In a separate experiment, the effect of retinoic acid on the amount of immunoprecipitable ODC protein was determined by immuno-blot using monoclonal antibody to ODC followed by horseradish peroxidase conjugated IgG fraction rabbit anti-mouse IgG (Cappel Scientific Division, Malvern, PA) and 4-chloro-1-naphthol (45-47). In this experiment, partially purified ODC (35-55% ammonium sulfate) fractions were subjected to SDS-polyacrylamide gel electrophoresis and electrophoretically transferred to nitrocellulose (45, 46). The nitrocellulose sheet onto which proteins had been transferred was treated with monoclonal antibody to ODC and peroxidase conjugated rabbit anti-mouse IgG (45, 46). Finally, ODC bands were stained with 4-chloro-1-naphthol (47). As was concluded from the intensity of stain, retinoic acid treatment depressed the amount of immunoprecipitable ODC protein. Recently (48) it has also been shown that increases in epidermal ODC activity caused by application of TPA to mouse skin correlate quantitatively with increases in the amount of enzyme protein measured immunologically.

Retinoic acid may suppress the amount of immunoprecipitable ODC protein either by inhibiting the synthesis or by enhancing the degradation of ODC. To substantiate the conclusion that retinoic acid may inhibit the synthesis of ODC caused by TPA, we determined the effect of retinoic acid application on TPA-caused increased level of ODC RNA in mouse skin. As shown in Figure 4, a single application of 10 nmol of TPA to mouse skin led to an increase in hybridizable RNA species-containing regions of ODC mRNA at 4 hr after TPA treatment. This TPA-caused increased level of ODC RNA was depressed by application of 17 nmol of retinoic acid 1 hr prior to 10 nmol of TPA to mouse skin. The dot intensity corresponds to the amount of ODC RNA. In a separate experiment, application of 17 nmol of retinoic acid 1 hr before application of 10 nmol of TPA to mouse skin inhibited ODC induction. ODC (nmol CO_2/30 min/mg protein) values were: acetone-acetone, 0.1; retinoic acid (RA)-acetone, 0.0; acetone-TPA, 12.5; RA-TPA, 0.3.

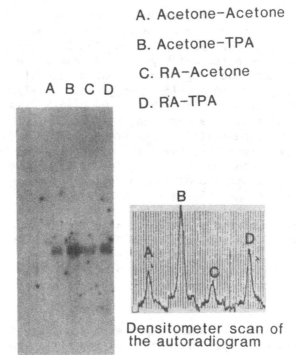

A. Acetone–Acetone

B. Acetone–TPA

C. RA–Acetone

D. RA–TPA

A B C D

B

A

C

D

Densitometer scan of
the autoradiogram

Northern Blot of RNA from mouse skin

Figure 4. Effect of application of retinoic acid on mouse
skin ODC mRNA. Acetone or 17 nmol of retinoic acid in
acetone was applied 1 hr before application of acetone or
10 nmol of TPA in acetone to mouse skin and mice were
killed 4 hr after the second treatment. Skin was excised,
placed immediately in liquid nitrogen and pulverized in a
morter. Total cellular RNA was prepared from the ground
skin by urea extraction and CsCl gradient centrifugation
method of Ross (49) with minor modifications. RNAs were
washed 4 times with 3.0 M sodium acetate (pH 5.0)
containing 5 mM EDTA, and twice with 100% ethanol; RNA was
then desiccated, dissolved in sterile distilled water, and
stored at -70°C. Poly (A) containing mRNA was fractionated by affinity chromatography on agarose poly(U) column
(P.L. Biochemicals, Inc., NJ). ODC RNA was identified by
the Northern blot method (50, 51) by means of DNA-RNA
hybridization analysis using a radiolabeled complementary
DNA (cDNA) probe pOD48 (52). RNA bands containing ODC
mRNA homology were visualized by exposing Kodak X-Omat AR
film to the washed nitrocellulose filter at -70° with
intensifying screens.

The answer to the question about the mechanism by which retinoic acid inhibits the transcription of ODC is impossible unless the mechanism by which TPA leads to the transcription for epidermal ODC is defined. TPA binds specifically to mouse epidermal fractions and [^{3}H]TPA-binding activity co-purifies with Ca^{2+}-activated phospholipid-dependent protein kinase (PK-C) (53-57). Our recent results indicate the phosphorylation of both histone (H1) and nonhistone proteins (Mr x 10^{-3} = 115, 112, 66, 62, 58 and 54) at about 3 hr following TPA treatment to mouse skin (data not shown). We have also shown that the level of available Ca^{2+} may be required for ODC induction by TPA (58). The possibility should be examined that Ca^{2+}-dependent processes may be involved in the transcription of ODC caused by TPA.

SUMMARY AND CONCLUSIONS

Direct evidence was sought that the tumor promoter TPA caused increased mouse epidermal ODC activity involves both increased messenger RNA and de novo protein synthesis. Application of 10 nmol of TPA to mouse skin led to a dramatic induction of soluble epidermal ODC activity which was accompanied by enhanced binding of [^{3}H]DFMO and [^{35}S]methionine incorporation into ODC protein as determined by gel electrophoresis of ODC immunoprecipitated with monoclonal antibodies to ODC. Also, TPA treatment to mouse skin resulted in an increased ODC messenger RNA as quantitated by means of DNA-RNA hybridization analysis using radiolabeled complementary DNA (cDNA) probe. Application of 17 nmol of retinoic acid 1 hr prior to application of 10 nmol of TPA to skin resulted in inhibition of the induction of ODC activity which accompanied inhibition of [^{3}H]DFMO binding and [^{35}S]methionine incorporation into ODC protein and a decreased level of ODC RNA. Retinoic acid inhibition of the induction of epidermal ODC activity was not the result of nonspecific cytotoxicity, production of a soluble inhibitor of ODC, or direct effect on ODC activity. In addition, inhibition of TPA-caused increased ODC activity does not appear to be due to enhanced degradation and/or post-translational modification of ODC by transglutaminase-mediated putrescine incorporation. Inhibition of ODC synthesis was not the result of the inhibitory effect of retinoic acid on general protein synthesis. The results indicate that retinoic acid

possibly inhibits TPA-caused synthesis of ODC protein
selectively. It is now concluded that the mechanism of
inhibition of mouse skin tumor promotion by retinoic acid
and certain of its analogs involves the property of
retinoids to inhibit the induction of ODC by TPA, and
retinoic acid inhibits TPA-caused de novo synthesis of ODC
at the transcriptional level.

REFERENCES

1. DeLuca, H.F. Retinoic acid metabolism. Fed. Proc.
    38:2519-2523, 1979.
2. Dowling, J.E., and Wald, G. The biological function
    of vitamin A acid. Proc. Natl. Acad. Sci. USA
    46:587-608, 1960.
3. Wolbach, S.B., and Howe, P.R. Tissue changes follow-
    ing deprivation of fat soluble A vitamin. J. Exp.
    Med. 42:753-777, 1925.
4. DeLuca, H.F. The metabolism of vitamin A and its
    functions. In: Nutritional Factors in the Induction
    and Maintenance of Malignancy (eds. E.C. Butterworth,
    Jr. and M.L. Hutchinson), pp. 149-167, Academic
    Press, Inc., New York, 1983.
5. Mettlin, C., Graham, S., and Swanson, M. Vitamin A
    and lung cancer. J. Natl. Cancer Inst. 62:1435-1438,
    1979.
6. Hinds, M.W., Kolonel, L.N., Hankin, J.H., and
    Lee, J. Dietary vitamin A, carotene, vitamin C and
    risk of lung cancer in Hawaii. Am. J. Epidemiol.
    119:227-237, 1984.
7. Moore, T. Effects of vitamin A deficiency in
    animals: pharmacology and toxicology of vitamin A.
    In: The Vitamins (ed. Sebrell and Harris), 2nd edi-
    tion, no. 1, pp. 245-266 and 280-294, Academic Press,
    New York, 1967.
8. Sporn, M.B., and Newton, D.L. Chemoprevention of
    cancer with retinoids. Fed. Proc. 38:2528-2534,
    1979.
9. Pawson, B.A., Ehmann, C.W., Itri, L.M., and
    Sherman, M.I. Retinoids at the threshold: Their
    biological significance and therapeutic potential.
    J. Medicinal Chem. 25:1270-1277, 1982.
10. Mayer, H., Bollag, W., Hänni, R., and Rüegg, R.
    Retinoids, a new class of compounds with prophylactic
    and therapeutic activities in oncology and derma-
    tology. Experientia 34:1105-1119, 1978.

11. Moon, R.C., McCormick, D.L., and Mehta, R.G. Inhi-
     bition of carcinogenesis by retinoids. Cancer Res.
     (suppl.) 43:2469s-2475s, 1983.
12. Sporn, M.B., and Roberts, A.B. Role of retinoids in
     differentiation and carcinogenesis. Cancer Res.
     43:3034-3040, 1983.
13. Bollag, W. Therapy of epithelial tumors with an
     aromatic retinoic acid analog. Chemotherapy 21:236-
     247, 1975.
14. Hill, D.L., and Grubbs, C.J. Retinoids as chemo-
     preventive and anticancer agents in intact animals
     (review). Anticancer Res. 2:111-124, 1982.
15. Elias, P.M., and William, M.L.: Retinoids, cancer
     and the skin. Arch. Dermatol. 117:160-180, 1981.
16. Yuspa, S.H. Retinoids and tumor promotion. In:
     Diet, Nutrition and Cancer (ed. Daphne A. Roe), pp.
     95-109, Alan R. Liss, Inc., New York, 1983.
17. Kummet, T., and Meyskens, F.L. Vitamin A: A poten-
     tial inhibitor of human cancer. Seminars in Oncology
     10:281-289, 1983.
18. Ong, D.E. A novel retinol-binding protein from rat,
     purification and partial characterization. J. Biol.
     Chem. 259:1476-1482, 1984.
19. Jetten, A.M. Modulation of cell growth by retinoids
     and their possible mechanism of action. Fed. Proc.
     43:134-139, 1984.
20. Sani, B.P., Dawson, M.I., Hobbs, P.D., Chan, R.L.,
     and Schiff, L.J. Relationship between binding
     affinities to cellular retinoic acid binding protein
     and biological potency of a new series of retinoids.
     Cancer Res. 44:190-195, 1984.
21. Goldstein, S.M., Moskowitz, M.A., and Levine, L.
     Inhibition of stimulated prostaglandin biosynthesis
     by retinoic acid in smooth muscle cells. Cancer Res.
     44:120-125, 1984.
22. Verma, A.K. Biochemical mechanism of modulation of
     skin carcinogenesis by retinoids: In: Retinoids
     (eds., Orfanos, Braun-Falco, Farber, Grupper, Polano,
     Schuppli), pp. 117-131, Springer-Verlag, New York,
     1981.
23. Verma, A.K., Conrad, E.A., and Boutwell, R.K. Dif-
     ferential effects of retinoic acid and 7,8-benzo-
     flavone on the induction of mouse skin tumors by the
     complete carcinogenesis process and by the
     initiation-promotion regimen. Cancer Res. 42:3519-
     3525, 1982.

24. Verma, A.K., Shapas, B.G., Rice, H.M., and
    Boutwell, R.K. Correlation of the inhibition by
    retinoids of tumor promoter-induced mouse epidermal
    ornithine decarboxylase activity and of skin tumor
    promotion. Cancer Res. 39:419-425, 1979.
25. Verma, A.K., and Boutwell, R.K. Inhibition of tumor
    promoter-induced mouse epidermal ornithine decarboxy-
    lase activity and prevention of skin carcinogenesis
    by vitamin A analogs (retinoids). In: Polyamines in
    Biomedical Research (ed. Gaugas), pp. 185-202, John
    Wiley & Sons, Ltd., England, 1980.
26. Verma, A.K., Rice, H.M., Shapas, B.G., and
    Boutwell, R.K. Inhibition of 12-O-tetradecanoyl-
    phorbol-13-acetate-induced ornithine decarboxylase
    activity in mouse epidermis by vitamin A analogs
    (retinoids). Cancer Res. 38:793-801, 1978.
27. Verma, A.K. Mouse skin carcinogenesis. In: Models
    in Dermatology (eds., Maibach, Lowe), vol. 2,
    Dermatopharmacology and Toxicology, pp. 313-321,
    Karger, Basel, 1985.
28. Boutwell, R.K. The function and mechanism of
    promoters of carcinogenesis. CRC Critical Rev.
    Toxicol. 2:419-443, 1974.
29. Verma, A.K., and Boutwell, R.K. Effects of dose and
    duration of treatment with the tumor-promoting agent,
    12-O-tetradecanoylphorbol-13-acetate on mouse skin
    carcinogenesis. Carcinogenesis 1:271-276, 1980.
30. Murray, A.W., and Fitzgerald, D.J. Tumor promoters
    inhibit metabolic cooperation in coculture of
    epidermal and 3T3 cells. Biochem. and Biophys. Res.
    Commun. 91:395-401, 1979.
31. Blumberg, P.M. In vitro studies on the mode of
    action of the phorbol esters, potent tumor promoters:
    Part I. CRC Crit. Rev. Toxicol. 8:153-197, 1980.
32. Boutwell, R.K., Verma, A.K., Ashendel, C.L., and
    Astrup, E. Mouse skin: A useful model system for
    studying the mechanism of chemical carcinogenesis.
    In: Carcinogenesis, A Comprehensive Survey (eds.
    Hecker, Fusenig, Kunz, Marks and Thielmann), vol. 7,
    pp. 1-12, Raven Press, New York, 1982.
33. Weinstein, I.B., Gattoni-Celli, S., Kirschmeier, P.,
    Hsiao, W., Horowitz, A., and Jeffrey, A. Cellular
    targets and host genes in multi-stage carcino-
    genesis. Fed. Proc. 43:2287-2294, 1984.
34. O'Brien, T.G. The induction of ornithine decarboxy-
    lase as an early, possibly obligatory, event in mouse
    skin carcinogenesis. Cancer Res. 36:2644-2653, 1976.

35. Takigawa, M., Verma, A.K., Simsiman, R.C., and
    Boutwell, R.K. Inhibition of mouse skin tumor promo-
    tion and of promoter-stimulated epidermal polyamine
    biosynthesis by α-difluoromethylornithine. Cancer
    Res. 43:3732-3738, 1983.
36. Weeks, C.E., Herrmann, A.L., Nelson, F.R., and
    Slaga, T.J. α-Difluoromethylornithine, an irrevers-
    ible inhibitor of ornithine decarboxylase, inhibits
    tumor promoter-induced polyamine accumulation and
    carcinogenesis in mouse skin. Proc. Natl. Acad. Sci.
    USA 79:6028-6032, 1982.
37. Jänne, J., Pösö, H., and Raina, A. Polyamines in
    rapid growth and cancer. Biochim. Biophys. Acta.
    473:241-293, 1978.
38. Raina, A., and Jänne, J. Polyamines as cellular
    regulators. Medical Biology 59:269-461, 1981.
39. Seely, J.E., and Pegg, A.E. Changes in mouse kidney
    ornithine decarboxylase activity are brought about by
    changes in the amount of enzyme protein as measured
    by radioimmunoassay. J. Biol. Chem. 258:2496-2500,
    1983.
40. Metcalf, B.W., Bey, P., Danzin, D., Jung, M.J.,
    Casara, P., and Vevert, J.P. Catalytic irreversible
    inhibition of mammalian ornithine decarboxylase (E.C.
    4.1.1.17) by substrate and product analogues. J. Am.
    Chem. Soc. 100:2551-2553, 1978.
41. Verma, A.K., and Boutwell, R.K. Vitamin A acid
    (retinoic acid), a potent inhibitor of 12-O-tetra-
    decanoyl-phorbol-13-acetate-induced ornithine
    decarboxylase activity in mouse epidermis. Cancer
    Res 37:2196-2201, 1977.
42. Pritchard, M.L., Seeley, J.E., Pösö, H.,
    Jefferson, L.S., and Pegg, A.E. Binding of radio-
    active α-difluoromethylornithine to rat liver
    ornithine decarboxylase. Biochem. Biophys. Res.
    Commun. 100:1597-1603, 1981.
43. Matsufuji, S., Fujita, K., Kameji, T., Kanamoto, R.,
    Murakami, Y., and Hayashi, Shin-ichi. A monoclonal
    antibody to rat liver ornithine decarboxylase. J.
    Biochem. 96:1525-1530, 1984.
44. Laemmli, U.K. Cleavage of structural proteins during
    the assembly of the head of bacteriophage T4. Nature
    (Lond.) 227:680-685, 1970.
45. Towbin, H., Staehelin, T., and Gordon, J. Electro-
    phoretic transfer of proteins from polyacrylamide
    gels to nitrocellulose sheets: procedure and

applications. Proc. Natl. Acad. Sci. USA 76:4350-
4354, 1979.

46. Glass, W.F., Briggs, R.C., and Hnilica, L.S.
    Identification of tissue-specific nuclear antigens
    transferred to nitrocellulose from polyacrylamide
    gels. Science 211:70-72, 1981.

47. Bio-Rad Immuno-Blot Assay Kit Instruction Manual.
    GAR-HRP (Goat Anti-Rabbit IgG) or GAM-HRP (Goat Anti-
    Mouse IgG).

48. O'Brien, T.G., Madara, T., and Ponsell, K. Changes
    in ornithine decarboxylase (ODC) activity caused by
    tumor promoters are due to changes in the amount of
    enzyme protein. Proc. Am. Assoc. Cancer Res. 25:77,
    1984.

49. Ross, J. Precursor of globin messenger RNA. J. Mol.
    Biol. 106:403-420, 1976.

50. Thomas, P.S. Hybridization of denatured RNA and
    small DNA fragments transferred to nitrocellulose.
    Proc. Natl. Acad. Sci. USA 77:5201-5205, 1980.

51. Wahl, G.M., Stern, M., and Stark, G.R. Efficient
    transfer of large DNA fragments from agarose gels to
    diazobenzyloxymethyl-paper and rapid hybridization by
    using dextran sulfate. Proc. Natl. Acad. Sci. USA
    76:3683-3687, 1979.

52. McConlogue, L., Gupta, M., Wu, L., and Coffino, P.
    Molecular cloning and expression of the mouse
    ornithine decarboxylase gene. Proc. Natl. Acad. Sci.
    USA 81:540-544, 1984.

53. Ashendel, C.L., and Boutwell, R.K. Direct measure-
    ment of specific binding of highly lipophilic phorbol
    diester to mouse epidermal membranes using cold
    acetone. Biochem. Biophys. Res. Commun. 99:543-549,
    1981.

54. Solanki, V., and Slaga, T.J. The down-modulation of
    receptors for phorbol ester tumor promoter in primary
    epidermal cells. Carcinogenesis 3:993-998, 1982.

55. Kikkawa, U., Takai, Y., Tanaka, Y., Miyake, R., and
    Nishizuka, Y. Protein kinase C as a possible
    receptor protein of tumor promoting phorbol esters.
    J. Biol. Chem. 258:11442-11445, 1983.

56. Niedel, J.E., Kuhn, L.J., and Vandenbark, G.R.
    Phorbol diester receptor copurifies with protein
    kinase C. Proc. Natl. Acad. Sci. USA 80:36-40, 1983.

57. Ashendel, C.L., Staller, J.M., and Boutwell, R.K.
    Solubilization, purification, and reconstitution of a
    phorbol ester receptor from the particulate protein

fraction of mouse brain. Cancer Res. <u>43</u>:4327-4332, 1983.

58. Verma, A.K., and Boutwell, R.K. Intracellular calcium and skin tumor promotion: calcium regulation of the induction of epidermal ornithine decarboxylase activity by the tumor promoter 12-0-tetradecanoyl-phorbol-13-acetate. Biochem. Biophys. Res. Commun. <u>101</u>:375-383, 1981.

ACKNOWLEDGEMENTS

We thank Deborah Erickson for capable technical assistance. The work was supported by NIH grants CA-35368 and CA-36323.

THE EFFECTS OF ANTIOXIDANTS ON THE INDUCTION OF MALIGNANT

TRANSFORMATION IN VITRO.

Ann R. Kennedy

Department of Cancer Biology

Harvard School of Public Health
665 Huntington Avenue, Boston, MA 02115

Abstract

There is now much evidence to suggest that free radicals play a role in malignant transformation. Several of the agents which suppress malignant transformation in vivo and in vitro may do so by inhibiting free radical reactions, either by prevention of free radical induction/formation (presumably, the action of protease inhibitors) or by the detoxification of free radicals through a variety of mechanisms. The agents we've studied which have effects on radiation induced transformation in vitro and are known to have a role in free radical detoxifying reactions include: catalase, superoxide dismutase, selenium, vitamin E, dimethylsulfoxide and several copper containing compounds such as CuDIPS (Cu II) (3,5-diisopropyl-salicylate$_2$), cuprous chloride and cupric chloride.

There is currently much interest in the role of free radicals in tumor promotion in vivo and in vitro. Several of the known biological effects of the potent tumor promoter, 12-0-tetradecanoyl-phorbol-13-acetate (TPA), are known to be antagonized by agents which interact with free radicals, such as antioxidants. We have observed that in vitro promotion by TPA can be enhanced by the presence of ferrous ions (Fe^{2+}) in the cellular medium. It is known that TPA treatment of cells results in the production of $O_2^{\cdot}$ and H_2O_2. As ferrous ions (Fe^{2+}) are necessary for the conversion of H_2O_2 to OH·, via a Fenton-type reaction, it is possible that at least some of the cellular effects attributable to TPA could be brought about by the interaction of hydroxyl radicals with cellular components. If OH· is the primary damaging free radical species leading to promotion, it is not surprising that agents such as antioxidants suppress promotion.

Introduction

There is much evidence that free radicals play a role in carcinogenesis induced by both physical and chemical carcinogens. The biological effects of ionizing radiation are known to be due to the interactions of free radicals with cellular components. Cellular damage leading to malignant transformation by chemical carcinogens may also result from free radical reactions, as many chemical carcinogens are converted into reactive electrophiles as well as other major metabolites which give rise to free radical intermediates and reactive reduced oxygen species as a result of autooxidative processes and oxidation-reduction cycles. These cycles are coupled with molecular oxygen to form reactive reduced oxygen species such as the superoxide anion radical (O_2^{-}) and hydrogen peroxide (H_2O_2) (1). Recently, there has been great interest in a role for free radicals in tumor promotion, as has been reviewed elsewhere (1,2).

There are many agents which can modify carcinogen-induced-malignant transformation in vitro and many of these modifying agents are known to play a role in free radical reactions, as has been recently reviewed (3,4). The experiments presented in this report were designed to gain further insight into the role that free radicals may play in the induction of transformation in vitro.

Materials and Methods

In all of the experiments reported here, the C3H10T½ in vitro transformation assay system was used: the system and detailed procedures for our studies on the modification of radiation and chemically induced transformation have been previously described (3-5).

Stock cultures were maintained in 60-mm Petri dishes and were passed by subculturing at a 1:20 dilution every 7 days. The cells used were in passages 9-14. They were grown in a humidified 5% CO_2 atmosphere at 37°C in Eagle's basal medium supplemented with 10% heat-inactivated fetal bovine serum and gentamycin. Plating efficiencies were determined from 3 dishes seeded with a cell density one fifth that of the dishes used for the transformation assay; these cultures were terminated at 10 days. The various treatment toxicities were considered in the design of the experiments such that all dishes used for the transformation assays contained approximately 300 viable cells per dish.

Results

Superoxide dismutase (SOD) and catalase are "antioxidant" enzymes which are part of the normal cellular defense system against active oxygen species; the particular reactions in which they play a role are shown in Fig. 1. The effects of superoxide dismutase and catalase on the initiation and promotion stages of radiation transformation in vitro are shown in Figs. 2-3; catalase has a highly significant suppressive effect on the enhancement of radiation transformation by TPA as well as a suppressive effect on the SOD enhancement of the initiation stage of radiation transformation (when both compounds are present at the time of the radiation exposure).

$$O_2^{\cdot -} + O_2^{\cdot -} + 2\ H^+ \longrightarrow O_2 + H_2O_2$$
$$\text{superoxide}$$
$$\text{dismutase}$$

$$2H_2O_2 \longrightarrow O_2 + 2H_2O$$
$$\text{catalase}$$

Figure 1. Reactions involving active oxygen species in which superoxide dismutase and catalase are known to be involved.

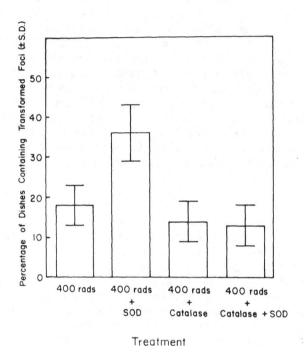

Figure 2. Effects on SOD and/or catalase on the initiation stage of radiation transformation induced by 400 rads of x-irradiation. When present at the time of the x-ray exposure, SOD enhances radiation transformation, while catalase is capable of suppressing the enhancement of radiation transformation by SOD. (Summary of data presented in reference 5).

We have also observed that several copper containing compounds can suppress radiation transformation when present during cellular irradiation. As shown in Fig. 4, CuDIPS, cupric chloride and cuprous chloride have an approximately equal ability to suppress transformation when present (at 5 μg/ml) at the time of the x-ray exposure.

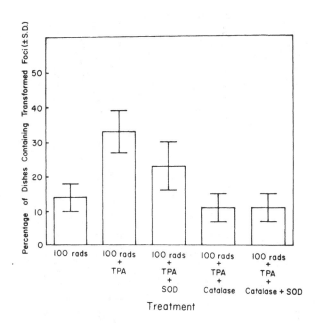

<u>Figure 3.</u> Effect of SOD and/or catalase on promotion <u>in vitro</u>. Radiation induced transformation was enhanced by TPA treatments; catalase or catalase + SOD significantly suppressed the enhancement of radiation transformation <u>in vitro</u> by TPA (Summary of data presented in reference 5).

In Table 1, the results of two experiments designed to determine whether cupric chloride could affect 3-methylcholanthrene (MCA)-induced transformation <u>in vitro</u> are shown. In these experiments, cupric chloride (at 5 µg/ml) was present either at the time of the cellular exposure to MCA or throughout the 6 week transformation assay period (beginning 48 hours after MCA exposure) or at both of these times. As can be observed in Table 1,

Table 1: Effect of cupric chloride (5 ug/ml) on methylcholanthrene (MCA) induced transformation in vitro[1]

Treatment Group	Plating Efficiency-% (average)	Total Number of Foci Observed		Fraction of Dishes Containing Transformed Foci	
		Type 3	Types 2+3	Type 3	Types 2+3[5]
1. Cupric Chloride	20.0	0	0	0/18	0/18
2. MCA	18.0	9	14	7/38=0.18	9/38=0.24
3. MCA + Cupric Chloride[2]	19.0	2	11	2/37=0.05	8/37=0.22
4. MCA + Cupric Chloride[3]	5.1	14	20	9/35=0.21	15/35=0.43
5. MCA + Cupric Chloride[4]	2.4	6	18	5/37=0.14	11/37=0.30

[1]Combined results of two separate experiments showing similar trends in the data. Cells were seeded such that there would be approximately 300 surviving cells/dish; 24 hrs. later, they were exposed to MCA (1.0 μg/ml) for a period of 24 hours.
[2]Treatment Group #3 - Cupric Chloride was given once per week throughout the assay period, beginning 48 hrs. post-MCA treatment.
[3]Treatment Group #4 - Cupric Chloride was only present during the 24 hr. MCA exposure.
[4]Treatment Group #5 - Cupric Chloride was present at the time of MCA treatment and given once per week throughout the assay period.
[5]Statistical Analysis Groups 2 vs. 3,4, or 5, p > 0.05.

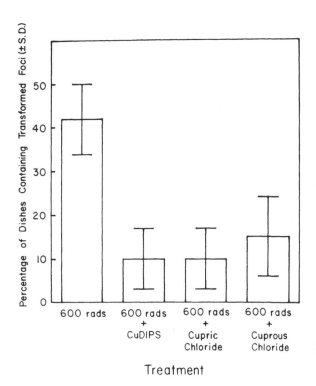

<u>Figure 4.</u> Suppressive effects of copper containing
compounds on the initiation phase of radiation
transformation <u>in</u> <u>vitro</u>. When CuDIPS, cupric
chloride or cuprous chloride (all at 5 µg/ml) were
present during the radiation exposure, they were
capable of suppressing radiation induced
transformation <u>in</u> <u>vitro</u> by comparable amounts.
(Summary of data presented in reference 5).

cupric chloride did not have a significant effect on MCA
induced transformation in C3H10T½ cells when present for
any of the time periods tested.

The results of two experiments in which Fe^{2+} was
added to irradiated cultures treated with the tumor

Table 2: Effect of Ferrous Ions on radiation
transformation enhanced by TPA treatments

Treatment	Plating Efficiency (%)	Total Number of Surviving Cells	Total Number of Foci Observed (Types 2+3 Foci)	Fraction of Dishes Containing Transformed Foci[1] (Types 2+3)
1. 100 rads	37.2	15387	0	2/46=0.04
2. 100 rads + TPA	26.5	12984	49	21/48=0.44
3. 100 rads + TPA + Fe^{2+}	34.0	14378	7	7/47=0.15

[1]Combined results of two separate experiments showing similar trends for the data.
[2]Statistical Analysis Group 2 vs. 3, $p < 0.01$.

promoting agent, TPA, are shown in Table 2. It can be observed that the presence of ferrous ions (FeCl$_2$, at 10µg/ml) enhanced the ability of TPA to promote radiation induced transformation in vitro. Two "radioprotective" agents, mannitol and cysteamine, were tested for their ability to affect radiation induced transformation (different concentrations of the compounds were present either ½ hr. before to ½ hr. after the x-ray exposure and/or throughout the 6 week transformation assay period [i.e., the compounds were added to cultures two times per week]). In none of these experiments did the radioprotective agents have a significant effect on radiation induced transformation in vitro (data not shown). For the transformation assays utilizing both of the radioprotective agents, both toxic and nearly toxic concentrations (to C3H10T½ cells) of the compounds were utilized in our studies as it is known that they must be present at such concentrations for their radioprotective effects to be observed (6).

Discussion

Our work has suggested that free radicals, presumably active oxygen species, may play a role in both the initiation and the promotion stages of transformation in vitro. We have observed that several compounds have the ability to affect the initiation stage of transformation in vitro. For example, we have observed that several copper containing compounds (including CuDIPS, cuprous chloride and cupric chloride [5]) are very effective at the inhibition of radiation transformation when they are present at the time of the radiation exposure, as shown in Fig. 4. It is known that such copper containing compounds have the ability to scavenge O$_2^-$ (5,7). In other studies reported here, we did not observe a suppressive effect of cupric chloride on 3-methycholanthrene induced transformation in vitro (Table 1). Our results suggest that the initiation of transformation in vitro by methylcholanthrene may not be as dependent on free radical/cellular interactions as is the initiation of transformation by ionizing radiation, although in many other respects, the initiation of transformation by polycyclic hydrocarbon chemical carcinogens (such as methylcholanthrene) and ionizing radiation appears to involve a similar process (reviewed in references 8,9).

We have also observed that SOD and catalase can affect the initiation stage of radiation transformation; the molecular reactions in which SOD and catalase play a role are shown in Fig. 1 (10). As observed in Fig. 2, when present at the time of the radiation exposure, SOD enhances radiation transformation, while catalase is capable of suppressing the enhancement of radiation transformation by SOD. These results suggest that H_2O_2 can play an important role in the initiation of radiation transformation in vitro. The enhancement of radiation transformation by SOD could lead to the conversion of superoxide anion radicals (O_2^{-}), formed in cells as a result of the radiation exposure, to higher levels of H_2O_2 (see Fig. 1) than would normally be present following the radiation exposure. Assuming that H_2O_2 can cause cellular damage resulting in transformation, higher concentrations of H_2O_2 could lead to higher yields of transformants. As catalase converts H_2O_2 to non-reactive species (see Fig. 1), its presence could reduce the H_2O_2 concentration and, by that mechanism, reduce the yield of transformed foci in cultures.

H_2O_2 as a cellular damaging agent has been previously studied extensively. There is much information to suggest that H_2O_2 can play a role in both the initiation and later stages of carcinogenesis and in causing cytogenetic changes thought to be related to cancer induction (reviewed in reference 5). The effects of H_2O_2 on cellular DNA are thought to be due to the conversion of H_2O_2 into the hydroxyl radical, OH· (11). It is known that ionizing radiation results in the production of OH· as well as other active oxygen species; it is widely thought that OH· is the primary DNA damaging free radical leading to the cytotoxic effects of radiation (12-16). Whether OH· is also responsible for the mutagenic and/or carcinogenic effects of radiation is controversial.

In the experiments reported here, we have attempted to determine whether OH· might be the active oxygen species leading to malignant transformation in vitro. The radioprotective aminothiol compound, cysteamine, is known to scavenge OH· (6) and mannitol is considered a reasonably specific scavenging agent for OH·. In our studies we observed no effects of cysteamine or mannitol in either the initiation or later stages of transformation in vitro. If we had observed that the presence of mannitol or cysteamine had an effect on radiation transformation, our results could have implicated OH· as a primary damaging active oxygen species leading to transformation in vitro. The characteristics of OH· could contribute to the negative findings in our mannitol and cysteamine studies; the extremely electrophilic OH· is so reactive as a free radical species that it is thought to be first encounter limited, with very little reaction specificity (mean path less than 0.001 microns). Thus, its cellular interactions are essentially limited to the site of its formation; if it is not present at a cellular site important for the induction of transformation, its effects will not be observed in a study such as ours. Active oxygen species such as H_2O_2 have quite different characteristics when compared to OH·; H_2O_2 has the ability to travel for relatively large distances (including through cellular membranes—H_2O_2 diffuses in and out of cells approximately as readily as does water [17]) before interacting with cellular components.

In the experiments reported here, there is some evidence that OH· may be important in the enhancement of radiation transformation by TPA. We observed that the promotional response brought about by TPA on radiation transformation could be enhanced by the presence of ferrous ions (Fe^{2+}) in the cellular medium. Fenton-type reagents [such as ferrous ions (Fe^{2+})] are known to be necessary for the conversion of H_2O_2 to OH· (Redox reaction in which Fe^{2+} can catalyse the decomposition of H_2O_2: $Fe^{++} + H_2O_2 \rightarrow Fe^{+++} + OH^- + OH·$). TPA is known to induce $O_2^{\cdot}$ and H_2O_2 in cells (18), with the conversion of H_2O_2 to OH· then occurring via a Fenton-type reaction. As Fe^{2+} enhances the promoting ability of TPA in vitro, our results suggest that OH· may be the active oxygen species responsible for the enhancement of transformation in vitro by TPA. These results are entirely consistent with the results presented for the effects of catalase (with or without SOD) on promotion in vitro; the suppressive effects of catalase on the enhancement of transformation by TPA could be due to its role in the removal of H_2O_2. With a lower level of H_2O_2, there will also be a reduced level of OH· to play a role in promotion by TPA in vitro.

Most of the studies discussed here have utilized
agents known to take part in specific chemical reactions
and were designed to gain information about the specific
molecular species involved in the induction of
transformation. While the exact molecular species
responsible for cancer induction is still unknown, our
work does suggest that carcinogen (and TPA) induced free
radical species may play a role in the development of a
transformed cell. Lowering the level of these induced
free radical species in cells may thus have a beneficial
effect in lowering the cancer incidence. There are many
naturally occurring dietary free radical quenching
compounds (discussed in references 2,4,19 and in this
volume) which have interactions with free radicals
similar to those described for the agents studied here;
it is conceivable that such naturally occurring
antioxidants could be useful in ultimately lowering the
incidence of cancer in human populations.

Acknowledgments

I thank Marilyn Collins and Babette Radner for
expert technical assistance in the studies reported here.
This research was supported by NIH Grants CA-22704 and
ES-00002.

References

1. Copeland, E.S.   A National Institutes of Health
   Workshop Report.   Free radicals in promotion - a
   chemical pathology study section workshop.   Cancer
   Res. 43: 5631-5637, 1983.

2. Cerutti, P.A.   Prooxidant states and tumor promotion.
   Science 227: 375-381, 1985.

3. Kennedy, A.R.   Promotion and other interactions
   between agents in the induction of transformation in
   vitro in fibroblasts.   In: Mechanisms of Tumor
   Promotion, Vol. III, "Tumor Promotion and
   Carcinogenesis In Vitro" edited by T.J. Slaga, CRC
   Press, Inc., Chapter 2, pp.13-55, 1984.

4. Kennedy, A.R.   Role of free radicals in the
   initiation and promotion of radiation-induced and

chemical carcinogen-induced cell transformation. In: Oxygen and Sulfur Radicals in Chemistry and Medicine (editor-A. Breccia), Proceedings of a Symposium organized by Instituto di Scienze Chimiche, University of Bologna, Italy and held as the Palazzo dei Priori, Fermo, Italy, Aug. 28-Sept. 5, 1984 (in press).

5. Kennedy, A.R., Troll, W. and J.B. Little. Role of free radicals in the initiation and promotion of radiation transformation in vitro. Carcinogenesis 5: 1213-1218, 1984.

6. Casarett, A.P. Radiation Biology. Prentice-Hall, Inc. Englewood Cliffs, New Jersey, 1968.

7. Brigelius, R., Spottl, R., Bors, W., Lengfelder, E., Saran, M. and U. Weser. Superoxide dismutase activity of low molecular weight Cu^{2+}-chelates studied by pulse radiolysis. FEBS Lett. 47: 72-75, 1974.

8. Kennedy, A.R. Evidence that the first step leading to carcinogen-induced malignant transformation is a high frequency, common event. In: Cell Transformation Assays: Application to Studies of Mechanisms of Carcinogenesis and to Carcinogen Testing (Barrett, J.C., editor) Raven Press, New York (in press).

9. Kennedy, A.R. and J.B. Little. Evidence that a second event in x-ray induced oncogenic transformation in vitro occurs during cellular proliferation. Radiation Res. 99: 228-248, 1984.

10. Fridovich, I. Superoxide dismutases. Adv. Enzymol. Relat. Areas Mol. Biol. 41: 35-97, 1974.

11. Lesko, S.A., Lorentzen, R.J. and P.O.P. Ts'o. Role of superoxide in deoxyribonucleic acid strand scission. Biochemistry 19: 3023-3028, 1980.

12. Roots, R. and S. Okada. Protection of DNA molecules of cultural mammalian cells from radiation-induced single strand scissions by various alcohols and SH

compounds. Int. J. Radiat. Biol. Relat. Stud.
Phys. Chem. Med. 21: 329-342, 1972.

13. Achey, P. and H. Duryea. Production of DNA strand
    breaks by the hydroxyl radical. Int. J. Radiat.
    Biol. Relat. Stud. Phys. Chem. Med. 25: 595-601,
    1974.

14. Ward, J.F. and I. Kuo. Deoxynucleotides—models for
    studying mechanisms of strand breakage in DNA. II.
    Thymidine 3'5' -diphosphate. Int. J. Radiat. Biol.
    Relat. Stud. Phys. Chem. Med. 23: 543-557, 1973.

15. Ward, J.F. Molecular mechanisms of radiation-induced
    damage to nucleic acids. Adv. Radiat. Biol. 5: 181-
    239, 1975.

16. Armel, P.R., Strniste, G.F. and S.S. Wallace.
    Studies on the Escherichia coli x-ray endonuclease
    specificity. Role of hydroxyl and reducing radicals
    in the production of DNA lesions. Radiation Res. 69:
    328-338, 1977.

17. Freeman, B.A. and J.D. Crapo. Biology of disease:
    free radicals and tissue injury. Lab. Invest. 47:
    412-426, 1982.

18. Goldstein, B.D., Witz, G., Amoruso, M., Stone, D.S.
    and W. Troll. Morphonuclear leukocyte superoxide
    anion radical (O_2^-) production by tumor promoters.
    Cancer Lett. 11: 257-262, 1981.

19. Doll, R. and R. Peto. The causes of cancer:
    Quantitative estimates of avoidable risks of cancer
    in the United States today. J. Natl. Cancer Inst.
    66: 1191-1308, 1981.

FREE RADICALS, DIETARY ANTIOXIDANTS AND MECHANISMS IN CANCER PREVENTION; IN VITRO STUDIES.

Carmia Borek

Departments of Pathology and Radiology
Columbia University
College of Physicians & Surgeons
New York, New York 10032

INTRODUCTION

It is frequently stated that 90% of the incidence of cancer in a population is due to environmental factors including food consumption and life style (2,32). The definition "environmental" implies non genetic factors though clearly, genetic predisposition plays a role in determining the susceptibility of an individual to becoming a victim of the disease (40).

Carcinogenesis is a multistage process as has been observed in vivo (6,47) and in vitro, in cell cultures, under defined conditions free from host mediated effects (4,14,41,44).

The initiation of the neoplastic process by physical or chemical agents takes place via irreversible DNA alterations. These may include mutations, methylation gene amplification, oncogene activation (31) or other genetic rearrangements, changes which under permissive physiological conditions (12) may lead to abnormal expression of cellular genes and transformation (14).

Initiation requires cell replication to fix the event as a hereditary property of the cell (26,27). Later events associated with expression of the transformed phenotype require additional cell replication (27,28) (Fig. 1).

65

The onset of neoplastic events can be triggered by radiation, the most ubiquitous carcinogen, measurable at low doses (10,14) and by a variety of environmental and dietary chemicals (2,49,24)) which provide a public threat worthy of attention.

The kinetics of events initiated by various carcinogens differ. Radiation imparts its oncogenic potential within a fraction of a second (1,10) while the effort of chemicals depend on their persistance in cells and tissues which in turn depends on the type of chemical, the target tissue, dose, period of exposure and the pharmacho kinetics associated with its metabolism and distruction (9). Given to the right target cell and tissue and administered in sufficiently high doses radiation and a variety of chemicals can act alone or in

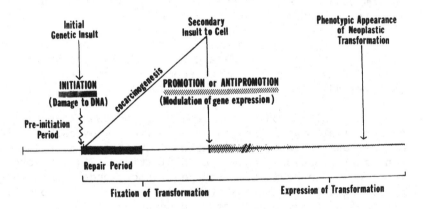

Fig. 1   Diagram of events which may occur at a cellular level in the course of induction and development of transformation.

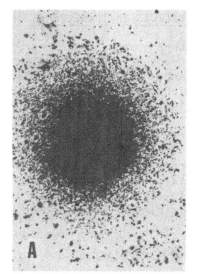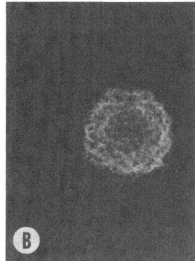

Fig. 2   A radiation transformed hamster   cell   clone   (A)
and its progeny growing in agar (B), indicating a
transformed phenotype (10,14).

synergism as complete   carcinogens,   producing   tumors   in
vivo   or   malignant colonies in vitro (8,10,14) (Fig.   2),
over the years evidence has been accumulating both in vivo
and   in   vitro   that chemicals which in themselves are non
carcinogenic can modulate the neoplastic process acting as
tumor promotors (6,29,30,47,52).   These cocarcinogens such
as TPA, a phorbol ester derivate (22,23,44) or   teleocidin
(18,34)   can   effectively   enhance   the   rate of malignant
transformation following initiation by   a   carcinogen   and
modify   the   neoplastic   expression   in a manner that is in
part reversible (18,30,44,47,50).

PERMISSIVE AND POTENTIATING FACTORS IN TRANSFORMATION

The actions of initiators and promotors in determining the onset, and frequency of the neoplastic process are controlled by a balance of cellular permissive and protective factors (12) which can be studied in vitro in cell culture systems (10,13,14).

Among the permissive factors thyroid hormones play a critical potentiating role. Their level in the cell determines in a dose related manner the ability of the cell to be transformed by radiation (37)or chemicals (20). Our recent findings also indicate that the effect of tumor promotors such as TPA and teleocidin are dependent on the presence of thyroid hormones (18).

Our results imply that the permissive action of thyroid hormones in transformation is mediated via a thyroid dependent cellular "transforming" protein(s) (20,37) as well as by the ability of the hormones to influence the oxidant state of the cell (18).

ANTIOXIDANT PROTECTIVE SYSTEMS

The cellular oxidant state is of utmost importance also in cellular protection against the oncogenic potential of radiation and chemicals, both in the initiation and promotion phases of transformation.

This has become apparent from our work (13,16,25,29) and others (2,46,47,53) underscoring the notion that free radicals play a role in carcinogenesis.

Inherent cellular factors comprised of enzymes, vitamins, micronutrients and low molecular weight substances are protectors. These include superoxide dismutase and catalase (33,45,53) peroxidases and thiols (5,3) vitamin A (30,36,39,44) vitamin C (5) and vitamin E (25,51) and the micronutrient selenium (16,25,43). These antioxidants serve to defend the cells against elevated levels of free radicals produced by radiation, chemical carcinogens and tumor promotors (1,2,10,14,36,53). The free radicals which include superoxides, hydroxyls, and fatty acid radicals vary in their half life but to varying degrees damage the cell. Both the radicals and their products cause lipid peroxidation mainly in the membrane, with resulting toxic products (25), inactivation of enzymes and cross linking of DNA (14,33,45,46).

Superoxide Dismutase and Catalase

Protective systems vary among species and within cells and tissue (29) Thus the effectiveness of adding nutritional or enzymatic antioxidants in cancer prevention will vary too (25,29).

For example we have found that superoxide dismutase (SOD) inhibits oncogenic transformation by radiation and bleomycin in hamster embryo cells and suppresses TPA action in enhancing transformation (25). By contrast catalase had little effect as an inhibiting transformation in this system but was an effective anticarcinogen in C3H10T1/2 mouse cells (53). An examination of enzyme levels in both systems indicated that hamster cells were rich in catalase suggesting that the inherent enzyme levels were high enough to detoxify peroxides formed in the course of exposure to x rays and bleomycin (25).

Protease Inhibitors

Protease inhibitors have been known to be effective inhibitors of carcinogenesis and tumor promotion in vivo (50).

In vitro where we can define stages of activity we find that the protease inhibitor antipain acts as a double edged sword in hamster and mouse cells (29) antipain has an anticarcinogenic effect on radiogenic transformation when added after exposure to radiation. Its effectiveness decreased with time (29) Fig. 3. However, antipain serves as a potentiator and markedly enhances transformation When added before radiation (29,35).

The activities of antipain as well as leupeptin were not reflected in a modification of sister chromatid exchanges (35). or in altered DNA synthesis and repair (17). The action of the protease inhibitors are probably imparted at the level of the cell membrane. Antipain added after radiation exerts its suppressive action by

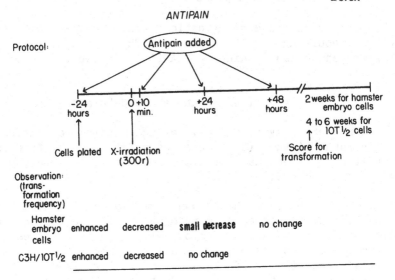

Fig. 3 General design of the experiments with antipain
and the observed results on its effects on
x-ray-induced transformation frequency at
scoring time. Cells were plated at time 0 and
irradiated 24 hr later. Antipain was added at
plating time or 10 min, 24 hr, or 48 hr after
irradiation. Transformed colonies were scored
after 2 weeks for hamster embryo cells or 6
weeks for the 10T1/2 mouse cells (23).

inhibiting cellular proteases associated with the
expression of transformation. It's potentiating activity
when added prior to irradiation is under study.

Retinoids

Retinoids have been known for some time to serve as
anticarcinogens *in vivo*, on chemically induced tumors
(30,42,48).

Our work has addressed the questions whether vitamin A analogs at non toxic concentration can affect early and late events in radiogenic transormation, and whether they can modulate cocarcinogenesis of radiation with chemical carcinogens or tumor promotors. If they do, what are the underlying mechanisms invovled.

Our finding indicate that retinol all trans-retinoc acid and trimethyl methoxyphenyl analog of ethyl retinamide inhibit radiogenic transformation as well as completely suppress the action of the tumor promotor TPA in an irreversible fashion (44) (Fig. 4). Retinoic acid also inhibited transformation by Trp-P-2 (11), a pyrolysis from protein foods (24,49) as well as suppressing the cocarcinogenic synergism between x rays and Trp-P-2 (11). The action of the retinoids and TPA, alone and in combination, was not reflected in DNA damage as ascertained by sister chromatid exchanges frequencies (44). Their antagonism was reflected at the cell membrane (11) as well as on cell morphology (Fig. 5).

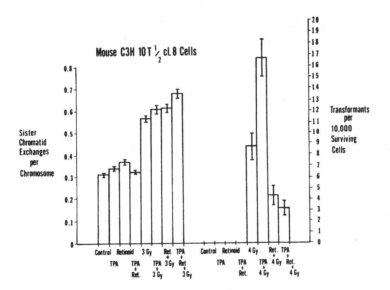

Fig. 4 Comparison of the effects of retinoid. TMMP-ERA and TPA on transformation (right) and sister chromatid exchange (left) (44) (1Gy = 100 rad.)

Retinoic acid reduced the activity of Na^+/K^+ ATPase though mg ATPase and 5' nucleotidase, other membrane associated enzymes, were unaffected (11). The antagonism between the retinoid and TPA was also reflected in Na/K ATPase levels. The retinoid suppressed a TPA mediated enhancement of Na^+/k^+ ATPase by bringing the enzyme back to control levels (11). underscoring the pleotropic effects of the tumor promotor. TPA inhibited the production of the transport retinol-binding protein (RBP) in liver cells in culture and this effect was suppressed by a concomitant addition of retinol (22). Clearly, the effect of tumor promotors is of broad scope. TPA effectively modulates cell transformation but at the same time it can regulate a protein which controls the transport of vitamin A, an inhibitor of TPA action on transformation.

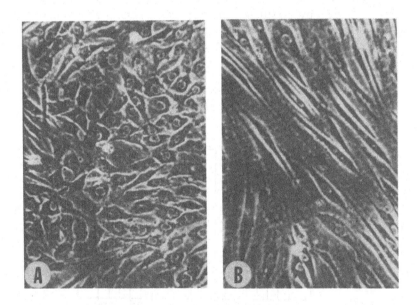

Fig. 5 C3H 10T1/2 cells (a), treated with retinoic acid
        (b) Note, the altered morphology.

Selenium

Selenium is a micronutirent in our diet and an inexcritable component of the enzyme glutathione peroxidase (25). As such, Se plays a role in detoxifying peroxides which are formed in normal metabolic processes in the cell (24,25) and are enhanced during cellular exposure to radiation and chemcials. Selenium has been found to have anticarcinogenic properties in vivo, to inhibit the growth of tumors induced by chemical carcinogens (43) but its role as an inhibitor of radiation carcinogenesis was unknown (25). Moreover, while both epidemiological and experimental data indicated an inverse relation of cancer incidence with selenium dietary intake the underlying mechanism of its action remained obscure (25).

Our recent work has addressed these problems and our findings indiate the following:

Pretreatment of mouse C_3H 10T1/2 cells with non toxic levels of sodium selenite inhibits the induction of malignant transformation by x rays, tryptophan pyrolysate (Trp-P-2) and by benzo(a)pyrene, three environmental carcinogens (11,16,25).

The action selenium as an anticarcinogen was mediated via its ability to induce high levels of free radical scavanging systems in the cells exposed to the oncogenic agents. These included the enzyme gluathione peroxidase, a selenium dependent enzyme, as well as catalase and non protein thiols (Tabel 1) (16,25). The induction of these protective systems resulted in a doubling of peroxide breakdown in the cells (25) Table 1. There is a close interrelation between selenium and vitamin E in their antioxidant actions (25). However, the role of vitamin E as an anticancer agent varies with the model studied (51) and probably depends on the tissue content of the vitamin (25) We found selenium to be a true protector. Its maximum effectiveness was imparted when cells were preincubated with the trace element. Thus, selenium can serve as a true radioprotective and chemoprotective agent in carcinogensis (16,25).

Table 6. Transformation, Glutathione Peroxidase (GSH), Catalase and Nonprotein Thiols (NPSH) in Selenium Pre-treated and Untreated C3H 10T1/2 Cells.

	Untreated	Selenium Treated (2.5μmNa,SeO_3Px)
Transformation by 400 rad X-ray	1.2×10^{-3}	6.1×10^{-4}
Transformation by B(a)P 1.2 μg/ml	1.1×10^{-3}	2.2×10^{-4}
GSH px*	5.2	10.0
Catalase*	4.3	6.0
NPSH[+]	1.0	2.1

*ṅ moles H_2O_2 reduced/min/mg protein.
+n moles/mg protein.

CONCLUSION

Cell systems in vitro offer powerful tools to study the role of free radicals in carcinogenesis. They afford us the opportunity to assess the role and mechanism of enzymatic and nutritional factors in their actions as antioxidants and their capacity as anticarcinogens acting to suppress different stages of the neoplastic process.

Free radicals are continuously produced by living cells. They are generated in the process of cell respiration and intermediary metabolism in both health and disease.

Under optimal cellular metabolic conditions cellular antioxidants are sufficient to impart protection against oxidant stress. However, under conditions of exposure to carcinogens or to unfavorable metabolic stress which enhance free radicals levels inherent protection may prove to be inadequate leading eventually to neoplastic transformation. This may be the underlying factor in our earlier findings that hepatocytes in culture can be transformed by nutritional stress into hepatoma like cells which lose cellular communication via permeable membrane junctions and acquire a variety of phenotypic changes associated with malignancy, including aneuploidity altered ganglioside. Composition capacity to grow in agar and tumorogenicity in animals (7).

Under stressful conditions cells require the external addition of antioxidants to enable them to cope with the excess load of free radicals and to minimize oxidative damage and oncogenic transformation (Fig 6).

Some nutrient antioxidants act directly, other agents such as selenium will impart their protection by inducing high levels of inherent protective enzyme systems which destroy peroxides (25), this enables the cell itself to increase its scavanging powers and to cope with the "overload" of free radicals and their toxic products thus preventing the onset and progression of malignant transformation.

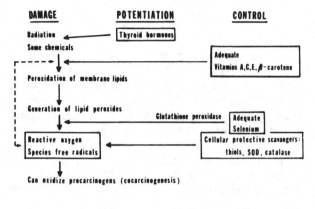

Fig. 6 A scheme illustrating the possible events induced
        by free radicals produced following cellular
        exposure to radiation or some chemical carcinogen
        and the antioxidant scavanging effects of some
        enzymes vitamins and micronutrients.

ACKNOWLEDGEMENT

This article and some of the work described were supported by a contract from The National Foundation for Cancer Research and by grant no. 12356 from the National Cancer Institute.

REFERENCES

1. Alexander, P. and Lett, J. Comprehensive Biochemistry, pp. 267-356. Florkin, M.Stots, E. (eds.) Elsevier, Amsterdam, 1968.
2. Ames, B. N. Dietary carcinogens and anticarcinogens. Oxygen radicals and degenerative diseases, Science 211: 1256-1264, 1983.
3. Arnott, M. S., Van Eys, J. and Wang, Y. M. Molecular Interactions of Nutrition and Cancer, pp. 1-474, Raven Press, New York, 1982.
4. Barrett, J. C. and Ts'o, P. O. P. Evidence for the progressive nature of neoplastic transformation In Vitro. Proc. Nat. Acad. Sci. U.S.A. 71: 3761-3765, 1978a.
5. Benedict, W. F., Wheatly, W. L. and Jones, P. A. Inhibition of Chemically Induced Morphological Transformation and Reversion of Transformed Phenotype by Ascorbic Acid in C_3H10T1/2 Cells. Cancer Res. 40 2796-2801, 1980.
6. Berneblum, I. Sequential Aspects of Chemical Carcinogenesis: sSin. In: Cancer; A Comprehensive Treatise. pp. 451-484, Becker, F. F., (ed.) Plenum Press, New York, 1982.
7. Borek, C. Neoplastic Transformation In Vitro of a Clone of Adult Liver Epithelial Cells into Differentiated Hepatoma-Like Cells under Conditions of Nutritional Stress. Proc. Nat. Acad. Sci. (USA) 69: 956-959, 1972.
8. Borek, C. X-ray Induced In Vitro Neoplastic Transformation of Human Diploid Cells. Nature 283: 776-778, 1980a.
9. Borek, C. Differentiation, Metabolic Activation and Malignant TransFormation in Cultured Liver Cells Exposed to Chemical Carcinogens. In: Advances in Modern Environmental Toxicology. Vol. 1. pp. 297-318. Mishra, N. Dunkel, V. and Mehlman, M. A. (eds) Senate Press, Princeton, New Jersey, 1980b.
10. Borek, C. Radiation Oncogenesis in Cell Culture. Adv. Cancer Res. 37: 159-232, 1982a.
11. Borek, C. Vitamins and Micronutrients Modify Carcinogenesis and Tumor Promotion In Vitro. In: Molecular Interrelations of Nutrition and Cancer,

PP. 337-350, Arnott, M. S., Van Eys, J.   and Wang.,
Y. M. (eds) Raven Press, New York, 1982b.

12. Borek, C.   Permissive and Protective Factors in
Malignant Transformation of cells in culture. In: The
Biochemical   Basis   of   Chemical   Carcinogenesis,
pp. 175-188, Greim.   H.,   Juna,   R.,   Kraemer,   M.,
Marquardt, H.   and Oesch, F. (eds) Raven Press, New
York, 1984a.

13. Borek, C. In Vitro Cell Cultures as Tools in the
Study of Free Radicals and Free Radical Modifiers in
Carcinogenesis. In: Methods In Enzymology, Volume on
Oxygen Radicals in Biological Systems, pp. 465-479.
Colowick C. P. Kaplan, N. O. and Packer, L.   (eds)
Academic Press, New York, 1984b.

14. Borek, C.   The Induction and Control of Radiogenic
Transformation In Vitro: Cellular and   Molecular
Mechanisms.   J.   Pharmach. and Therap.   1985, In
Press.

15. Borek, C. and Andrews, A.   Oncogenic Transformation
of Normal, XP and Bloom Syndrome Cells by X-Rays and
Ultraviolet Irradiation.   In: Human Carcinogenesis,
pp. 519-541, Harris, C. C.   and Antrup, H. (eds)
Academic Press, New York, 1983.

16. Borek, C. and Biaglow, J. E.   Factors Controlling
Cellular Peroxide Breakdown: Relevance to Selenium
Protection against Radiation and Chemically Induced
Carcinogenesis. Proc.   Am.   Ass. Cancer Res. 25:
125 (abstract), 1984.

17. Borek, C.   and Cleaver, J.E.   Protease Inhibitors
Neither Damage DNA nor Interfered with DNA in Human
Cells. Mutat. Res. 82: 373-380, 1981.

18. Borek, C., Cleaver, J. E. and Fujiki, H.   Critical
Biochemical   and   Regulatory   Events in Malignant
Transformation and Promotion In Vitro.   In: Cellular
Interaction by Environmental Tumor Promoters and
Relevance to Human Cancer, Fujiki, H.   et al.   (ed)
Japan Scientific Societies, Tokyo, 1984a, in press.

19. Borek, C.   and Guernsey, D. Membrane Associated Ion
Transport Enzymes in Normal and Oncogenically
Transformed Fibroblasts and Epithelial Cells. Studia
Biophysica 81 (1): 53-54, 1981.

20. Borek, C., Guernsey, D. L., Ong, A.   and Edelman,
I. S.   Critical Role Played by Thyroid Hormone in
Induction of Neoplastic Transformation by Chemical
Carcinogens in Tissue Culture. Proc. Natn. Acad.
Sci. U.S.A 80: 5749-5752, 1983a.

21. Borek, C., Higashino, S, and Loewenstein, W. R. Intercellular Communication and Tissue Growth-IV. Conductance of Membrane Junctions of Normal and Cancerous Cells in Culture. J. Memb. Biol. 1: 274-293, 1969.

22. Borek, C., Miller, R.C., Geard, C. R., Guernsey, D. L. and Smith, J. E. In Vitro Modulation of Oncogenesis and Differentiation by Retinoids and Tumor Promoters. In: Carcinogenesis. Vol. 7, pp. 277-284, Hecker, E. (ed) Raven Press, New York, 1982.

23. Borek, C., Miller, R., Pain, C. and Troll, W. Conditions for Inhibiting and Enhancing Effects of the Protease Inhibitor Antipain on X-Ray-Induced Neoplastic Transformation in Hamster and Mouse Cells. Proc. Natn. Acad. Sci. U.S.A. 76: 1800-1803, 1979.

24. Borek, C. and Ong, A. The Interaction of Ionizing radiation and Food Pyrolysis Products in Producing Oncogenic Transformation In Vitro. Cancer Lett. 12: 61-66, 1981.

25. Borek, C., Ong, A., Donohue, L. and Biaglow, J. E. Selenium Protects against In Vitro Radiation and Chemically Induced Transformation by Controlling Peroxide Breakdown. Proc. Natn. Acad. Sci. U.S.A., 1984C, in press.

26. Borek, C. and Sachs, L. In Vitro Cell Transformation by X-Irradiation Nature 210: 276-278, 1966a.

27. Borek, C. and Sachs, L. Cell Susceptibility to Transformation by X-Irradiation and Fixation of the Transformed State. Proc. Natn. Acad. Sci. U.S.A. 57: 1522-1527, 1967.

28. Borek, C. and Sachs, L. The Numbers of Cell Generations required to fix the transformed state in X-ray Induced Transformation. Proc. Natn. Acad. Sci. U.S.A. 59: 83-85.

29. Borek, C. and Troll, W. Modifiers of Free Radicals Inhibit In Vitro the Oncogenic Actions of X-Rays, Bleomycin, and the Tumor Promoter 12-0-tetradecanoylphorbol 13-Acetate. Proc. Natn. Acad. Sci. U.S.A. 80: 5749-5752.

30. Boutwell, R. K. Retinoids and Prostaglandin Synthesis Inhibitors as Protective Agents against Chemical Carcinogenesis and Tumor Promotion. In: Radioprotectors and Anticarcinogens, Nygaard, O. K. and Simic, M.G. (eds) A. P. New York, 557-566, 1983.

31. Cooper, G. M. Cellular Transforming Genes. Science 218: 801-806, 1982.
32. Doll, R. and Peto, R. The Causes of Cancer: Quantitative Estimates of Avoidable Risks of Cancer in the United States Today. J. Natn. Cancer Inst. 66: 1191-1308, 1981.
33. Fridovich, I. The Biology of Oxygen Radicals. Science 201: 875-880, 1978.
34. Fujiki, H., Mori, M., Nakayasu, M., Terada, M. and Sugimura, T. A Possible Naturally Occurring Tumor Promoter, Teleocidin B from Streptomyces. Biochem. Biophys. Res. Commun. 90: 976-983, 1979.
35. Geard, C. R., Freeman, M. R., Miller, R. C. and Borek, C. Antipain and Radiation Effects on Oncogenic Transformation and Sister Chromatid Exchanges in Syrian Hamster Embryo and Mouse C3H10T1/2 cells. Carcinogenesis 2: 1229-1235.
36. Goldstein, B. D., Witz, G., Amoruso, M., Stone, D.S. and Troll, W. Stimulation of Human Polymorphonuclear Leukocyte Superoxide Anion Radial Production by Tumor Promoters. Cancer Lett. 11: 257-262, 1981.
37. Guernsey, D.L. Borek, C. and Edelman, I. S. Crucial Role of Thyroid Hormone in X-Ray Induced Transformation in Cell Culture. Proc. Natn. Acad. Sci. U.S.A. 78: 5708-5711, 1981.
38. Guernsey, D. L., Ong, A. and Borek, C. Modulation of X-Ray Induced Neoplastic Transformation In Vitro by Thyroid Hormone. Nature 288: 591-592, 1980.
39. Harisiadis, L., Miller, R. C., Hall, E. J. and Borek, C. A Vitamin A Analogue Inhibits Radiation-Induced Oncogenic Transformation. Nature 274: 486-487, 1978.
40. Harnden, D. G. The Nature of Inherited Susceptibility to Cancer. Carcinogenesis 5: 1535-1537, 1984.
41. Kennedy, A. R., Murphy, G. and Little, J. B. Effect of Time and Duration of Exposure to 12-0-Tetradecanoylphorbol-13-Acetate on X-Ray Transformation of C3H 10T1/2 cells. Cancer Res. 40: 1915-1920, 1980b.
42. Lotan, R. Effects of Vitamin A and its Analogs (Retinoids) on Normal and Neoplastic Cells. Biochem. Biophys. Acta. 605: 33-91, 1980.
43. Medina, D. Selenium Mediated Inhibition of Mouse Mammary Tumorgenesis Cancer Lett. 8: 281-245, 1980.
44. Miller, R. C., Geard, C. R., Osmak, R. S., Rutledge Freeman, M., Ong, A., Mason, H., Napholtz, A., Perez, N., Harisiadis, L. and Borek, C. Modified

of Sister Chromatid Exhchanges and radiation-induced transformation in rodent Cells by the Tumor Promoter 12-O-Tetradecanoyl-Phorbol-13-Acetate and two retinoids, Cancer Res. 41: 655-659, 1981.

45. Pryor, W. A. The Role of Free Radical Reactions in Biological Systems. In: Free Radicals in Biology. Vol. 1, pp. 1-49, Pryor, W. A. (ed) Academic Press, New York, 1976.

46. Radioprotectors and Anticarcinogens, Nygaard O. F. and Simic, M. G. (eds), Academic Press, New York, 1983.

47. Slaga, T. G., Klein-Szanto, A. J. P., Triplett, L. L. and Yotti, P. C. Skin Tumor Promoting Activity of Benzoyl Peroxide, Science (Wash.) 213: 1023-1024, 1981.

48 Sporn, M. B., Dunlop, N. M., Newton, D. L. and Henderson, W. R. Relationships between structure and activity of retinoids. Nature 263: 110-113, 1976.

49. Sugimura, T. Tumor Initiators and Promoters Associated with Ordinary Foods. In: Molecular Interrelations of Nutrition and Cancer, pp. 3-24, Arnott, M.S. Van Eys, J. and Wang, Y. M. (eds) Raven Press, New York, 1982.

50. Troll, W., Witz, Gisela, Goldstein, B., Stone, D. and Sugimura, T. The Role of Free Oxygen Radicals in Tumor Promotion and Carcinogenesis. Carcinogenesis, Vol. 7: pp. 593-597, Raven Press, New York, 1982.

51. Wattenberg, L.W., Inhibition of Carcinogenic and Toxic Effects of Polycyclic Hydrocarbons by Phenolic Antioxidants and Ethoxygnin J. Nat. Cancer Inst. 48: 1425-1430, 1972.

52. Wigler, M. and Weinstein, I.B. Tumor Promoter Induces Plasminogen Activator. Nature 259: 232-233, 1976.

53. Zimmerman, R. and Cerutti, P. Active Oxygen Acts as a Promoter of Transformation in Mouse Embryo C3H 10T1/2C18 Fibroblasts. Proc. Natn. Acad. Sci. U.S.A. 81: 2085-2087, 1984.

ASCORBATE EFFECTS ON ENDOMEMBRANE ELECTRON TRANSPORT AND

MEMBRANE FLUX

D. James Morré, Iris Sun and F. L. Crane

Department of Medicinal Chemistry and Pharmacognosy, Cancer Center, and Department of Biological Sciences, Purdue University, West Lafayette, IN 47907

A central problem of cellular biology and biochemistry is how membrane translocations in cell motility, saltatory motion and vesicular transport (endocytosis/exocytosis) occur. Little is known about the mechanisms to transduce chemical energy into physical displacements of membrane sheets, vesicles or protrubances (1,2).

In this report, we summarize evidence for a role of ascorbic acid as an electron acceptor in a redox system involving the enzyme NADH-monodehydroascorbate reductase (MDAR) that may reside uniquely in those cellular membranes (plasma membrane, coated vesicles, secretory vesicles, endocytotic vacuoles) most often implicated in bulk translocations of cellular membranes and in membrane movements (3,4). Especially interesting in this regard are the so-called bristle- or spiny-coated vesicles involved both in exocytosis and in receptor-mediated and absorptive edocytosis (5). These vesicles are characterized by a polygonal surface architecture (seen in thin sections of electron microscope preparations as spines or bristles). The dominant surface protein contributing to this distinctive morphological feature is a single, large polypeptide chain called clathrin (6).

Fractions from rat liver that contain 80% + 5% of coated vesicles along with isolated Golgi apparatus from which some of the coated vesicles may be derived (7) were found to be enriched both in NADH-MDAR and in ascorbate. Activities of

83

coated vesicles depleted of coat proteins as well as those
of isolated membranes of Golgi apparatus are enhanced by the
addition of supernatant fractions enriched in coat proteins.
Quantative electron microscopy of cultured hepatocytes and
hepatoma cells treated with ascorbate showed increases in
coated vesicles and in coated membrane surfaces within the
Golgi apparatus zone. The results are consistent with a
role of monodehydroascorbate as an acceptor for electron
transport-mediated transfer of electrons from NADH perhaps
to oxygen by coated membranes as part of a mechanism to
drive membrane translocations via generation of a proton
gradient or of a membrane potential.

EVIDENCE FROM CYTOCHEMISTRY

    Our interest in ascorbate as a potential electron
acceptor for membrane-located energy transduction mechanisms
was stimulated initally by the chance observation from
cytochemical studies of the distribution of NADH-ferricyanide
oxidoreductase that clathrin-coated membrane surfaces were
much more reactive than adjacent uncoated membranes. This
was observed for coated membranes both at the Golgi apparatus
and at the cell surface (8). An NADH-ferricyanide oxidoreductase is distributed widely among endomembranes of
rodent liver (9) and other cells and tissues (10). A
component resistant to preparation of tissues for cytochemistry and to fixation with glutaraldehye is characteristic of
plasma membrane and mature Golgi apparatus elements in rat
(11) and mouse (9) liver.

    While reduction of monodehydroascorbate by NADH-cyto-
chrome b_5 reductase of endoplasmic reticulum has been proposed (12), an NADH-MDAR activity exists also that is distinct from NADH-cytochrome b_5 reductase (13). It has been
found especially concentrated in a light membrane fraction
(14, 15) that our results suggest may have contained coated
vesicles.

ISOLATION OF MEMBRANES AND COATED VESICLES FROM RAT LIVER

    Procedures for isolation of Golgi apparatus and of
reference fractions and for the criteria for determination
of purity of fractions were as described (16). Coated
vesicles were isolated from rat liver (3) in an approximate
yield of 1 to 2 mg protein per 40 g liver. Based on analyses of electron micrographs, the fractions were 80% $\pm$ 5%

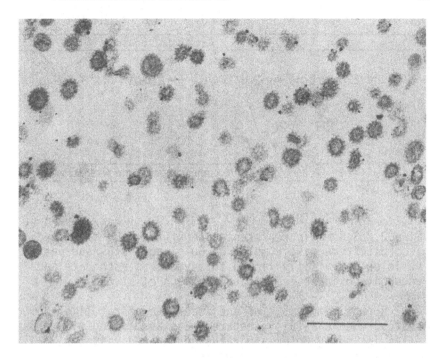

Fig. 1. Transmission electron micrograph of a coated vesicle fraction from rat liver representative of those prepared for use in this study. Vesicle surfaces were covered by the pentagonal-hexagonal patterns typical of clathrin coats. From Sun et al. (3). Bar = 0.5 μm.

coated vesicles (Fig. 1). This agreed closely with the 17% contamination by mitochondria, endoplasmic reticulum, plasma membrane and Golgi apparatus fragments determined from analyses of marker enzymes (3).

Among the enzymatic activities concentrated in the coated vesicle fractions were acid phosphatase (2 μmoles/h/ mg protein), oubain-sensitive Na^+, K^+, Mg^{2+}-ATPase (7.5 μmoles/h/mg protein), NADH-cytochrome c reductase (6 μmoles/h/mg protein) and NADH-ferrcyanide reductase (600 μmoles/h/mg protein) all with specific activities intermediate between those of the Golgi apparatus and of the plasma membrane (3). NADH-MDAR was concentrated in coated vesicles (6-fold compared to Golgi apparatus). Both ascorbic acid and ascorbic acid oxidase were present as well and were enriched approximately 2-fold compared to the total homogenate (3).

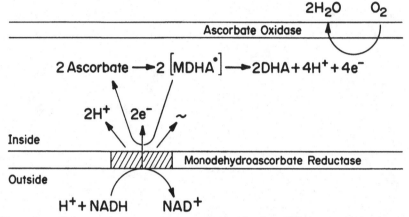

Fig. 2. Schematic representation of the NADH-monodehydroascorbate reductase complex of Golgi apparatus and coated
vesicles potentially linked to oxygen via ascorbate and
ascorbate oxidase. Modified from Sun et al. (3).

Approximately 50% of the ascorbate of rat liver homogenates, when carefully prepared, was associated with organ-
elles including Golgi apparatus and coated vesicles (3).
Despite the rather lengthy procedure involved in their
isolation, coated vesicles from rat liver contained nearly
10 micrograms ascorbic acid per mg protein, an amount about
twice that of the total homogenate. Ascorbate contained
within or supplied to either Golgi apparatus membranes or
coated vesicles can generate monodehydroascorbate (possibly
through the action of ascorbate oxidase also present in
the membranes). This is evidenced by the appearance of the
characteristic electron spin resonance signal of monodehydroascorbate. When NADH was added to the preparations, the
monodehydroascorbate was rapidly reduced by the NADH-MDAR
catalyzed reaction as evidenced by the rapid disappearance
of the electron spin resonance signal. Thus, monodehydroascorbate can serve as an electron acceptor for the NADH-
MDAR system of the Golgi apparatus-vesicle-plasma membrane
complex, perhaps with the ultimate transfer of electrons to
a suitable acceptor such as oxygen (Fig. 2).

One possibility to regulate NADH-NDAR activity and to
account for the cytochemical findings indicative of enhanced
ferricyanide reduction associated with coated membrane surfaces (8) would be that some combination of the membrane-
bound reductase with the coat protein clathrin resulted in
the activation of the reductase. This, in turn, would

Table 1. Subfractionation of coated vesicles and the
"activation" of NADH-MDAR of isolated and clathrin-depleted
membranes by addition of fractions enriched in clathrin.
Values are specific activities + standard deviations from
three different membrane preparations (3).

| Fraction | Specific activity (nmoles/min/mg protein) | | |
	NADH-MDA Reductase	Ascorbate Oxidase	NADH-Fe(CN)$_6$ Reductase
Coated vesicles	17.0 + 3.0	41 + 9	1031
Clathrin-depleted membranes	14.0 + 1.1	143 + 24	672 + 24
Clathrin-enriched supernatant	0.7 + 0.2	10 + 2	23 + 1
Membranes + supernatant			
Based on total pro.	15.2 + 3.7	57 + 9	22 + 22
Based on memb. pro.	30.4 + 7.4	114 + 18	750 + 40
Golgi apparatus (GA)	1.6 + 0.4	50 + 9	1771 + 5
GA + clathrin-enriched supernatant			
Based on total pro.	1.34 + 0.05		906 + 78
Based on memb. pro.	2.7 + 0.1		1892 + 156

provide for the enhanced electron transport to drive the
movement of the coated vesicles and coated regions during
both exo- and endocytosis as well as with intracellular
membrane translocations.

To test this hypothesis, coated vesicles from rat liver
were treated with 0.5 M tris(hydroxymethyl)methyl ammonium chloride, pH 7.2, to dissociate clathrin baskets. Stripped membranes
were removed by centrifugation for 1 h at 100,000 g and both
fractions, clathrin-depleted membranes and the clathrin-
enriched supernatant, were analyzed for content of clathrin
and membrane proteins by polyacrylamide gel electrophoresis
(3) and for enzymatic activities (Table 1).

Following removal of the clathrin coats, ascorbate
oxidase was enriched 3-fold in the membrane pellets as expected for a membrane-associated enzyme. However, neither
NADH-MDAR nor NADH-Fe(CN)$_6$ reductase showed enrichment, nor
did the supernatant containing the clathrin have activity.
However, when the coated vesicles were reconsitituted by
combining the two fractions, the final specific activity
based on total protein was nearer that of the starting
coated vesicles prior to extraction and approximately 3-fold

stimulated based on membrane protein for NADH-MDAR. Ascorbate oxidase was not so affected. NADH-Fe(CN)$_6$ reductase showed a similar, although not as striking, trend as NADH-MDAR. Addition of the clathrin-enriched fractions to Golgi apparatus membranes resulted in a nearly 2-fold stimulation of the NADH-MDAR as well (Table 1). Additionally, the activity of NADH-MDAR of coated vesicles and Golgi apparatus but not that of the endoplasmic reticulum was stimulated by calmodulin and was inhibited by drugs which are known inhibitors of calmodulin function (4).

To test for changes in membrane potential in the coated vesicles from rat liver in response to the addition of monodehydroascorbate and NADH as well as ascorbate, experiments were conducted using fluorescence of carbocyanine dyes to estimate relative changes in membrane potential (17). A response was noted (Table 2) and the combination of NADH plus monodehydroascorbate gave a greater response than either one alone. Ascorbate (1.5 mM) was similar to NADH alone.

The slow decline of fluorescence of the control vesicles was stopped by addition of KCl. Furthermore, if NADH was added with the KCl, the rate of fluorescence decline was increased. Monodehydroascorbate also increased the fluorescence decline in the presence of KCl. These exeriments, although reproducible in three trials, must still be regarded as preliminary and after suitable controls and calibrations are completed may indicate that a membrane potential in these vesicles can be modified by the redox systems present.

Table 2. Changes in charge across coated vesicle membranes measured by carbocyanine dye fluorescence (17).

Addition	Arbitrary units/min/mg protein
None	-2.2
+ 4 mM KCl	-0.7
45 µM NADH	-2.8
+ 4 mM KCl	-1.7
5 mM Monodehydroascorbate	-2.8
+ 4 mM KCl	-1.4
45 µM NADH + 5 mM Monodehydroascorbate	-3.3
+ 4 mM KCl	-1.1

Proton pumping to maintain an electrochemical gradient is well known in the major cell compartments including coated vesicles (18-20). Zang and Schneider (21) have found high ATPase activity in Golgi apparatus from rat liver. This ATPase could be inhibited by dicyclohexylcarbodiimide which also resulted in a 3-fold accumulation of newly synthesized proteins in Golgi apparatus. Thus, the implication is that energy for Golgi apparatus and, perhaps, of coated vesicle function is supported in part by an electrogenic proton gradient. Additionally, Glickman et al. have found a proton pump in Golgi apparatus that functions in parallel to chloride conductance (22).

In our own studies (23), we have found that Golgi apparatus membranes, isolated from mouse liver, pump protons inwards when supplied either with ATP or NADH. Acidification of Golgi apparatus cisternae was detected with neutral red, a permeant dye at neutral pH absorbing at 600 nm which becomes protonated to a non-permeant form absorbing at 550 nm within the interiors of acidified vesicles. Monensin, an ionophoric antibotic which catalyzes the exchange of mono-valent cations across biological membranes, disrupts the secretory function of Golgi apparatus (24) and has been related to acidification of the cisternal interiors as a prerequisiste for swelling and disruption of secretory activity (25). Monensin inhibits the acidification of Golgi apparatus mediated either by ATP or by NADH and at 20 μM strongly inhibits the activity of NADH semidehydroascorbate reductase activity in both coated vesicles and Golgi appara-tus (Table 3). This concentration of monensin had little or no effect on NADH-MDAR activity of endoplasmic reticulum and serves to indicate, along with other evidence (3), that the NADH-MDAR activity of Golgi apparatus and of coated vesicles

Table 3. Inhibition by monensin of NADH semidehydroascorbate reductase activity in membranes. Units of specific activity are nmoles NADH oxidized/min/mg protein. From Sun et al. (3).

| Monensin (μM) | NADH-monodehydroascorbate reductase specific activity | | |
	Golgi apparatus	Coated vesicles	Endoplasmic reticulum
0	4.3	15.5	24
5	4.5	14	22
10	3.9	13.5	22
20	0.8	9.5	21

is different from that of the classical cytochrome b_5
reductase complex of endoplasmic reticulum (12).

In a first attempt to relate the biochemical observations to a functional role for ascorbate in living cells, we
examined the response of coated vesicles of rat hepatocytes
and hepatomas to ascorbate supplied in the medium (27). The
results show a quantitative response in the number of coated
vesicles visible in the Golgi apparatus zone (Fig. 3).

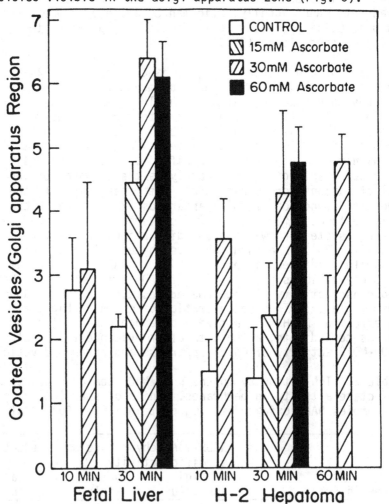

Fig. 3. Quantitation of numbers of coated vesicles per Golgi
apparatus region comparing fetal liver and H-2 hepatoma cells
(27). Ascorbate was added to the culture medium at t = 0.

As summarized in Figure 3, cultured hepatocytes and hepatoma cells when treated for 10-30 min with 30 mM ascorbate responded by a 2- to 3-fold increase in the numbers of coated vesicles of the Golgi apparatus zone as determined by quantitation from electron micrographs. At a near optimal concentration of 30 mM ascorbate, the effect was reproduced under a variety of different conditions of specimen preparation for electron microscopy (27). Coated vesicles of the cell surface may have been affected similarly but no increases due to ascorbate were obvious and were not quantitated due to lack of localization of coated vesicles of the cell surface to well defined cellular regions. Based on measurements of vesicle diameters, coated vesicles of liver cells distribute into different populations (7). Those at the cell surface have the greatest diameters and are distinct from those at the Golgi apparatus with the smallest diameters. However, the increase in numbers of coated vesicles of the Golgi apparatus zone may indicate some functional relationship between ascorbic acid and coated vesicle activity in agreement with our biochemical observations.

SUMMARY

Coated vesicles isolated from rat liver in about 80% fraction purity were enriched in NADH-monodehydroascorbate reductase activity, ascorbate oxidase, and ascorbic acid. The NADH-monodehydroascorbate reductase (and ascorbate oxidase) of the Golgi apparatus and coated vesicles differed from that of the endoplasmic reticulum in being inhibited by the sodium selective ionophore, monensin. Activities of both coated vesicles and Golgi apparatus fractions depleted of the coat protein, clathrin, were activated by the addition of clathrin-rich supernatant fractions. This activation was demonstrated both from cytochemistry in vivo and in vitro in reconstitution experiments with both coated vesicles and isolated Golgi apparatus. More than 60% of the ascorbic acid of rat liver homogenates was contained within membrane-bound compartments. Golgi apparatus and coated vesicles especially were enriched. The transmembrane redox activity involving the NADH-monodehydroascorbate reductase/ascorbic acid oxidase/ascorbic acid complex (Fig. 2) appeared to be able to generate a proton gradient or membrane potential capable of energizing membranes of cell components. Ascorbate administered to hepatocytes or hepatoma cells increased the numbers of coated vesicles associated with the Golgi apparatus regions. Supported in part by grants from Hoffman-LaRoche.

1. Morrē, D.J. (1977) Intern. Cell Biol. 1976-77. Brinkley, B.R. and Porter, K.R., eds. Rockefeller Univ. Press. pp. 293-303.
2. Palade, G.E. (1983) Methods Enzymol. 96, xxix-lv.
3. Sun, I.L., Crane, F.L., and Morrē, D.J. (1983) Biochem. Biophys. Res. Commun. 115, 952-957.
4. Sun, I.L., Morrē, D.J., Crane, F.L., Safranski, K. and Croze, E.M. (1984) Biochim. Biophys. Acta 797, 266-275.
5. Pearse, B.M.F. (1980) Trends. Biochem. Sci. 111, 131-134.
6. Pearse, B.M.F. (1976) Proc. Natl. Acad. Sci. 73, 1255-1259.
7. Croze, E.M., Morrē, D.M., and Morrē, D.J. (1983) Protoplasma 117, 45-52.
8. Morrē, D.J. (1981) Intern. Cell Biol. 1980-81. Schweiger, H., ed., Springer-Verlag, Berlin. pp. 622-632.
9. Goldenberg, H., Crane, F.L., and Morrē, D.J. (1979) J. Biol. Chem. 254, 2491-2498.
10. Crane, F.L., Goldenberg, H., and Morrē, D.J. (1979) Subcell. Biochem. 6, 345-399.
11. Morrē, D.J., Vigil, E.L., Frantz, C., Goldenberg, H., and Crane, F.L. (1978) Cytobiologie 18, 213-230.
12. Hara, T. and Minakami, S. (1971) J. Biochem. 69, 325-330.
13. Schulze, H.-U., Gallenkamp, H., and Staudinger, Hj.)1970) Hoppe-Seyler's Z. Physiol. Chem. 351, 809-817.
14. Schulze, H.-U. and Staudinger, Hj. (1971) Hoppe-Seyler's Z. Physiol. Chem. 352, 1659-1674.
15. Geiß, D. and Schulze, H.-U. (1975) FEBS Letters 60, 374-379.
16. Morrē, D.J. (1973) Mol. Tech. and Approaches in Devel. Biol., Chrispeels, M.J., ed. John Wiley, New York, pp. 1-27.
17. Sims, P.J., Waggoner, A.S., Wang, C.H., and Hoffman, J.F. (1974) Biochemistry 13, 3315-3330.
18. Stone, D.K., Xie, X.-S., and Racker, E. (1983) J. Biol. Chem. 258, 4059-4062.
19. Xie, X.-S., Stone, D.K., and Racker, E. (1983) J. Biol. Chem. 258, 14834-14838.
20. Forgac, M., Cantley, L., Wiedemann, B., Altstiel, L., and Branton, D. (1983) Proc. Natl. Acad. Sci. 80, 1300-1303.
21. Zang, G. and Schneider, D.L. (1983) Biochem. Biophys. Res. Commun. 114, 620-625.
22. Glickman, J., Croen, K., Kelly, S., and Al-Awquati, Q. (1983) J. Cell Biol. 97, 1303-1308.
23. Barr, R., Safranski, K., Sun, I.L., Crane, F.L. and Morrē, D.J. (1984) J. Biol. Chem. 259, 14604-14607.
24. Tartakoff, A.M. (1983) Cell 32, 1026-1028.
25. Boss, W.F., Morrē, D.J., and Mollenhauer, H.H. (1984) European J. Cell Biol. 34, 1-8.
26. Minnifield, N. and Morrē, D.J. (1984) Cell Biol. Intern. Rpts. 8, 215-219.

MODIFICATION OF TUMOR CELL RESPONSE

IN VITRO BY VITAMIN E

Kedar N. Prasad, Bhola N. Rama, and
Richard M. Detsch
Center for Vitamins and Cancer Research
Department of Radiology
University of Colorado Health Sciences Center
Denver, Colorado   80262

Introduction

The transformation from normal cells to cancer cells as a result of ionizing radiation, chemical carcinogens (tumor initiators and promoters), viruses, any combination of these agents, or random genetic error during replication probably occur frequently in the body; however, these transformed cells do not always establish themselves in the host as a clinical cancer. This suggests that the host exerts considerable selection pressure against the first or the first few transformed cells. The transformed cells probably escape the selection pressure of the host when the level of selection pressure is reduced. The transformed cells then acquire additional mutations and eventually become clinically detectable. Recent studies have identified several components of the host's selection pressure. These include certain vitamins, selenium, cAMP (adenosine 3',5'-cyclic monophosphate), and the host's immune system. Among vitamins, alpha-tocopherol (vitamin E) is one of the important components of the host's selection pressure against transformed cells. Since the transformed cells escape the selection pressure exerted by vitamin E at lower concentrations, this vitamin at higher concentrations should exert its antitumor activities either by inducing normal phenotype and/or by causing growth inhibition. Indeed, recent experimental results confirm the above anticancer activities of vitamin E.

Vitamin E in Cancer Prevention

Alpha tocopherol (vitamin E) has been shown to reduce chemically-induced tumors in animals (1-14). In a recent human prospective study (15), lower plasma vitamin E levels were associated with a higher risk of breast cancer. A recent case-control study (16) has also indicated that the plasma level of vitamin E is inversely related to the risk of lung cancer. The exact mechanisms of cancer protection provided by vitamin E are unknown. However, it has been reported that vitamin E may influence the processes of carcinogenesis at several levels. For example, vitamin E blocks the formation of cancer-causing agents such as nitrosamine and mutagenic substances in the gastrointestinal tract (13,17-22), prevents the action of tumor promoters (1-2) and initiators, and stimulates cellular immunity (23-29). Vitamin E has also been shown to stabilize the cellular membrane (30-34). This observation may be important in evaluating the role of vitamin E in regulating cell differentiation and malignancy. All these actions of vitamin E are important for cancer protection.

We have unraveled yet another mechanism of action of vitamin E in cancer prevention and treatment which involves induction of differentiation in certain established tumor cells in culture (35). This finding suggests that the presence of higher levels of vitamin E in the body may also reverse some newly transformed cells back to normal phenotype. This mechanism of cancer prevention may not be applicable to all types of cancer cells.

Vitamin E and Cell Differentiation

The phenomenon of differentiation of tumor cells is important not only from the prevention point of view but also from the perspective of treating cancer. In recent years several naturally occurring and nontoxic differentiating agents such as adenosine 3',5'-cyclic monophosphate (cAMP) (36-41), vitamin A (42-44), nerve growth factor (45-46), and butyric acid (47) have been identified. A more recent study (48) suggests that vitamin E succinate also enhances the level of differentiation of murine NB cells induced by cAMP stimulating agents. This suggests for the first time that vitamin E may regulate at least some effect of cAMP. The role of vitamin E in the differentiation of tumors cells is discussed below.

Neuroblastoma cells. The first report that vitamin E may induce differentiation in tumor cells appeared in 1979; it was demonstrated that dl-alpha tocopheryl acetate treatment of murine neuroblastoma (NBP_2) cells in culture induces morphological differentiation associated with the inhibition of cell division (49). However, in a later study (35), the vitamin E acetate solvent was found to be toxic for several types of tumor cells in culture. Since several toxic agents such as x-rays (50), adriamycin (51), bleomycin (51) and cytosine arabinoside (52) are known to cause morphological changes in NB cells in culture, the effect of vitamin E was re-investigated using dl-alpha tocopheryl succinate which is readily soluble in ethanol. It was found that vitamin E succinate by itself did not cause morphological differentiation (53); however, vitamin E succinate-treated cells were larger and did not grow in clumps. In addition, vitamin E succinate enhanced the differentiating effects of cyclic AMP stimulating agents (48) and γ-irradiation (54) on NB cells in culture. Vitamin E succinate was found to be more potent than dl-alpha tocopherol free alcohol, dl-alpha tocopheryl acetate and dl-alpha tocopheryl nicotinate (35) on the criteria of growth and survival inhibition. Therefore, vitamin E succinate has been routinely used in the studies of differentiation of tumor cells in culture.

Melanoma cells. D-alpha tocopheryl succinate induces morphological differentiation in murine B16 melanoma cells in culture (35) as evidenced by the fact that soma increase in size, the cytoplasmic processes elongate, and the cells arrange themselves in parallel with each other. These changes resemble those observed in cultures of normal melanocytes. Untreated melanoma cells form clumps during growth and exhibit mostly round

cell morphology. It should be pointed out that about 25%
of the cells were unaffected by vitamin E succinate
treatment. Vitamin E succinate-induced morphological
differentiation is associated with growth inhibition, and
both phenomena are primarily irreversible, i.e., when
vitamin E is removed after four days of treatment, the
differentiated phenotype is not reversed. Further
studies show that vitamin E succinate-induced
morphological differentiation of melanoma cells is also
expressed in hormone-supplemented serum-free medium;
however, the concentration of vitamin E succinate needed
to produce the effect is five times less. This suggests
that the effect of vitamin E succinate on melanoma cells
is not due to the involvement of any serum factors. The
exact mechanisms of action of vitamin E succinate on
differentiation of melanoma cells are unknown. In
addition to vitamin E succinate some other physiological
substances, such as cAMP (55-57), have been shown to
induce differentiation of B16 melanoma cells in culture.
It would be important to determine whether or not vitamin
E succinate mediates its effect on melanoma cells by a
cAMP-dependent mechanism or by some unique effect of
vitamin E succinate. It would be equally important to
investigate whether or not vitamin E succinate modulates
the effect of cAMP on melanoma cells. The above studies
would help in designing prevention and treatment studies
of melanoma in a selective and nontoxic manner.

Myeloid leukemia cells. Results of studies of the
differentiating effects of vitamin E on myeloid leukemia
cells have been controversial. One study (58) reports
that dl-alpha tocopherol induces morphological
differentiation in murine myeloid leukemia cells in
culture. Others (59), however, have shown that alpha
tocopherol prevents spontaneous and chemically-induced
differentiation of myeloid leukemia cells in culture.
Some of these differences may be due in part to
differences in solvents. Some solvents of alpha
tocopherol are very toxic to cells in culture (35), which
may account for the differences in results. In a recent
study (60), it has been reported that vitamin E enhances
the level of DMSO-induced differentiation of murine
myeloid leukemia cells in culture.

Glioma and prostate cells. Vitamin E succinate inhibits the growth of rat glioma (C6) cells (53) and human prostate cells (Webber and Prasad, unpublished observation) in culture without inducing cell differentiation.

Significance of vitamin E-induced differentiation in cancer prevention and treatment. The studies discussed above have been performed in vitro and cannot be extrapolated to in vivo phenomena. However, they do suggest that vitamin E succinate may reverse newly transformed cells back to normal phenotype, possibly an important mechanism for preventing certain tumors. The fact that vitamin E succinate induces differentiation in some established tumor cells suggests that this mechanism of action may be equally important in the treatment of some tumors with vitamin E succinate.

Modification of the Effect of Chemicals by Vitamin E

Most of the currently used chemotherapeutic agents are immunosuppressive, toxic and not naturally present in the body. These agents kill normal cells as well as tumor cells. It has been reported that dl-alpha-tocopheryl acetate in combination with vincristine, 5-fluorouracil, adriamycin or chlorozotocin produced a synergistic effect, whereas vitamin E in combination with bleomycin, 1-(2--chlorethyl)-3-cyclo-heyxyl-1-nitrosourea (CCNU), 5-3-dimethyl-1-triazeno-imidazole-4-carboxamide (DTIC), mutamycin or cis-diamine dichloro-platinum II produced an additive effect on NB cells in culture on the criterion of growth inhibition. In glioma cell cultures, vitamin E acetate in combination with vincristine or CCNU produced a synergistic effect, whereas vitamin E in combination with bleomycin, 5-fluorouracil, adriamycin, DTIC, mutamycin and cis-platinum produced an additive effect on the criterion of growth inhibition. These studies suggest that modification of the effect of chemotherapeutic agents on tumor cells depends upon tumor form and type of chemotherapeutic agent.

Our studies show that dl-alpha-tocopheryl acetate markedly enhances the antitumor effect of naturally occurring substances on NB, glioma and melanoma cells in

culture. For example, vitamin E and vitamin E succinate
enhance the effect of cAMP-stimulating agents (PEG$_1$ and
PGA$_2$, stimulators of adenylate cyclase, and RO20-1724, an
inhibitor of cyclic nucleotide phosphodiesterase) and
sodium butyrate (a four-carbon fatty acid). The extent
of vitamin E enhancement depends upon the form of tumor
cell and the type of naturally occurring substances. For
example, vitamin E in combination with PGE$_1$, RO20-1724 or
sodium butyrate produced a synergistic effect on NB
cells, whereas in glioma cell cultures, vitamin E in
combination with RO20-1724 produced a synergistic effect
on the criterion of growth inhibition. Vitamin E failed
to enhance the effect of PGE$_1$ and sodium butyrate on
glioma cells. Extensive studies are needed to test the
above concepts on animal tumors before applying them to
human tumors.

Modification of Radiation Effect by Vitamin E

Several studies have reported that vitamin E
protects normal tissue in vitro and in vivo against
radiation damage (64-71), whereas others have shown that
vitamin E is ineffective in protecting normal or tummor
tissue (72-75). Recent studies suggest that vitamin E
succinate at high concentrations, which by themselves
inhibit the growth of cells, enhances the effect of
radiation on murine NB cells in culture in an additive
manner (76). Vitamin E-induced enhancement of radiation
effect has also been observed on transplanted rat tumor
(77-78).

The exact mechanisms of vitamin E-induced
enhancement of radiation effects on tumor cells are
unknown; however, it has been reported (54) that
butylated hydroxyanisole (BHA), a lipid-soluble
antioxidant, also enhances the effect of radiation on NB
cells in culture. This suggests that the part of the
mechanisms of action of vitamin E may involve
antioxidation.

Our recent study (76) shows that vitamin E
succinate, at concentrations which do not affect the
growth of NB cells in culture, protects cells against
radiation damage. Vitamin E succinate increases the

survival of irradiated cells when added to culture immediately after irradiation for the entire observation period (7 days) or immediately before irradiation for the entire observation period. The presence of vitamin E succinate during irradiation alone was ineffective. Thus vitamin E succinate can be defined as a radiotherapeutic agent rather than as a radioprotective agent, since it appears to help the repair of post-irradiation damage. The radiotherapeutic effect of vitamin E succinate on NB cells in culture is primarily due to the effect of succinic acid, because sodium succinate also increased the survival of irradiated cells in a similar manner. Vitamin E succinate under certain experimental conditions may be slightly more effective than sodium succinate. To our knowledge, vitamin E succinate and sodium succinate are the first non-toxic chemicals which help the repair of post-irradiation damage.

Since the type and extent of the effects of vitamin E succinate are dependent upon the concentration of vitamin E succinate, radiation dose, form of tumor and type of chemotherapeutic agents, any pre-clinical or clinical study using vitamin E succinate must take into consideration all of these variables; otherwise, the efforts to modify tumor cell response with vitamin E may be ineffective.

Modification of the Effect of Hyperthermia by Vitamin E

We have reported (79,80) that vitamin E succinate, at concentrations which inhibit the growth of NB cells in culture, enhanced the effect of heat on the criteria of growth and survival in an additive manner. The presence of vitamin E during heat treatment and during the entire experimental period of observation was necessary for the above effects. BHA, a lipid soluble antioxidant, also enhanced the effect of heat, but to a lesser degree than that produced by vitamin E succinate. The fact that the vitamin E succinate in combination with heat produced only an additive effect suggests that the mechanisms of action of these agents on tumor cells are different.

Mechanisms of Action of Vitamin E Succinate

The exact mechanisms of action of vitamin E succinate on tumor cells are unknown. Two lipid-soluble antioxidants, butylated hydroxyanisole (BHA) and butylated hydroxytoluene (BHT), which share only antioxidant properties with vitamin E, produce morphological changes in some tumor cells in culture similar to those produced by vitamin E succinate (53). Thus the mechanisms of action of vitamin E succinate on tumor cells may partly involve antioxidation. The current view of the metabolism of vitamin E esters (vitamin E acetate and vitamin E succinate) is that they are hydrolyzed in the gut by esterases and form vitamin E free alcohol, which is then absorbed via the lymphatic system and intestinal mucosal cells. It is believed that only vitamin E free alcohol acts as an antioxidant (81-83). Vitamin E esters cannot act as an antioxidant until they are converted to the free alcohol form.

We have reported that vitamin E succinate is more potent than vitamin E acetate and vitamin E free alcohol (35) in causing cell differentiation and growth inhibition of tumor cells in culture. The higher potency of vitamin E succinate has also been reported by other investigators. For example, vitamin E succinate prevents radiation-induced transformation of hamster embryo cells in culture, whereas vitamin E free alcohol or vitamin E acetate does not (Dr. Ann Kennedy, personal communication). Vitamin E succinate is more effective in protecting adriamycin-induced skin ulcer than vitamin E acetate. The exact reasons for this are unknown; however, we have tested a hypothesis that the greater potency of vitamin E succinate is related to its higher uptake by tumor cells. To test this hypothesis, the uptake of vitamin E succinate in NB cells in culture was compared with that of vitamin E acetate and vitamin E free alcohol. Confluent NB cells were incubated in the presence of 8 μg/ml of vitamin E succinate. After 10,20,40 and 80 hours of incubation, cells were washed with serum-free medium three times and the levels of vitamin E succinate and free alcohol were determined by a HPLC, using vitamin E acetate as an internal standard. Results showed that untreated control cultures did not have any detectable levels of vitamin E succinate or vitamin E free alcohol. In treated cultures only vitamin E succinate was detected. When the cells were similarly treated with vitamin E acetate or vitamin E free alcohol for 20 hours, no uptake of either was detected. Thus, the greater potency of vitamin E succinate may be due to the fact that tumor cells pick up this form of vitamin E more readily.

The fact that only vitamin E succinate was detectable during the entire three days indicates that vitamin E succinate was either not hydrolyzed to vitamin E free alcohol within the cells or the amounts of converted vitamin E free alcohol were too small to be detected by our methodology. At this time it is unknown whether all the effects of vitamin E succinate on tumor cells are mediated by itself, by vitamin E free alcohol or by both forms of vitamin E.

Conclusions and Comments

The fact that vitamin E induces differentiation in some tumor cells and inhibits the growth and survival of all tumor cells in culture studies suggests that this mechanism of action of vitamin E may be important not only in cancer therapy but also in cancer prevention. We have observed that vitamin E succinate is more potent than the other forms of vitamin E (vitamin E free alcohol, vitamin E acetate and vitamin E nicotinate) on tumor cells. This is because vitamin E succinate is readily picked up by tumor cells, whereas other forms of vitamin E are not. Vitamin E succinate may act as a radiotherapeutic agent or radiosensitizing agent depending upon the concentrations of vitamin E. The radiotherapeutic effect of low concentration of vitamin E succinate is primarily due to the effect of succinic acid. Vitamin E succinate, at concentrations which inhibit the growth of tumor cells in culture, also enhance the effect of chemicals in an additive or synergistic manner, depending upon the type of chemicals and the form of tumor cells. High concentrations of vitamin E succinate also enhanced the effect of heat on NB cells in an additive manner. Further studies are needed to evaluate the role of vitamin E in cancer prevention and treatment.

REFERENCES

1. Boutwell, R.K. Biology and biochemistry of the two-step model of carcinogenesis. In F.L. Meyskens and K.N. Prasad (eds.), Modulation and mediation of cancer by vitamins, pp. 2-9, Basel:Karger Press, 1983.

2. Slaga, T.J. Multistage skin carcinogenesis and specificity of inhibitors. In F.L. Meyskens and K.N. Prasad (eds.), Modulation and mediation of cancer by vitamins, pp. 10-23, Basel:Karger Press, 1983.

3. Cook, M.G. and McNamara, P. Effect of dietary vitamin E on dimethylhydrazine induced colonic tumors in mice. Cancer Res., 40:1329-1331, 1980.

4. Ellison, N.M. and Londer H. Vitamin E and C and their relationship to cancer. Prog. Cancer Res. Therap., 17:233-241, 1981.

5. Haber, S.L. and Wissler, R.W. Effect of vitamin E on carcinogenicity of methylcholanthrene. Proc. Soc. Exp. Biol. & Med., 111:774-775, 1962.

6. Jaffe, W. The influence of wheat germ oil in the production of tumors in rats by methylcholanthrene. Exp. Med. Surg., 4:278-282, 1964.

7. Weerapdist, W. and Shklar, G. Vitamin E inhibition of hamster buccal pouch carcinogenesis. Oral Med. Oral Path. Oral Surg., 54:304-312, 1982.

8. Harman, D. Dimethylbenzanthracene-induced cancer: Inhibiting effect of dietary vitamin E. Clin. Res., 17:125a, 1969.

9. Lee, C. and Chen, C. Enhancemment of mammary tumorigenesis in rats by vitamin E deficiency. Proc. Am. Assoc. Cancer Res., 20:132a, 1979.

10. Ip, C. Dietary vitamin E intake and mammary carcinogenesis in rat. Carcinogenesis, 3:1453-1456, 1982.

11. Newberne, P.M. and Suphakarn, V. Nutrition and cancer: A review with emphasis on the role of vitamin C and E and selenium. Nutri. and Cancer 5:107-119, 1983.

12. Wang, Y-M, Howell, S.K., Kimball, J., Tsai, C.C., Sato, G., and Gleiser, C.A. Alpha-tocopherol as a potential modifier of daunomycin carcinogenecity in Sprague-Dawley rats. In Arnott, Van Eys, Y-N Wang (eds.), Molecular interrelation of nutrition and cancer, pp. 369-379, Raven Press:New York, 1982.

13. Newmark, J.L. and Mergens, W.J. Alpha-tocopherol (vitamin E) and its relationship to tumor induction and development. In Zedecik, Lipkins (eds.), Inhibition of tumor induction and development, pp. 127-168, Plenum:New York, 1981.

14. Odukoya, O., Hawach, F. and Shaklar, G. Retardation in experimental oral cancer by topical vitamin E. Nutri. and Cancer 6:98-104, 1984.

15. Wald, N.J., Boreham, J., Hayward, J.L., and Bulbrook, R.D. Plasma retinol, beta-carotene and vitamin E levels in relation to the future risk of breast cancer: Prospective studies involving 5,000 women. Brit. J. Cancer 49:321-324, 1984.

16. Menkes, M. and Comstock, G. Vitamin A and E and lung cancer. Am. J. Epidem. 120:490a, 1984.

17. Newmark, H.L. and Mergen, W.J. Application of ascorbic acid and tocopherols as inhibitors of nitrosamine formation and oxidation in food. In Solms, Hall (eds.), Criteria of food acceptance, pp. 379-390, Forster Publishing:Zurich, 1981.

18. Astill, B.D. and Mulligan, L.T. Phenolic antioxidants and the inhibition of hepatoxicity from N-diemthyl-nitrosamine formed in situ in the rat stomach. Food Cosm. Toxicol. 15:167-171, 1977.

19. Kamm, J.J., Dashman, T., Conney, A.H., et al. Effect of ascorbic acid on amine-nitrite toxicity. Ann. N.Y. Acad. Sci. 258:69-174, 1975.

20. Kamm, J.J., Dashman, T., Newmark, H., et al. Inhibition of amine nitrite hepatoxicity of alpha-tocopherol. Toxicol. Appl. Pharmacol. 41:575-583, 1977.

21. Bruce, W.R. and Dion, P.W. Studies relating to a fecal mutagen. Am. J. Clin. Nutr. 35:2511-2512, 1981.

22. Bright-See, E. and Newmark, H.L. Potential and probable role of vitamin C and E in the prevention of carcinogenesis. In F.L. Meyskens and K. N. Prasad (eds.), Modulation and mediation of cancer by vitamins, pp. 95-103, Karger:Basel, 1983.

23. Nockels, C.F. Protective effects of supplemental vitamin E against infection. Fed. Proc. 38:2134-2136, 1978.

24. Sheffy, B.E. and Schultz, R.D. Influence of vitamin E and selenium on immune response mechanisms. Fed. Proc. 38:2139-2143, 1979.

25. Tengerdy, R.P. Effect of vitamin E on immune response. In Machlin (ed.), Vitamin E, pp. 429-443, Dekker:New York, 1980.

26. Tanaka, J., Fujiwara, H. and Toriso, M. Vitamin E and immune response enhancement of helper-T-cell activity by dietary supplementation of vitamin E in mice. Immunology 38:727-734, 1979.

27. Yasunaga, T., Kato, H., Ohgaki, K., Inamota, T. and Hgikasa, T. Effect of vitamin E as immunopotentiation agent for mice at optimal dosage and its toxicity at high dosage. J. Nutr. 112:1075-1084, 1982.

28. Kurek, M.P. and Corwin, L.M. Vitamin E protection against tumor formation by transplanted murine sarcoma. Nutr. Cancer 4:128-139, 1982.

29. Black, M.M., Zachrau, R.E., Dion, A.S. and Katz, M. Stimulation of prognostically favorable cell-mediated immunity of breast cancer patients by high dose vitamin A and vitamin E. In K.N. Prasad (ed.), Vitamins, nutrition and cancer, pp. 134-143, Karger:Basel, 1984.

30. Molenar, I., Vos, J. and Hommmes, F.A. Effect of vitamin E deficiency on cellular membrane. Vitamins Horm. Res. 30:45-82, 1972.

31. Huang, C. Configuration of fatty acyl chains in EGG phosphatidylcholine-cholesterol mixed bilayer. Chem. Phys. Lipids 191:150-158, 1977.

32. Lucy, J.A. Structural interactions between vitamin E and polyunsaturated phospholipids. In deDuve, Hyaishi (eds.), Tocopherol, oxygen and biomembranes, pp. 109-120, Elsevier-North-Holland Medical Press, New York, 1978.

33. Maruschi, W.L. Vitamin E as in vivo lipid stabilizer and its effect on flavor and storage properties of milk and meat. In Machlin (ed.), Vitamin E, pp. 445-46, Dekker:New York, 1980.

34. Olcott, H.S. and Matill, H.A. Constituents of fats and oils affecting the development of rancidity. Chem. Res. 29:257-268, 1941.

35. Prasad, K.N. and Edwards-Prasad, J. Effect of
     tocopherol (vitamin E) acid succinate on
     morphological alterations and growth inhibition in
     melanoma cells in culture. Cancer Res. 42:550-555,
     1982.
36. Puck, T.T. Cyclic AMP, the microtubule-
     microfilament system and cancer. Proc. Natl. Acad.
     Sci., USA, 74:4491-4495, 1977.
37. Pastan, I. and Johnson, G.S. Cyclic AMP and the
     transformation of fibroblasts. Adv. Cancer Res.
     19:303-329, 1974.
38. Prasad, K.N.: Involvement of cyclic nucleotide in
     transformation. In Cameron, Pool (eds.), The
     transformation, pp. 236-266, 1981.
39. Ryan, W.L. and Heidrick, M.L. Role of cyclic
     nucleotide in cancer. Adv. Cyclic Nuc. Res. 4:87-
     116, 1974.
40. Granner, D.K. Protein kinase: Altered regulation
     in a hepatoma cell line deficient in adenosine
     3',5'-cyclic monophosphate binding proteins.
     Biochem. Biophys. Res. Commun. 46:1516-1522, 1972.
41. Prasad, K.N. Differentiation of neuroblastoma cells
     in culture. Biol. Rev. 50:129-165, 1975.
42. Lotan, R., Thein, R. and Lotan, D. Suppression of
     the transformed cell phenotype expression by
     retinoids. In F.L. Meyskens and K.N. Prasad (eds.),
     Modulation and mediation of cancer by vitamins, pp.
     211-222, Karger:Basel, 1983.
43. Sidell, N., Worth, G.D. and Seeger, R.C. Evidence
     for the ability of retinoic acid to regulate the
     phenotypic expression of human neuroblastoma. In
     F.L. Meyskens and K.N. Prasad (eds.), Modulation and
     mediation of cancer by vitamins, pp. 228-235,
     Karger:Basel, 1983.
44. Speers, W.C., Zimmerman, B. and Altmann, M.
     Transplantation of retinoic acid differentiated
     murine embryonal carcinomas. In K.N. Prasad (ed.),
     Vitamins, nutrition and cancer, Karger:Basel, 1984.
45. Goldstein, M.N., Land, V. and Bradshaw, R.
     Stimulation of human neuroblastoma in vitro with
     nerve growth factor. Proc. Am. Assoc. Cancer Res.
     13:89a, 1972.

46. Waris, T., Rochardt, L. and Waris, P. Differentiation of neuroblastoma cells induced by nerve growth factor in vitro. Experientia 29:1128, 1973.
47. Prasad, K.N. Butyric acid: A small fatty acid with diverse biological functions. Life Sci. 27:1351-1358, 1980.
48. Rama, B.N. and Prasad, K.N. Effect of dl-alpha tocopheryl succinate in combination with sodium butyrate and cAMP stimulating agent on neuroblastoma cells in culture. Int. J. Cancer 34:863-867, 1984.
49. Prasad, K.N., Ramanujam, S. and Gaudreau, D. Vitamin E induces morphological differentiation and increases the effect of ionizing radiation on neuroblastoma cells in culture. Proc. Soc. Exp. Biol. and Med. 161:570-575, 1979.
50. Prasad, K.N. X-ray induced cell morphological differentiation of mouse neuroblastoma cells in vitro. Nature 234:471-474, 1971.
51. Prasad, K.N., Edwards-Prasad, J., Ramanujam, S., and Sakamoto, A. Vitamin E increases the growth inhibitory and differentiating effects of tumor therapeutic agents in neuroblastoma and glioma cells in culture. Proc. Soc. Exp. Biol. Med. 164:158-163, 1980.
52. Katis, J.R., Winterton, R., and Schlesinger, K. Induction of acetylcholinesterase in mouse neuroblastoma tissue culture cells. Nature 229:345-346, 1971.
53. Rama, B.N. and Prasad, K.N. Studies on specificity of alpha-tocopheryl (vitamin E) acid succinate effects on melanoma, glioma and neuroblastoma cells in culture. Proc. Soc. Exp. Biol. & Med. 174:302-307, 1983.
54. Sarria, A. and Prasad, K.N. DL-alpha tocopheryl succinate enhances the effect of γ-irradiation on neuroblastomma cells in culture. Proc. Soc. Exp. Biol. & Med. 175:88-91, 1984.
55. Johnson, G.S. and Pastan, I. N^6O^2-Dibutyryl adenosine 3',5'-monophosphate induces pigment production in melanoma cells. Nature New Biol. 237:267-268, 1972.

56. Krieder, J.W., Rosenthal, M. and Linngle, N. Cyclic adenosine 3',5'-monophosphate in the control of melanoma cell replication and differentiation. J. Natl. Cancer Inst. 50:555-558, 1973.

57. Prasad, K.N. Role of prostaglandins in differentiation of neuroblastoma cells in culture. In Powels, Bockman, Honn, Ramwell (eds.), Prostaglandins and cancer, pp. 437-451, Alan R. Liss:New York, 1982.

58. Sakagami, H., Asaka, K., Abe, E., Miyaura, C., Suda, T., and Konno, K. Effect of dl-alpha tocopherol (vitamin E) on the differentiation of mouse myeloid leukemia cells. J. Nutr. Sci. Vitaminol. 27:291-300, 1981.

59. Takenag, K., Honma, Y. and Hoxumi, M. Inhibition of differentiation of mouse myeloid leukemia cells by phenolic antioxidants and α-tocopherol. Gann. 72:104-112, 1981.

60. Ohno, Y., Tokuma, T., Asashi, K., and Isono, K. Differentiation induction of murine erythroid leukemic cells by butylated hydroxytoluene. FEBS Letters 165:277-279, 1984.

61. Tappel, A.L. Vitamin E and free radicals perioxidation of lipids. Ann. N.Y. Acad. Sci. 203:12-27, 1972.

62. Diplock, A.T. and Lucy, J.A. The biological modes of action of vitamin E and selenium: A hypothesis. FEBS Letters 29:205-210, 1973.

63. McCay, P.C. and King, M.M. Vitamin E: Its role as a biological free radical scavenger and its relationship to the microsomal mixed-function oxidase system. In Machlin (ed.), Vitamin E, pp. 289-317, Dekker:New York, 1980.

64. Srinivasan, V., Jacobs, A.L., Simpson, S.A., and Weiss, J.F. Radioprotection by vitamin E. Effect on hepatic enzymes, delayed type hypersensitivity and post-irradiation survival of mice. In F.L. Meyskens, Jr. and K.N. Prasad (eds.), First international conference on the modulation an dmediation of cancer by vitamins, pp. 119-131, Basel:Karger, 1983.

65. Bacq, Z.M. and Herve A. Protection of mice against a lethal dose of x-rays by cyanide, azide and malononitrile. Brit. J. Radiol. 24:617-621, 1951.

66. Huber, R. and Schroeder, E. Anntioxydantien and Uberlbenstrate ganzkorperbestrahlter Mause. Strahlentherapie 119:308-315, 1962.

67. Sakamoto, K. and Sakka M. Reduced effect of irradiation on normal and malignant cells irradiated in vivo in mice pretreated with vitamin E. Brit. J. Radiol. 46:538-540, 1973.

68. Malick, M.A., Roy, R.M. and Sternberg, J. Effect of vitamin E on post-irradiation death in mice. Experientia 34:1216-1217, 1978.

69. Londer, H.M. and Myers, C.E. Radioprotective effect of vitamin E. Amer. J. Clin. Nutr. 31:705, 1978.

70. Prince, E.W. and Little, J.B. The effects of dietary fatty acids and tocopherol on the radiosensitivity of mammalian erythrocytes. Radiat. Res. 53:49-64, 1973.

71. Hoffer, A. and Roy, R.M. Vitamin E decreases erythrocyte fragility after whole-body irradiation. Radiat. Res. 61:439-443, 1975.

72. Furth, F.W., Coutler, M.P. and Howland, J.W. Failure of alpha tocopherol to protect against radiation injury in the rat. Univ. Rochester Atomic Energy Rep. 152:34, 1951.

73. Haley, T.K., McCulloh, E.F. and McCormick, W.G. Influence of water-soluble vitamin E on survival time in irradiated mice. Science 119:126-127, 1954.

74. Ershoff, B.H. and Steers, C.W. Jr. Antioxidants and survival time of mice exposed to multiple sublethal doses of -irradiation. Proc. Soc. Exp. Biol. Med. 104:274-276.

75. Rostock, R.A., Stryker, J.A. and Abt, A.B. Evaluation of high-dose vitamin E as a radioprotective agent. Radiology 136:763-765, 1980.

76. Rama, B.N., Detech, R.M. and Prasad, K.N. Combined effect of dl-alpha tocopheryl succinate, γ-irradiation and hyperthermia on neuroblastoma cells in culture. Journal of American Medical College of Nutrition, 3(3):252, 1984.

77. Kagerud, A., Holm. G., Larsson, H., and Peterson, H.I. Tocopherol and local x-ray irradiation of two transplantable rat tumors. Cancer Lett. 5:123-129, 1978.

78. Kagerud, A. and Peterson, H.I. Tocopherol in irradiation of experimental neoplasms. Influence of dose and administration. Acta Radiol. Oncol. 20:97, 1981.
79. Rama, B.N. and Prasad, K.N. Modification of the effect of hyperthermia on neuroblastoma cells in culture by DL-alpha tocopheryl succinate. Journal of Nutrition, Growth and Cancer 1:155-163, 1983.
80. Rama, B.N. and Prasad, K.N. Effect of hyperthermia in combination with vitamin E and cAMP on neuroblastoma cells in culture. Life Sciences 34, 21:2089-2097, 1984.
81. Diplock, A.T. and Lucy, J.A. The biochemical modes of action of vitamin E and selenium. A hypothesis. FEBS Lett. 29:205-210, 1973.
82. McCay, P.B. and King, M.M. Vitamin E: Its role as a biological free radical scavenger and its relationship to the microsomal mixed function oxidase system. In I.J. Machlin (ed.), Vitamin E, pp. 289-317, Dekker, 1980.
83. Tappel, A.L. Vitamin E and free radical peroxidation of lipids. Ann. N.Y. Acad. Sci. 203:12-27, 1972.

Acknowledgment

This work was supported by a grant from the Hill Foundation, the Henkel Corporation, The John F. Shafroth Memorial Fund and Eastman Chemical Products, Inc.

CHEMOPREVENTION (PRECLINICAL)

NUTRIENTS AND OTHER RISK FACTORS ASSOCIATED WITH CANCER

Paul M. Newberne, Thomas F. Schrager and
Michael W. Conner

Massachusetts Institute of Technology

Cambridge, MA 02139

The winds of change are sweeping across the face of cancer research and there is some exciting new information becoming available on risk factors and prevention of some forms of neoplasia. Studies about viral carcinogenesis, represented by the sophisticated studies with respect to AIDS; chemoprevention with retinoids, selenium and other substances; and the general aspects of lifestyle, including diet, are all encouraging, pointing toward eventual prevention.

We are gradually accepting the fact that epidemiology, while it offers interesting potential approaches to some problems, leaves much to be desired with respect to causal relationships between dietary nutrients and some forms of cancer. It is one thing to identify a subset of the population who smoke cigarettes and link this habit to lung cancer. It is quite a different matter to link green and yellow vegetables to carotene and thus to prevention of some forms of cancer. We must continue to question epidemiologic approaches, whether population based, case-control or cohort, when the results are to be used as a basis for intervention in some subsets of the population with far-reaching implications.

Perhaps we should use well-designed, rigidly controlled animal studies to guide epidemiologists, rather than vice versa. The diet of the American public is very heterogeneous and there are many confounding variables. Table 1,

taken from the HANES report (1979), illustrates this point.
In any case, the entire area of diet, nutrition and cancer
is yielding to increasingly sophisticated, elegant methodology and we can expect to see even more promising directions
for prevention in the future.

Table 1
Nutrient Intake by Percentiles of the US Population

	Percentile of Population								
	5th	10th	20th	50th	75th	90th	95th	X	SD
Daily protein(g)									
8813 males	36	46	62	84	114	153	179	93	45
11930 females	25	31	43	59	79	102	119	64	31
Daily vitamin A (IU)									
8813 males	801	1184	2057	3503	5951	9796	13770	5138	7245
11930 females	575	872	1548	2714	4781	8581	12625	4431	8016

(From DHEW Publication #79-1221, 1979).

This presentation will discuss epidemiological
suggestions and results of experimental studies relative to
a few specific sites for cancer.

I. CANCER OF THE ESOPHAGUS

A. Epidemiologic Evidence

An early observation of an association between esophageal cancer and nutrition was made nearly 50 years ago. It
was observed that Swedish women suffering from cancer of the
hypopharynx, frequently had anemia; this appeared to be
secondary to iron deficiency and perhaps multiple vitamin
deficiencies (Jacobson, 1961). This syndrome, named the
Plummer-Vinson syndrome, has since that time greatly
decreased in incidence along with general improvement in
iron and vitamin nutrition in that area.

Esophageal cancer represents the most striking
geographic variation, of any tumor site. There is a
wide disparity in incidence of this type tumor from country
to country and from region to region within countries,
suggesting environmental influences. Some of the highest
incidence rates in the world are found in South-Central Asia
in the region between Turkey, Iran, China, and the Soviet
Union. Investigations of this region have shown that these

areas have diets comprised mainly of bread and tea, and are severely deficient in vegetables (Joint Iran-International Agency for Research on Cancer Study Group, 1977). There is also a suggestion that opium ingestion may also be high in these regions. Because the habit is illegal, it is difficult to study this factor with any degree of confidence in a survey design. In a case-control study conducted in Iran as part of the large WHO effort to study esophageal cancer in this area, Cook-Mozaffari et al. (1979) confirmed that cases in Northern Iran tended to ingest lower levels of vitamins and fruits as well as lower levels of animal protein, compared to controls. This confirmed suggestions from the ecological study that deficiencies of vitamins in foods in these areas might be important in the etiology of the unusually high rate of esophageal cancer. Samples of food taken from the typical diets of cases and controls, showed no apparent differences in the levels of carcinogenic aflatoxins in the diet, thus diminishing the liklihood of contamination as a significant factor in esophageal cancer of the area.

The high rate of esophageal cancer observed in blacks in the United States are thought to be associated with alcohol as a risk factor (Pottern et al., 1981). Case-control studies conducted in Europe and North America have shown that alcohol and tobacco are risk factors probably interacting to increase susceptibility to esophageal cancer (Day and Munoz, 1982). On the other hand, in local geographic areas that experience particularly high incidence rates of esophageal cancer, alcohol and tobacco seem to be weak risk factors and probably significant. It was suggested as early as 1961 in a case-control study (Wynder and Bross, 1961) that nutrition was a factor in esophageal cancer. Milk and vegetable consumption was diminished in cases, compared to controls. Ziegler et al. (1981b) studying blacks in the Washington, D.C. area also found that diets deficient in meat, fish, fruits, vegetables, and dairy products were reported more often for cases as compared to controls. Mettlin et al. (1981), in Roswell Park Memorial Institute studies conducted between 1957 and 1964, observed that cases more frequently reported diets deficient in vitamin A than did controls.

Lin et al. (1977) reported low levels of zinc in serum, hair and esophageal tissue with this form of cancer (table 2) which led to some interesting experimental studies reported later in this chapter.

Table 2
Zinc Levels in Serum, Hair and Esophageal
Tissues From Patients With Esophageal Cancer,
Other Types of Cancer or Other Diseases

| | Zinc Concentrations (g/100 l or g) | | Esophageal | |
	Serum	Hair	Tumor	Esophagus
Normal Subjects	102.7+18.5	195.0+29.0	110.0+22.4	160.0+28
Patients With:				
Esophageal Cancer	78.0+14.9	162.0+33.0	---	---
Other Cancers	114.4+31.8	169.0+37.0	---	---
Other Disorders	96.2+15.0	212.0+48.0	149.0+18	248.0+17.0

(From Lin et al., 1977, abridged).

A massive screening program for esophageal cancer has
been initiated in Northern China (Yang, 1980). This will
provide additional valuable information regarding the determinants and natural history of this disease.

B. Experimental Evidence

The association of nutrients with esophageal cancer have
been, for the most part, inferential. In collaboration with
colleagues at the University of Hong Kong, we observed low
concentrations of zinc in serum and tissues of esophageal
cancer, obtained at or shortly after diagnosis. Table 2
lists some of the pertinent data. Based on these observations we have conducted extensive investigations using
experimental animals deficient in zinc (Fong et al., 1978)
with or without other risk factors. Table 3 lists results
typical of many studies. These data clearly imply that
interactions of dietary deficiencies of nutrients and exposure to toxins (alcohol) can significantly enhance esophageal cancer in animals (Gabrial et al., 1982).

An indication of mechanisms of zinc deficiency effects
on the esophagus is the markedly enhanced DNA synthesis and
mitosis in the zinc deficient esophagus. Table 4 lists
selected observations typical of several studies. Cell proliferation is significantly increased in the deficient

Table 3
Induced Tumor Incidence in Rats Deficient in Zinc;
Ethyl Alcohol and 13-cis Retinoic Acid Are Added Factors

Treatment, Zinc Content	MBN	4% Alcohol in Drinking Water	13-cis Retinoic Acid	No. Rats With Tumors	%
Control,60 ppm	-	-	-	0/12	0
Control,60ppm	+	-	-	14/35	40.0
Deficient, 7 ppm	+	-	-	25/33	75.7
60 ppm Control, Deficient 7 ppm to Post Dosing	+	-	-	18/35	51.4
Deficient	+	+	-	29/34	85.3
Deficient	+	+	+	33/35	94.3

(From Gabrial et al., 1982, abridged).

esophageal epithelium; this is temporarily depressed by
treatment with the esophageal carcinogen, MBN. Within three
weeks after carcinogen treatment, however, zinc deficient
epithelium was back to the same rate of DNA synthesis as the
untreated, zinc deficient epithelium while the control,
MBN-treated epithelium was still depressed. The interpretation of these data is that, at time of carcinogen exposure,
the zinc deprived esophagus has many more cells in division
compared to controls; these may be more vulnerable to the
carcinogen.

Table 4
Mitotic Counts and ^{3}H-thymidine in Esophageal
Epithelium of Zinc Deficient Rats

Treatment	^{3}H-thymidine DPM/ug DNA (untreated)	Mitotic Counts % of Counted	
		untreated	+MBN
Control Diet	58+7	2.1+1.5	5.8+1.6
Zn Deficient Diet	152+8	6.9+3.0	2.1+1.3

(Schrager, Busby and Newberne, 1985, unpublished).

We have recently examined the capacity of the esophageal
to incorporate ^{3}H-thymidine into DNA and for the epithelium
to undergo mitosis, when low in zinc (Schrager et al.,
1983). After a single initiating dose of MBN, levels of the
promutagenic bases O^6 methylguanine and 7-methylguanine were
greater in esophageal DNA than non-target hepatic DNA. The
ratio of O^6 methylguanine: 7-methylguanine was greater in

the zinc deficient group than the two control diet groups.

After six (carcinogenic) doses of MBN the levels of both methylated bases increased in both the esophagus and liver, with the greatest increase in the esophagus. Repair was greatest in the pair-fed group and least in the zinc deficient group.

These data suggest that zinc deficient enhancement of MBN esophageal carcinogenesis may be mediated by increased levels of the promutagen 0^6 methylguanine in DNA and a reduced ability to remove it.

Esophageal cancer has been associated with riboflavin deficiency in epidemiological investigations (Cook-Mozaffari, 1979). Oral and esophageal tissue damage has been associated with riboflavin deficiency in primates (Foy and Kondi, 1984). We have shown (Newberne, 1984) that riboflavin deficiency injures the oral and esophageal epithelium in the rat and, also, increases susceptibility and severity of esophageal cancer induced by MBN. Table 5 illustrates characteristic observations.

Table 5
Riboflavin (B_2) Deficiency in the Rat:
Enhanced Esophageal Carcinogenesis

Treatment	Incidence of Neoplasms	
	No.	%
Control Diet	0/10	0.0
Control Diet + MBN*	8/20	40.0
B_2 Deficiency	0/20	0.0
B_2 Deficiency + MBN	23/26	88.0

*Methylbenzylnitrosamine. Newberne, 1984.

II. CANCER OF THE STOMACH

A. Epidemiologic Evidence

Experimental studies in animals have clearly shown that alkylnitrosoureas can induce stomach cancer. There has been research into the biochemistry of the related nitrosamines and nitrosamides, which are capable of being formed within the stomach in conjunction with nitrites and which are found in human saliva (Tannenbaum, 1983). Nitrates, which are commonly added to foods for preservation, have been found to be readily convertible to nitrites when foods are stored at room temperature but not when they are refrigerated or when vitamin C, BHT, or BHA are added to the food. These data led to the working hypothesis that derivatives of nitrates, found in foods may be etiologically significant in human gastric cancer.

Migrant studies have shown that migration from high-incidence areas to low-incidence areas results within two generations in the migrants in gastric cancer rates very similar to those of their new country. Japanese immigrants to Hawaii (Haenszel and Kurihara, 1968) and Eastern European immigrants to the United States (Haenszel, 1961), have provided sound evidence for the conclusions that environment is important, and, perhaps foods and nutrition contribute significantly to the incidence of gastric cancer.

Ecological studies in Chile (Armijo and Coulson, 1975) showed a strong correlation between the use of nitrate fertilizers for agricultural purposes and regional mortality rates for gastric cancer, further suggesting an important role for nitrates in this disease. Similar positive ecological studies have been conducted in Columbia (Cuello et al., 1976) and England (Hill et al., 1973) where nitrate levels in drinking water positively correlated with gastric cancer mortality rates.

Many case-control studies have been conducted of diet and gastric cancer. Stocks (1957) found fried foods to increase risk; Pernu (1960) found that meat and animal fat consumption increased risk. Hirayama (1967) reported salted foods to be a risk factor, and milk to be apparently protective. On the other hand, Meinsma (1964), reported bacon as a risk factor and citrus fruits as protective, and Higginson (1966) suggested that cooked fats are a risk factor. However, other studies by Dunham and Brunschwig (1946), Wynder et al. (1963b), Acheson and Doll (1964), and Graham et al. (1967) reported essentially negative findings. Bjelke (1971) reported the apparent protective effect of fruit and vegetable consumption, and Haenszel et al. (1972) also reported an apparent protective effect of raw vegetable consumption, although pickled vegetables and salted fish increased risk in Japanese in Hawaii. In a later replication of this study of Japanese in Japan, this finding was not reproduced, although lettuce and celery were found to decrease risk (Haenszel et al., 1976). Bjelke (1973) found cereals and smoked fish to increase risk and vegetables and fruits to decrease risk in a second case-control study conducted in Minnesota, and Modan et al. (1974) found that starchy foods increased risk in a case-control study in Israel. A large Japanese cohort study (Hirayama, 1979a) showed that milk consumption and green and yellow vegetable consumption were associated with decreased risk, while smoking was associated with increased risk of subsequent stomach cancer. In a later analysis of data from this cohort (Hirayama, 1982) soybean paste soup was found to be associated with lower risk, thus supporting the hypothesis that protease inhibitors may protect against gastric cancer. Hirayama points out, however, the possible confounding effects of vegetable consumption.

Considering all case-control and prospective studies together, it is difficult to identify any consistent pattern of foods which seems to increase risk.

B. Experimental Evidence

A majority of the experimental evidence for various risk factors in gastric cancer has used the rat as the experimental animal and N-methyl-N'-Nitro-N-Nitrosoguanidine (MNNG) as the carcinogen. These studies have attempted to identify risk factors and elucidate mechanisms by which gastric cancer is initiated and promoted. Some of the factors considered include induced uclers (Shirai et al., 1978; Nagar et al., 1984); a broad variety of nutrients (Mirvish, 1983); mucosal concentrations of thiols (Wiestler, 1983); aspirin (Tsung-Hsien, et al., 1983); salt (Tatematsu, 1975) among others. Most of these have been concerned with the chronic effects of MNNG and selected risk factors; not much in the way of correlative studies have been published linking early gastric mucosal changes with the ultimate neoplasms. We have conducted a series of studies addressing the problem of risk factors, using the MNNG rat model and superimposing additional factors, some of which are considered risks and others not. We have thus linked gastric cancer with early changes in the mucosa which appear to be important in the early incipient stages of carcinogenesis. This model appears to offer a screening potential as well as a means for furthering our understanding of the mechanisms of the

carcinogenesis process. A brief resume of some of the
results are described here.

Rats were given MNNG from weaning, 75 mg/liter of
drinking water for 3-months. Additional agents were
superimposed, as shown in table 6. At the end of 12 months
the rats were sacrificed and examined for gastric lesions.
Data listed in table 6 illustrate the response to the
various risk factors.

Table 6
Effects of Putative Risk Factors on MNNG-induced
Gastric Cancer in Rats

Group and Treatment	Duration (months)	Proliferative Lesions in Stomach			
		Forestomach		Glandular Stomach	
		Papil-lomas	Carcin-omas	Dys-plasia	Adeno-carcinoma
Untreated	12	0/10	0/10	0/10	0/10
MNNG	12	3/14	8/14	9/14	5/14
MNNG+NaCl	12	3/9	6/9	2/9	7/9
MNNG+DFMO	12	3/14	2/14	3/14	2/14
MNNG+NaCl+DFMO	12	1/5	2/5	3/5	2/5
MNNG+Bile	12	6/13	7/13	4/13	7/13
MNNG+DEM	12	5/15	10/15	8/15	1/15

(Newberne et al., 1985, abridged. <u>Carcinogenesis</u>, in press).

We have examined a number of factors which appear to
modify risk for stomach cancer in rats treated with MNNG.
Table 6 lists some of the more significant findings. After
twelve months on study, both salt and bile acids had an
enhancing effect on carcinogenesis. Forestomach benign and
malignant tumors were present in some animals of all groups
after 12 months, except for untreated controls. Bile and
sodium chloride increased the incidence of neoplasia overall
in both forestomach and glandular stomach, when the two
tumor sites are combined. DFMO, an inhibitor of ornithine
decarboxylase, depressed tumor development to some extent
when bile and salt were added as risk factors; this was less
marked in the case of salt, which appeared to cause more
injury to the stomach than did bile. Diethylmaleate (DEM),
a thiol depleter, appeared to have an inhibitory effect on
glandular carcinoma.

In a subchronic, 3-month study there were a number of
observations of significance. First, the morphologic evidence for injury to the stomach was greatest for salt and

bile, which correlates well with the incidence of cancer.
aspirin was similar to salt and bile, in this regard, but we
do not yet have the chronic exposure data on aspirin, alcohol, nitrite or BHA for comparison. Both DFMO and DEM
tended to inhibit gastric injury; this correlated with the
observed long-term effects. BHA caused mild changes in the
mucosa, but less severe than the others.

^{3}H-thymidine labeling and mitotic figure counts agreed
with the other early observations.

Based on epidemiologic studies and on experimental animal investigations it appears that there are a number of
factors which can increase the risk for gastric cancer.
This is particularly the case with agents or conditions
which chronically injure the mucosa, setting off cell necro-
sis and continued hyperplasia. These alterations permit a
larger number of cells to be exposed to real or potential
carcinogen, DNA is damaged and repair is inadequate, and
neoplasia is the end result.

The overall conclusions which may be drawn from the
results of this study, combined with other data, are that
cancer is a multistage process, that continued insult of a
tissue from whatever cause increases risk, particularly
where cell turnover is increased, and that
activation/deactivation and macromolecular binding are
significant events in carcinogenesis.

III. CANCER OF THE LIVER

Liver cell cancer, or hepatocellular carcinoma (HCC), is
not a major tumor in most of the Western world, but it is
the major primary liver cancer when the world in its
entirety is considered; it differs in many respects from
cholangiocellular carcinoma, which is much less common. In
the human, HCC is the most common malignancy among black
populations in Africa residing south of the Sahara, but it
is one of the least common liver tumors among Northern
European populations, suggesting environmental factors in
its etiology.

HCC is one of the most malignant human neoplasms in
terms of response to treatment, progression, and outcome.
Cancer registries indicate that the incidence of HCC is now

increasing in some countries. Since prospects for treatment
of HCC are not encouraging, the ultimate goal is prevention.
This will require the identification and validation of carcinogens and other factors involved in the process and the
development of means for prevention of exposure to such
agents or factors. Effective methods for intervention will
be needed.

Careful epidemiologic studies in several countries where
HCC is prevalent have demonstrated a close association between chronic hepatitis B virus infection and HCC in man.
These observations have provided important clues as to
etiology and, combined with remarkable progress in molecular
biology in recent years, the study of HCC has entered a new
era in which research on liver cancer has moved ahead of
research on cancer of most other organ sites. Much of the
detailed work on HCC has been done using analogues of this
tumor induced by chemicals in laboratory animals. In addition, valuable information has been derived from observations on spontaneous HCC in rodents and in domestic
animals. Virus-associated HCC has been identified in the
woodchuck and in the domestic duck. These observations,
together with the close association of hepatitis B virus to
HCC in man, have resulted in enormous interest and markedly
broadened research activity in the area of viral-associated
HCC (Okuda and Mackay, 1982).

While epidemiological studies have strongly implicated
hepatitis B virus (HBV) infection as a major risk factor in
HCC (Beasley 1982; Mason et al., 1984); other observations
provide equally convincing data which clearly point to a
multifactorial etiology for this type of cancer. The differences in hepatitis B surface antigen carrier rates in
urban and rural populations could not account for the differences in the incidence of HCC in these two groups, as
noted by a number of studies (Harris and Sun, 1984; Kew et
al., 1983; Sun and Wang, 1983).

Integration of HBV DNA in both normal and in neoplastic
liver cells has been demonstrated (Shafritz et al., 1981;
Mason et al., 1984) but additional risk factors must be
given due consideration. In those areas of the world where
HCC occurs in highest incidence there is most often a triad
of interacting problems: 1) HBV antigen (HBs-Ag) carriers,
2) malnutrition, and 3) food contamination with aflatoxins
and other environmental contaminants (Rogers and Newberne,

1980; Harris and Sun, 1984; IARC Monographs 1-29, 1976;
1982) or self-imposed hepatotoxins including alcohol (Lieber
et al., 1979; Purtilo and Gottlieb, 1973; Keen and Martin,
1971; Lieber and Martini, 1980). Malnutrition appears to
represent a major force for increased sensitivity for HCC
(Newberne and McConnell, 1980; Newberne et al., 1983;
Newberne, 1984).

In a series of studies, we have established that
lipotropic factors (methionine, choline, folate, B_{12}) have a
profound effect on sensitivity to a number of chemical carcinogens (Rogers and Newberne, 1980) and that a deficiency
of lipotropes alone, results in a significant incidence of
HCC in mice and rats, without superimposing carcinogens
(Newberne et al., 1983). These observations have been
reported from other laboratories (Ghoshal and Farber, 1983;
Mikol et al., 1983) generated considerable interest in the
scientific community concerned with cancer research. Taking
something out of the diet, rather than putting something
into it to induce cancer is a new concept. The following
data illustrate some new and fascinating aspects of hepato-
carcinogenesis.

Rodents can be depleted of lipotropes and become pro-
foundly susceptible to carcinogens. Table 7 illustrates the
remarkably enhanced sensitivity to chemical carcinogens of a
broad variety of structure and reactivity.

In the lipotrope deficient rat, as liver fat increases,
the number of cells labeled by [^{3}H]-thymidine also increases
(Newberne et al., 1982). In addition, we found that lipotrope deficiency alone causes a sharp increase in cell
death, as others have reported (Ghoshal et al., 1983).
There is increased DNA synthesis and increased cell turnover, both of which are essential components of hyperplasia
of the liver parenchyma.

The dietary effect is similar to that produced by a partial hepatectomy; a key difference however is that cell
death and compensatory hyperplasia of the parenchyma continues as long as the choline deficient diet is fed.
Partial hepatectomy causes only a temporary wave of
hyperplasia and this returns to normal when the prehepatec-
tomy liver volume is approximated. Lipoperoxidation has
been considered by some to be related to the initiation of
transformation of hepatocytes and promotion of hepatocar-

Table 7
Chemical Carcinogenesis in
Lipotrope Deficiency[a]

Carcinogen[b]	Tumor Site	Tumor Incidence(%)	
		Control	Deprived
AFB$_1$	Liver	15	87
DEN	Liver	70	80
DMN	Liver	28	27
	Kidney	16	3
AAF	Liver	19	41
	Mammary	80	79

[a] From Rogers and Newberne (1980).
[b] AFB$_1$, aflatoxin B$_1$; DEN, N-nitrosodiethylamine; DMN,
nitrosodimethylamine; AAF, N-2-Fluorenylacetamine.

cinogenesis (Perera et al., 1984; Ghoshol et al., 1984). It
is interesting that our laboratory published such a relationship more than 15 years ago (Newberne et al., 1969) and
confirmed the observations with more sophisticated techniques a few years later (Wilson et al., 1973). The synthetic antioxidants BHA and BHT protected the kidney and liver
from choline deficiency and largely returned serum and
tissue lipids to near control values. Furthermore, our
later observations confirmed the probable relationship between lipid peroxidation and choline deficiency injury.
Table 8 indicates TBA values and the free radical index
(FRI) of the lipotrope deficient liver.

Table 8
Lipotrope Deficiency and Liver Lipids

Parameter	Chow Diet	Treatment	
		Choline Deficient	Choline Supplemented
Hepatic Lipid			
% dry wt.	22.2+ 0.5	44.6+ 2.1	24.0+ 1.8
Free Radical Index	464 $\overline{+}$71	553 $\overline{+}$85	303 $\overline{+}$ 22
Liver TBA	129 $\overline{+}$ 4.2	21 $\overline{+}$ 9.6	6.2$\overline{+}$ 2.3

From Wilson et al., 1973, abridged. Values are mean $\pm$ S.E.,
9 liver samples.

Poirier's laboratory (table 9) and our own investigations (table 10) point toward hypomethylation. Wilson et
al. (1984) observed 10-15% decrease in the
5-methyldeoxycytidine in the deficient liver, but only after
about six months on diet. Our studies (Punyarit and

Newberne, 1985) essentially confirm the data of Wilson et
al. (table 10) although our methods were slightly different.
We maintained rats on diet for up to six months, performed a
partial hepatectomy to generate new DNA (and accompanying
methylation) and two weeks later sacrificed the animals for
DNA analyses. In agreement with Wilson et al., (1984) it
was only after 6 months of continuous exposure to the
lipotrope deficient diet that we found a modest hypomethylation of cytosine. This indicates that it is a slow process
and, if, involved with carcinogenesis, hypomethylation very
likely requires chronic derangement of liver genetic
material over long periods of time.

Table 9
Lipotrope Deficiency, 5-Methyldeoxycytidine
Content of Hepatic DNA
% Deoxycytidine Residues as 5-Me deoxycytidine

Treatment	8 Weeks	22 Weeks
Control	3.33+0.03	3.27+0.04
Deficient	3.13+0.05	2.81+0.04

(From Wilson et al., 1984, abridged).

Table 10
Lipotropes and 5'-Methylcytosine in Liver DNA
5-methylcytosine as % of cytosine

Time on Diet	Control	Deficient
3 weeks	4.8+0.09	4.5+0.11
3 months	4.4+0.13	4.7+0.20
6 months	4.5+0.10	3.3+0.06

(Punyarit and Newberne, 1985; unpublished). Two weeks prior
to sacrifice a 2/3 partial hepatectomy was performed. We
are indebted to Dr. Ronald Shank, University of California,
Irvine for some of the DNA analyses listed in table 10.

Gene activity frequently correlates with hypomethylation
(Doerfler, 1983). In addition to the data reported above it
should be noted that Wainfan (1985) has found that liver
tRNA, isolated from rats fed a lipotrope deficient diet is
hypomethylated and that there is an increase in the activity
of N^2-guanine tRNA methyltransferase (NMG2), mimicing the
effects of the liver carcinogen, ethionine. Thus, not only
is DNA hypomethylated but tRNA critical to normal cell proliferation, is also hypomethylated in the choline deficient
liver.

It seems quite likely that means are at hand for dissecting out the basic role of dietary induced injury which contributes to the enhancing effect of lipotrope deficiency hepatocellular carcinoma. This will move our efforts in understanding carcinogenesis in general considerably ahead and contribute to the ultimate goal of preventing liver cell neoplasia and, perhaps, other types of cancer.

IV. CANCER OF THE COLON/RECTUM

Industrialized societies eat diets which are very high in fat, compared to nonindustrialized societies. Colon cancer rates are particularly high in North America and Europe, whereas in Africa, South America, and Asia, rates are relatively low. This observation, in conjugation with animal studies, to be described later, have, in some instances, linked fat to human colon cancer. Hill et al. (1979) found that high socioeconomic status (SES) groups in Hong Kong experienced over twice the colon cancer rates as low SES groups. Dietary surveys showed that the high SES group ate more meat, but also more of almost every other type of food as well, than the low SES group. Ecological studies in the United States also suggest meat to be a risk factor. Colorectal cancer is much lower in Seventh-Day Adventists, who are often lacto-ovo-vegetarian, as compared to nonadventists (Enstrom, 1980). Similarly, Mormons also have relatively low rates, yet a special dietary survey in Southern Utah which is almost entirely Mormon, showed meat consumption levels to be virtually identical to the remainder of the United States suggesting that factors other than low meat consumption may be important in explaining the low colon cancer rates in this area. Similarly, a comparative study by Kinlen (1982) of strict religious orders in Britain showed that colon cancer mortality was not lower in an order which ate no meat as compared to one which did. In addition, there are some ecological patterns which are not entirely consistent with the fats hypothesis. Dietary fat intake is very high in Finland, yet colon cancer rates are relatively low, and within the United States there is no correlation between regional beef fat consumption and colorectal cancer rates (Enstrom, 1975).

Case-control studies have not always confirmed the suspicion generated from experimental and ecological studies that fat is a risk factor for colon cancer. This

particularly fits with the recent observations from
Newberne's laboratory (Nauss et al., 1983; 1984) and from
the observations in Hawaiian studies (Stemmerman et al.,
1984). Higginson (1966) reported no case-control differences in diet as measured. In a study in Norway, Bjelke
(1971) found that vegetables and vitamin C apparently reduce
risk; this was also found in a similar study conducted in
Minnesota (Bjelke, 1973), but no association was seen with
dietary fat. Haenszel et al. (1973) found only that
starches and legumes were positively associated with risk in
a case-control study conducted on Japanese in Hawaii, a
finding which was not replicated in a later study of
Japanese in Japan (Haenszel et al., 1980). Dales et al.
(1978), however, reported higher risk for those who ate
diets that were both high in fat and low in fiber, and Jain
et al. (1980) reported a study in Canada in which cases
reported eating more fat than controls.

Burkitt (1971,1978) proposed that dietary fiber is protective against colon cancer. This hypothesis was based on
the observation that dietary fiber intake was considerably
greater in areas of the world where colon cancer rates are
low. Low fiber in the diet, he proposed, led to physical,
chemical, and bacteriological aberrancies in stool composition which in turn could cause colon cancer. The ecological data are certainly consistent with this hypothesis, as
are some case-control studies. In a case-control study in
Israel, Modan et al. (1975) observed that colon cancer
patients tended to report less frequent ingestion of foods
high in fiber. Dales et al. (1978) reported increased risk
with diets high in fat and low in fiber in a study of blacks
in the San Francisco area. A study by Graham et al. (1978),
however, found no relationship between fiber or fat
ingestion and cancer risk; instead cases tended to eat fewer
cruciferous vegetables (e.g., cabbage, broccoli, and
brussels sprouts). This led to the hypothesis that perhaps
chemicals contained within the cruciferous vegetables, which
have been found by Wattenberg and Loub (1978) to be capable
of inducing arylhydrocarbon hydroxylase (AHH) activity in
the gut, might thus be protective against colon cancer.
Haenszel et al. (1980), in studying colon cancer in Japan,
was unable to replicate his earlier findings of increased
risk with starches and legumes from the Hawaiian study, but,
consistent with the AAH hypothesis, he found that cabbage
ingestion tends to decrease risk.

The large Japanese prospective study (Hirayama, 1979a) did not demonstrate any apparent relationship between the frequency of meat intake and colorectal cancer risk. Hirayama (1979a) did however demonstrate a strong positive correlation among 29 health centers between percentages of individuals who eat meat daily and the standardized mortality ratio for colon cancer in the district. In sum, case-control studies have shown inconsistent results.

Important activity in current research is in the area of metabolic epidemiology of colon cancer. Examination of stools of small numbers of individuals on various diets has purported to show that there is a relationship between the level of fat ingestion and the amount of bile acids and fecal sterols, as well as the fecal flora found in the stools (Reddy, 1981). Japanese in Hawaii have more deoxycholic acid in the stools than Japanese in Japan (Mower et al., 1979). Furthermore, Seventh-Day Adventists in New York City have more mutagens in the stool than non-Seventh-Day Adventists (Reddy et al., 1980a). Comparing the stools of New York City residents to those of residents of Umea, Sweden, where colon cancer rates are lower, there were no differences in the total amount of bile acids, neutral sterols, and B-glucuronidase activity, although the stool concentrations were lower in the Swedes (Domellof et al., 1982). It may be that higher levels of dietary fiber intake in Sweden serves to dilute the concentrations of potential carcinogens in the stool.

Although there is a fourfold difference in colon cancer rates between Denmark and Finland, fecal sterols, bile acids, and oral-to-anal transit times are not different in the two populations (Jensen and MacLennan, 1979). In addition, such metabolic studies are usually based on a small number of subjects who are not always randomly selected from the populations being compared. Despite this, work in metabolic epidemiology of feces may nonetheless be important in understanding the determinants of colon cancer, particularly with respect to the significance of various mutagens found in the stool, their sites of action (Hill, 1981), and the determinants of fecal microbial activity (Mackowiak, 1982). Such biological markers of adverse dietary effects are much more sensitive indicators than cancer and may be useful in understanding the determinants of disease and the effectiveness of interventions.

     In the case of animal studies with colon carcinogenesis,
there are equally disquieting observations, none of which
have been adequately explained. For example, there are
those (Reddy et al., 1978; 1980) who suggest that dietary
fat and fiber, and the consequences of these on such parameters as bile acids and other contributory factors are the
key to colon carcinogenesis. These hypotheses are still
being tested and preliminary results should be regarded with
caution. The animal data, detailed below, will point out
both encouraging and discouraging aspects of state of the
art experimentation. Some of the earlier, significant
publications on the role of dietary fat in experimental
colon cancer are those of Reddy et al., 1974; 1977; 1979;
1980. These investigators reported that rats fed 5% corn
oil diets had a higher tumor incidence and a larger number
of tumors per animal than those fed a 5% lard diet. Tumor
incidence and multiplicity increased with higher (20%) fat
levels but the incidence and multiplicity of tumors were
comparable with corn oil or lard. Table 11 illustrates some
of their observations.

Table 11
Colon Tumor Incidence With Two Levels
and Types of Dietary Fat

Diet	Colon Tumors(%)	Total Tumors Per Rat
Corn oil, 5%	36	0.77
Lard, 5%	17	0.22
Corn oil, 20%	64	1.55
Lard, 20%	67	1.50
Purina® Chow	25	0.25

     One hypothesis linking dietary fat to colon cancer is
that cholesterol is converted to bile acids which act as
promoters of carcinogenesis (Kritchevsky, 1982).
Epidemiological studies have shown however, (Enstrom, 1975)
that when beef consumption in the United States doubled
(between 1940-1970) the incidence of colon cancer mortality
was virtually unchanged. In addition, the incidence of
colon cancer is the same in Seventh Day Adventists, who eat
meat sparingly (Phillips, 1975) and Mormons, who consume a
conventional diet (Lyon et al., 1976).

     These epidemiological observations have suggested a
metabolic clue to the effect of fats which may be through
fecal steroid metabolism and excretion. Steroids have been
measured in populations at high and at low risk for colon

cancer. Table 12 lists results of one such investigation.
The absolute amount of steroids excreted is much lower in
control subjects but this could reflect the health status of
the individuals. In the neutral sterol fraction the ratio
of cholesterol to its metabolites is higher in colon cancer
patients, perhaps indicating inability to metabolize cholesterol. Comparisons of fecal steroids in populations of
varying susceptibility to colon cancer have also given
variable results.

Table 12
Fecal Steroids in Three Groups of Subjects
mg/g Dry Feces

Steroid	Control (40)*	Adenomatous Polyps(15)*	Colon Cancer(35)*
Neutral			
Cholesterol	3.2	6.4	12.6
Coprostanol	12.9	19.6	18.7
Coprostanone	1.9	4.0	3.9
Acidic			
Cholic	0.4	0.4	0.5
Chenodeoxycholic	0.2	0.3	0.5
Deoxycholic	3.7	0.3	7.0
Lithocholic	3.1	5.4	6.5

From Reddy, 1979, abridged.   *Number subjects.

If bile acids are, in fact, a risk factor in colon carcinogenesis, substances which enhance excretion of bile
acids should inhibit the development of colon tumors. This
has been tested in experimental animals. Bran and cellulose
inhibit DMH-induced colon tumors in rats (Barbolt et al.,
1978; Freeman et al., 1980). Despite tumor inhibition,
neither of these fibers bind bile acids to any appreciable
extent (Story and Kritchevsky, 1976). Moreover, Nigro et
al., (1973) have shown that cholestyramine, a bile acid-
binding resin, when added to the diet of rats given one of
three carcinogens significantly increased tumor incidence
(Table 13). These data argue against any direct effect of
bile acids on colon tumorigenesis.

The influence of dietary fiber on colon cancer has been
the subject of extensive investigations by epidemiologists
and experimental oncologists (Doll and Peto, 1986). Results
from human population studies have been variable; animal investigations have been variable as well but, in general, the
results point to an effect of fiber on induced colon tumors.

Table 13
Cholestyramine and Colon Cancer

Carcinogen	Diet	Number of Colon Tumors Proximal	Distal
1,2-Dimethylhydrazine	Normal Diet (ND)	15	1
	Normal Diet + Cholestyramine(NDC)	31	29
Azoxymethane	ND	19	8
	NDC	33	36
Methylazoxymethanol	ND	4	2
	NDC	18	15

From Nigro et al., 1973, abridged.

Table 14 taken from the work of Watanabe et al. (1979) illustrates results characteristic of many studies. These authors suggest that the effects are related to bile acid binding capacity and that this correlates with severity of mucosal damage. Thus, the bile acid and fiber effects may be mechanical rather than because of metabolic aberrations.

Table 14
Dietary Fiber and Colon Cancer in Rats Induced
by Two Carcinogens

Fiber (15% of Diet)	Carcinogen and Tumor Incidence(%) Azoxymethanol (AOM)	Methylnitrosourea (NMU)
Control	57.7	69.0
Alfalfa	53.3	83.3
Pectin	10.0	58.6
Bran	33.0	60.0

From Watanabe et al., 1979, abridged.

In contrast to some of the results referred to above where increased dietary fat enhanced experimentally induced colon cancer in rats, we have failed to observe an effect of either quality or quantity of fat on induced tumor incidence (Nauss et al., 1983; 1984). Table 15 lists results of studies with three different fats and two different colon carcinogens. The negative nature of these two carefully conducted studies, one of which (DMH) has been repeated with similar results, casts doubt on the significance of dietary fat on colon carcinogenesis. The conflicting data between epidemiological and experimental studies might be explained in a number of ways. Most logical would be the diversity of exposures of humans to environmental factors, compared to a single variable in animal studies.

Table 15
Quality and Quantity of Dietary Fat and Colon
Carcinogenesis With Two Colon Carcinogens

Dietary Fat		Carcinogen/%	Colon Tumors
% (Wt)	Type	DMH	NMU
5	Mixed	77	55
24	Beef Tallow	68	63
24	Corn Oil	63	55
24	Crisco®	55	38

From Nauss et al., 1983; 1984; abridged. Each group
comprised of 40 rats each.

SUMMARY

The available evidence from epidemiological and experimental studies support the view that nutrients, interacting
with other factors, either as lifestyle, or as non-nutrient
dietary components do, indeed, influence susceptibility to
cancer. Esophageal cancer is associated with malnutrition
in some populations as a result of dietary deficits; in
others with excessive smoking and drinking, which may, in
fact, precipitate a deficiency of nutrients. Nutrients
which appear to be important include protein, riboflavin,
zinc and perhaps selenium. Toxic materials which appear to
be involved include alcohol, mycotoxins and nitrosamines.

Gastric cancer, and particularly, the high incidence in
Japan and in parts of central and South America have been
associated with nitrates, nitrites and nitrosamines, where a
lack of vitamin C may be important. In addition, risk factors include salty, pickled foods, aspirin, alcohol and
other traumatizing agents.

Liver cancer is in highest incidence where a triad of
disease exists. Infection with hepatitis B virus (HBV),
malnutrition, and contamination with mycotoxins in staple
food products, may all interact to result in greater susceptibility to liver cancer. This is most evidence in sub-
populations of South America, Southeast Asia, India, and
East and South Africa. In western populations alcohol and,
to a lesser extent, infection and chronic hepatitis may be
important risk factors.

Finally, colon cancer is an enigma. While it seems to
be slowly creeping up in western, industrialized

populations it has not clearly been shown to be associated with any single dietary nutrient or factor. The attractive hypothesis that fiber is a major factor has not been confirmed; the same is true for fat quality or quantity.

We are left with the strong suggestions from epidemiologic and animal studies that diet and nutrition are involved with human cancer. Except for breast cancer and dietary fat however (not covered in this review) there is no single dietary nutrient, acting in isolation, that can be pointed to as a major contribution. Moderation and variation in dietary nutrients would appear to be the best recommendation at this point in time. The elucidation of factors and mechanisms in diet and cancer is as complex as the foods upon which such proposals are based.

ACKNOWLEDGMENTS

The work reported here from our laboratory, and the preparation of this manuscript were supported in part by USPHS Contract No. 1-CP33238, NCI and grant ES 00597, NIEHS.

REFERENCES

Acheson, E.D., and Doll, R. (1964). Gut 5:126-131.
Barbolt, T.A., and Abraham, R. (1978). Proc. Soc. Exp. Biol. Med. 157:656-659.
Beasley, R.P. (1982). Hepatology 2:215-224.
Bjelke, E. (1971). In "Oncology 1970" (R.L. Clark, R.W. Cumley, J.E. McCay, and M. M. Copeland, eds.), Vol. 5, p. 320-34. Yearbook Medical Publ. Chicago, Illinois.
Bjelke, E. (1973). Ph.D. Thesis, University of Minnesota. (University Microfilms. Ann Arbor, Michigan).
Burkitt, D.P. (1971). Cancer 28:3-13.
Burkitt, D.P. (1978). Am. J. Clin. Nutr. 31:558-564.
Cook-Mozaffari, P.J., Azordegan, F., Day, N.E., Ressicand, A., Sabai, C., and Aramesh, B. (1979). Br. J. Cancer 39:293-309.
Cuello, C., Correa, P., Haenszel, W., Gordillo, G., Brown, C., Archer, M., and Tannenbaum, S. (1976). J. Natl. Cancer Inst. 57:1015-1020.
Dales, L.G., Friedman, G.D., Ury, H.K., Grossman, S., and Williams, S.R. (1978). Am. J. Epidemiol. 109:132-144.

Day, N., and Munoz, N. (1982). In "Cancer Epidemiology and Prevention" (D. Schottenfeld and J. Fraumeni, eds.), pp. 606-609. Saunders, Philadelphia, Pennsylvania.

Doerfler, W. (1983). Ann. Rev. Biochem. 52:93-124.

Department of Health, Education, and Welfare. (1979). DHEW Publ. #(PHS) 79-1221. Hyattsville, Maryland.

Domellof, L., Darby, L., Hanson, D., Mathews, L., Simi, D., and Reddy, B.S. 91982). Nutr. Cancer 4:120-127.

Dunham, L.J., and Brunschwig, A. (1946). Gastroenterology 6:286-293.

Enstrom, J.E. (1975). Br. J. Cancer 32:432-439.

Enstrom, J.E. (1980). In "Cancer Incidence in Defined Populations" (J. Cairns, J.L. Lyon, and M. Skolnick, eds.), pp. 69-90. Cold Spring Harbor Laboratory, Cold Spring Harbor, New York.

Fong, L.Y.Y., Sivak, A., Newberne, P.M. (1978). J. Natl. Cancer Inst. 61:145-150.

Foy, H., and Kondi, A. (1984). JNCI 72:941-948.

Freeman, H.J., Spiller, G.A., and Kim, Y.S. (1980). Cancer Res. 40:2661-2665.

Gabrial, G.N., Schrager, T.F., and Newberne, P.M. (1982). J. Natl. Cancer Inst. 68:785-789.

Ghoshal, A.K., and Farber, E. (1983). Proc. Am. Assoc. Cancer Res. 24:98 (abst.).

Ghoshal, A.K., Rushmore, T., Lim, Y., and Farber, E. (1984). Cancer Res. 25:94 (abst.).

Graham, S., Lilienfeld, A.M., and Tidings, J.E. 91967). Cancer 20:2224-2234.

Graham, S., Dayal, H., Swanson, M., Mittelman, A., and Wilkinson, G. (1978). J. Natl. Cancer Inst. 61:709-714.

Haenszel, W. (1961). J. Natl. Cancer Inst. 26:37-132.

Haenszel, W., and Kurihara, M. (1968). J. Natl. Cancer Inst. 40:43-68.

Haenszel, W., Kurihara, M., Segi, M., and Lee, R.K.C. (1972). J. Natl. Cancer Inst. 49:969-988.

Haenszel, W., Berg, J.W., Segi, M., Kurihara, M., and Locke, F.B. (1973). J. Natl. Cancer Inst. 51:1765-1779.

Haenszel, W., Kurihara, M., Locke, B., Shimuzu, K., and Segi, M. (1976). J. Natl. Cancer Inst. 56:265-274.

Haenszel, W., Locke, F.B., and Segi, M. (1980). J. Natl. Cancer Inst. 64:17-22.

Harris, C.C., and Sun, T. (1984). Carcinogenesis 5:697-701.

Higginson, J. (1966). J. Natl. Cancer Inst. 37:527-545.

Hill, M.J. (1981). Cancer Res. 41:3778-3780.

Hill, M.J., Hawkworth, G., and Tattersall, G. (1973). Br. J. Cancer 28:562-567.

Hill, M., MacLennan, R., and Newcombe, K. (1979). Lancet
    1:436.
Hirayama, T. (1967). Proc. Int. Cancer Congr. 9th, Tokyo
    October 1966; UICC Monogr. Ser. 10:37-48.
Hirayama, T. (1982). Nutr. Cancer 3:223-233.
IARC Monographs 1-29, Lyon, (1976).
IARC/IPCS (1982). IARC Tech. Rpt. 82/001.
Jacobson, F. 91961). In "Neoplastic Disease at Various
    Sites: Tumors of the Esophagus" (N.C. Tanner and D.W.
    Smithers, eds.), Vol. 4, pp. 53-60, Linvingstone,
    Edinburgh.
Jain, M., Cook, G.M., Davis, F.G., Grace, M.G., Howe, G.R.,
    and Miller, A.B. (1980). Int. J. Cancer 26:757-768.
Jensen, O.M., and MacLennan, R. (1979). Int. J. Med. Sci.
    15:329-334.
Joint Iran-International Agency for Research on Cancer Study
    Group. (1977). J. Natl. Cancer Inst. 59:1127-1138.
Kew, M.C., Rossouri, E., Hodkinson, J. et al (1983).
    Hepatology 3:65-68.
Kinlen, L.J. (1982). Lancet 1:946-949.
Kritchevsky, D. (1982). In "Molecular Interrelations of
    Nutrition and Cancer" (Arnott, M.S., VanEys, J., Yang,
    Y.M., eds.), Raven Press: New York, pp. 209-217.
Lieber, C.S., Seltz, H.K., Garro, A.J., Worner, T.M. (1979).
    Cancer Res. 39:2869-2876.
Lin, H.J., Chan, W.C., Fong, L.Y.Y., and Newberne, P.M.
    (1977). Nutr. Rpts. Internat. 15:635-643.
Mackowiak, P.A. (1982). N. Engl. J. Med. 307:83-93.
Martini, G.A. (1980). In "Cancer Detection and Prevention"
    (Nieburgs, H.E., ed.), vol. 2, pp. 1303-1312.
Mason, W.S., Halpern, M.S., and Thomas, W. (1984). Cancer
    Surveys 3:1-11.
Meinsma, L. (1964). Voeding 25:357-365.
Mettlin, C., Graham, S., Priore, R., Marshall, J., and
    Swanson, M. (1981). Nutr. Cancer 2:143-147.
Mikol, Y.B., and Poirier, L.A. (1981). Cancer Lett.
    13:195-201.
Modan, B., Lubin, F., Barell, V., Greenberg, R.A., Modan,
    M., and Graham, S. (1974). Cancer 34:2087-2092.
Modan, B., Barell, V., Lubin, F., Modan, M., Greenberg,
    R.A., and Graham, S. (1975). J. Natl. Cancer Inst.
    55:15-18.
Mower, H.F., Ray, R.M., Shoff, R., Stemmerman, G.D., Nomura,
    A., Glober, G.A., Kamiyama, S., Shimada, A., and
    Yamakawa, H. (1979). Cancer Res. 39:328.

Nauss, K.M., Locniskar, M., and Newberne, P.M. (1983). Cancer Res. 43:4083-4090.

Nauss, K.M., Locniskar, M., Sondergaard, D., and Newberne, P.M. (1984). Carcinogenesis 5:225-260.

Newberne, P.M. (1982). In "Trace Substances in the Environment. A Handbook, Vol. II, pp. 1-45.

Newberne, P.M. (1984). In "The Toxicologist" The Society of Toxicology: Akron.

Newberne, P.M. (1984). Seminars in Liver Disease 4:122-135.

Newberne, P.M., Bresnahan, M.R., and Kula, N.S. (1969). J. Nutr. 97:219-231.

Newberne, P.M., Charnley, G., Adams, K., Cantor, M., and Roth, D. (1985). Carcinogenesis (in press).

Newberne, P.M., deCamargo, J.L.V., and Clark, A.J. (1982). Tox. Path. 2:95-109.

Newberne, P.M., and McConnell, R. (1980). J. Env. Path. & Tox. 3:323-356.

Newberne, P.M., Rogers, A.E., and Nauss, K.M. (1983). In "Nutrition Factors in the Induction and Maintenance of Malignancy" Academic Press:New York, pp. 247-271.

Newberne, P.M., and Schrager, T. (1983). Environ. Health Perspectives 50:71-83.

Nigro, N.D., Bhadrachari, N., and Chomchai, C. (1973). Dis. Colon Rectum 16:438-443.

Okuda, K., and Mackay, I. (eds.) (1982). Report No. 17, UICC Technical Report Series, Vol. 74, Geneva.

Perera, M., Demetris, A., Katyal, S., and Shinozuka, H. (1984). Cancer Res. 25:141 (abst.)

Pernu, J. (1960). Ann. Med. Intern. Fenn. (Suppl.) 33:1-117.

Pottern, L.M., Morris, L.E., Blot, W.J., Ziegler, R.G., and Fraumeni, J.F. (1981). J. Natl. Cancer Inst. 67:777-783.

Punyarit, P., and Newberne, P.M. (1985). Unpublished.

Reddy, B.S. (1979). Adv. Nutr. Res. 2:199-218.

Reddy, B.S. (1981). Cancer Res. 41:3700-3705.

Reddy, B.S., Narisawa, T., Vukusich, D., Weisburger, J.H., and Wynder, E.L. (1976). Proc. Soc. Exp. Biol. Med. 151:237-239.

Reddy, B.S., Mastromarino, A., and Wynder, E. (1977). Cancer 39:1815.

Reddy, B.S., Sharma, C., Darby, L., Laakso, K., and Wynder, E.L. (1980a). Mutat. Res. 72:511-522.

Reddy, B.S., Cohen, L.A., McCoy, G.D., Hill, P., Weisburger, J.H., and Wynder, E.L. (1980b). Adv. Cancer Res. 32:237-345.

Rogers, A.E., and Newberne, P.M. (1980). Nutr. Cancer
    2:104-112.
Schrager, T., Busby, W.J. Jr., and Newberne, P.M. (1985).
    unpublished.
Shafritz, D.A., Shouval, D., and Sherman, H. et al. (1981).
    New Eng. J. Med. 305:1067-1073.
Stemmerman,   (1984).
Stocks, P. (1957). Supplement to Part II of British Empire
    Cancer Campaign 35th Annual Report covering the Year
    1957.
Story, J.A., and Kritchevsky, D. (1976). J. Nutr.
    106:1292-1294.
Sun, T., and Wang, N. (1983). In "Human Carcinogenesis"
    (C.C. Harris, and H.N. Autrup, eds.), Academic Press:
    New York, pp. 757-780.
Tannenbaum, S.R. (1983). Lancet 1:629-631.
Wainfan, E., Diznik, M., Hluboky, M., and Balis, M.E.
    (1985). FASEB Abst. No.
Wattenberg, L.W., and Loub, W.D. (1978). Cancer Res.
    38:1410-1413.
Wilson, R.B., Kula, N.S., Newberne, P.M., and Conner, M.W.
    (1973). Exper. & Mol. Pathol. 18:357-368.
Wilson, M.J., Shivapurkar, N., and Poirier, L.A. (1984).
    Biochem. J. 218:987-994.
Wynder, E.L., and Bross, I.J. (1961). Cancer 14:389-413.
Wynder, E.L., Kmet, J., Dungal, N., and Segi, M. (1963b).
    Cancer 16:1461-1496.
Yang, C.S. (1980). Cancer Res. 40:2633-2644.
Ziegler, R.G., Morris, L.E., Blot, W.J., Pottern, L.M.,
    Hoover, R., and Fraumeni, J.F. (1981b). J. Natl. Cancer
    Inst. 67:1199-1206.

SUPPLEMENTAL CAROTENOIDS PREVENT SKIN CANCER BY BENZO(a)PYRENE, BREAST CANCER BY PUVA, AND GASTRIC CANCER BY MNNG. Relevance in human chemoprevention.

L. Santamaria[1], A. Bianchi[2], A. Arnaboldi[1], L. Andreoni[1], G. Santagati[3], C. Ravetto[1], L. Bianchi[1], R. Pizzala[1], P. Bermond[4].

[1] C. Golgi Institute of General Pathology, Centro Tumori; [2] Institute of Pharmacology II; [3] Medical Clinic; University of Pavia, 27100 Pavia, Italy. [4] Centre Hospitalier, 51100 Reims, France.

INTRODUCTION

In 1980, the results of an experiment carried out on female mice with the methodology used to show a photoenhancement of benzo(a)pyrene (BP) carcinogenicity, demonstrated that supplemental dietary carotenoids prevent BP skin cancer, both following long UV irradiation and in the dark (29). Such experiment was stimulated by the fact that carotenoids produce a reduction in the UV-B induced sunburn erythema response (14,15) and delay skin tumor induction in hairless mice exposed to UV-B (16).

Since BP must be activated to oxidative derivatives to perform its carcinogenic activity (42), the above results pointed out that the mechanism of carotenoids protection was most probably consistent with their activities as oxyradical scavengers and/or singlet oxygen ($^1O_2$) quenchers (10), rather than as pro-vitamin A precursors.

139

Later, in 1984, the same experimental procedure was applied to photocarcinogenesis by 8-methoxypsoralen (8-MOP), a drug used in photochemotherapy, whose photodynamic mechanism is questionable, as far as oxygen requirement is concerned (19,17).

In such experiment, supplemental dietary carotenoids protected female mice against the onset of a mammary carcinoma (32).*In vitro* investigations on photomutagenesis on *Salmonella typhimurium* , TA 102 by 8-MOP in the presence of carotenoids, indicated a two-step photoreaction by this drug; namely, an anoxic 8-MCP-DNA photobinding followed by an oxygen dependent enhancement of genotoxicity, which can be prevented by carotenoids (33).

Finally, in 1985, an experimental attempt was completed on gastric carcinogenesis induced in rats by the direct carcinogen N - methyl - N' - nitro - N - nitrosoguanidine (MNNG) , to verify whether supplemental carotenoids can affect such carcinogenesis, where neither light excitation nor oxidative metabolic processes were presumably involved. The results demonstrated that supplemental carotenoids did not affect any dysplasia arising from the glandular part of rat gastric mucosa, but dramatically prevented the progression of dysplasias to infiltrating gastric carcinomas (34).

All the above data are presented here in different sections (each one carrying the initials of the responsible authors) with reference tc both methodology and results to put forward possible applications in human cancer chemoprevention.

I. BENZO(a)PYRENE CARCINOGENICITY AND ITS PREVENTION BY SUPPLEMENTAL DIETARY CAROTENOIDS
(L.S., A.B., A.A., L.A., P.B.)

In the last decade, carotenoids were demonstrated to produce a reduction in the UV-B (290-320 nm) induced sunburn erythema response (14,15). Then, experimental attempts proved that injection or peroral administration of such pigments produces a delay of skin tumor induction in hairless mice exposed to UV-B irradiation (5,16).

To perform a study on the possible modulation of skin cancer induction by carotenoids in animals, with reference to human pathology, an experimental study was carried . out in which the photo-enhancement of BP carcinogenicity (BP-PCE), as demonstrated previously (27), had to be adopted as a model to closely reproduce the actual skin cancer pathogenesis occurring in humans. Furthermore, the property of carotenoids to quench free radicals and singlet oxygen states (14,10) suggested a role of these pigments as preventive rather than therapeutic agents against cancer, according to its modern pathogenetic view (40).

The methodology of this leading experiment was as follows. β-carotene (BC) and canthaxanthine (CX) were perorally administrated to female Swiss albino mice, strain 955, with daily diet (2.5 mg of BC or CX in 5 g of pellets). One month later, the mice were given additional administrations of BC and CX, dissolved in arachidic oil, by catheter, twice a week (100 mg per 1 Kg of body weight). Two hours after BC and CX administration by catheter, the mice were painted with BP (100 μg) acetone solution on a clipped mid-dorsum area and were either exposed to long UV light (Philips bulb HPW 125 W, 300-400 nm with maximum output at 365 nm, and a negligible emission at 313 nm, with flux at animal level: 5.89×10^3 erg cm^{-2} sec^{-1}) for two hours or kept in the dark. In this experiment, 16 groups of animals, 75 per group, were employed. Of these, 6 groups were used to investigate the activity of BC and CX on BP photocarcinogenesis. The other groups were controls with respect to light, solvent and carotenoids, and were either exposed to UV or kept in the dark. For each experimental group the cumulative percentage of mice bearing one or more tumors was calculated using conventional statistical methods based on adjustment for mice that died during each two-week period of observation.

As shown in Fig. 1, BP-PCE was evident soon after the beginning of tumor onset. It was at its maximum at 28-36 weeks after initial UV exposure, when the percentage of mice with tumors in the irradiated group was in the range of 50. At this stage, BP-PCE was also clearly inhibited to the same extent by BC and CX treatments. In the dark, at the beginning, BC and CX did not show any significant inhibition of carcinogenesis. From the 44th to the 60th week, BC and CX completely blocked the kinetics of BP-PCE at tumor incidence values of 40% and 54-64%, respectively. Thus, BC was more active than CX. Furthermore, BC and CX exerted a significant inhibitory activity also on carcinogenesis in the dark. In this case, CX was more efficient ($p = <0.01$) than BC ($p = < 0.05$). No one of the control animal groups showed any tumor onset except for the group exposed to light without BP or carotenoids; 8% of mice had tumors (papillomas + some epitheliomas) at the end of the experiment. This was expected, on the basis of previous data (28), although long UV light is generally considered to be non carcinogenic.

In this connection, it should be pointed out that the above experimental skin cancer initiated from the effects of a carcinogen associated with the action of UV-A light (320-400 nm), which is generally considered non tumorigenic, and a negligible 313 nm tumorigenic

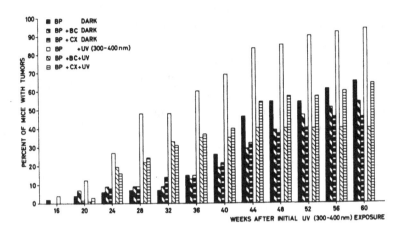

Fig. 1. BC and CX protective effect on BP-PCE and BP carcinogenesis in the dark. (After Santamaria et al,
Experientia, 1983).

band (2.6% of the total light) which is present in the
sun spectrum at earth level. The energy output of such
tumorigenic band during the experiment was 100 times
less than the minimum UV (< 320 nm) energy requirement
for skin carcinogenesis (1). Therefore, the low
incidence of skin neoplastic growth observed in the
control group without BP or carotenoids exposed to
light, can be considered a long term effect of near UV
light, perhaps by exciting endogenous photodynamic
substances.

The data reported in Fig. 1 were original in
demonstrating that carotenoids, with and without
pro-vitamin A activity, have antitumorigenic properties.
The mechanism of this skin cancer protection can be
explained assuming that BP initiates a carcinogenic
process by oxyradical formation, that is the metastable

species first observed in hematoporphyrin aerated saline solution excited by light (> 320 nm) (41,26). Indeed, both these substances behave in the same fashion in a photodynamic reaction (26) and are photocarcinogenic in mice (2,27). Such metastable states, however, are considered also possible in the dark by excitation via interaction of molecules with endogenously produced free radicals such as O_2^- OH·, or singlet oxygen (40). Thus, the properties of carotenoids as free radical scavengers and singlet oxygen quenchers (10), rather than as UV screening agents (12,35), fit into their antitumorigenic activity (30,31). Apart from prevention, BC may also exert a therapeutic action on tumor transplanted mice (25,36).

II. SUPPLEMENTAL CAROTENOIDS PREVENT BREAST CARCINOMA IN SWISS MICE BY PHOTOINDUCTION OF 8-METHOXYPSORALEN (8-MOP)
(L.S., A.B., L.A., G.S., A.A., P.B.)

The above results suggested that a similar methodology should be applied also in an attempt to prevent a photocarcinogenic process induced by 8-methoxypsoralen (8-MOP), a photodynamic drug which is equally active in aerated and anoxic media (19,20). Later on, however, it was found that in 8-MOP photoreactions the possibility cannot be excluded that O_2 is generated by triplet energy transfer (23) and that, next to the photo-cross-linking reaction with DNA, $^1O_2$ is produced playing a role in photosensitization effects on bacteria (39).

Female Swiss albino mice, strain 955, were painted with 8-MOP (10 μg) absolute ethanol solution on a clipped mid-dorsum area and exposed for 45 min to long UV light (300-400 nm) twice a week (26). The general experimental scheme was exactly the same as that used for BP *in vivo* studies.

TABLE I

Tumor incidence in mice painted 8-methoxypsoralen (8-MOP), fed β-carotene (BC) or canthaxanthine (CX), kept in the dark or exposed to UV (300 - 400 nm) light, at 80th week after initial UV exposure.

Experimental animal group (75 mice each group)	UV light exposure	Percent mice with tumors
8-MOP	–	0
8-MOP+BC	–	0
8-MOP+CX	–	0
8-MOP	+	38
8-MOP+BC	+	16
8-MOP+CX	+	18
Control groups	– +	0
No drug	+	9
No drug	–	0
Carotenoids	– +	0
Arachidic oil	– +	0

The picture of results at the 80th week after initial UV exposure is reported in Table I. Carcinogenicity was expressed by the production of subcutaneous malignant tumors classified predominantly as mammary adenocarcinomas (with lung metastases), and a few skin appendages carcinomas. These tumors occurred in different regions, but no one within the painted areas as it was previously observed (28).

Our data demonstrated that both carotenoids (with and without pro-vitamin A activity) prevent 8-MOP photocarcinogenicity to the same extent, up to about 50-55%. The long UV light exposure, however, exerted *per se* 9% carcinogenic induction, independently of the negligible energy delivered by 313 nm, as it was also observed in a previous experiment (28). Noteworthily, also this UV-A carcinogenic effect is prevented by supplemental carotenoids.

As far as the mechanism of action is concerned, one should consider that BC and CX yielded results similar to those observed in the inhibition of photocarcinogenic enhancement by BP. Therefore, the properties of carotenoids as radical scavengers and/or singlet oxygen quenchers must play a role. This is important to assume that the photocarcinogenic effect of 8-MOP must imply the involvement of oxygen.

III. PHOTOMUTAGENICITY BY 8-MOP IN *SALMONELLA TYPHIMURIUM* TA 102 AND ITS PARTIAL PREVENTION BY CAROTENOIDS (L.S., L.B., A.B., R.P., G.S., P.B.)

The findings of protection by carotenoids in breast photocarcinogenesis produced by 8-MOP, suggested, as it was just pointed out, that an oxygen involvement in this mechanism should take place. Therefore, the action of BC on photomutagenicity in a UV-A irradiated 8-MOP bacteria system was investigated. Such experimental attempt was carried out using a strain of *S. Typhimurium* , TA 102, sensitive to oxidative mutagens irradiated in a medium under normal atmospheric conditions or bubbled with nitrogen (33).

The assay procedure was similar to that described by Jose (8). 8-MOP and BC, dissolved in DMSO, were added to bacteria suspensions at different concentrations; the suspensions were pre-incubated for 20 min at room temperature and then exposed to UV-A radiation, in normal atmospheric conditions, or pre-bubbled for 60 min with nitrogen to obtain an anoxic medium.

As shown in Fig. 2, under normal atmospheric conditions (in the presence of air) 8-MOP proved to be mutagenic after UV-A irradiation at a concentration of

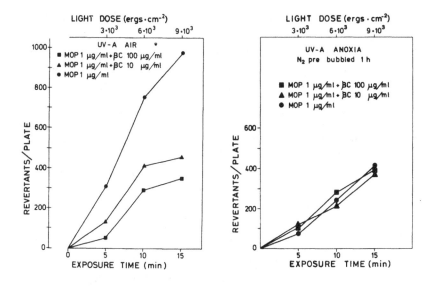

Fig. 2. 8-MOP photomutagenesis in air and its inhibition
by BC; photomutagenesis in anoxia with no BC protection. Evidence for a diphasic photoreaction.
(After Santamaria et al. Med. Biol. Env., 1984).

1 µg/ml (4.6 µM) confirming previous findings on *E. coli*
(18). Such mutation is prevented by BC 10 and 100 µg/ml
(18.6 - 186 µM) up to about 50% and 7C%, respectively.
The mechanism of this phenomenon was not due to an
umbriferous screen effect, but rather to a
physiochemical action of the drug. Indeed, the
absorption of UV-A light by BC solution in the same
experimental conditions was negligible. UV-A light and
BC were found to have no mutagenic effect *per se*; BC was
not found to be a photomutagenic substance.

The same experiment carried cut in a medium
saturated with nitrogen (Fig. 2) showed that
photomutagenesis by 8-MOP does occur, but to an extent
up to about 65% lower than in the presence of air. In
this case BC did nct play any protective role. The same
experimental picture was obtained with CX.

The above results may be somehow considered complementary to the data reported by de Mol et al. (18) which demonstrated that oxygenation enhances 8-MOP photomutagenesis in *E. coli* especially when D_2O is used as a medium where $^1O_2$ has a longer life time.

Actually, our findings proved that 8-MOP photomutagenesis occurs in anoxia, but is greatly enhanced in the air through an oxygen effect which is thoroughly eliminated by BC or CX. This clearly demonstrated a two-step photoreaction.

BC was not used by de Mol et al. in their experiment where formation of $^1O_2$ was demonstrated (17), because this compound was believed to be unsuitable for several photochemical reasons. Nevertheless, our data showed that BC is effective also in an *in vitro* system; this suggests the proper interpretation of the mechanism of action of photocarcinogenesis prevention by 8-MOP. Indeed, it is possible to figure out that 8-MOP displays also *in vivo* a two-step photoreaction (33) as follows: first, an oxygen independent photoadduct with pyrimidine bases of DNA (3), secondly, an *in situ* generation of $^1O_2$ (7) or activated oxyradical species, which are quenched when tissues are saturated with carotenoids.

The fact that 8-MOP is photomutagenic also in anoxic conditions, although to a lesser extent, does not disprove the original statement that photosensitizing properties of furoccumarins are oxygen independent (19).

IV. SUPPLEMENTAL CAROTENOIDS PREVENT GASTRIC CANCER INDUCED BY N-METHYL-N'-NITRO-N-NITROSOGUANIDINE (MNNG) IN RATS
(L.S., A.B., C.R., A.A., G.S., L.A.)

The antitumorigenic activity of carotenoids,

described in the previous sections, concerned substances
listed as indirect carcinogenic agents, being dependent
on light excitation and/or metabolic oxidation. Hence,
it was worth trying to test supplemental carotenoids
upon a carcinogenic process induced by MNNG, a direct
carcinogen active independently of light and,
presumably, oxidative processes. MNNG was administrated
to rats, according to Kunze et al. (11) at low doses and
over a limited period of time to develop gastric cancer
stepwise via several successive stages of transformation
with varying biological potential, expressed by
dysplasia grade I (mild), II (moderate), and III
(severe).

Adult female Wistar rats (initial weight between
180 and 200 g) were perorally given BC or CX, according
to methods described in the above chapters. One month
later, all rats of the experimental groups received MNNG
continuously for 250 days (time of exposure) in their
drinking water at a dosage of 83 mg/1000 ml; MNNG
treatment was then discontinued, according to Kunze et
al. (11). Supplemental administration of BC or CX
continued throughout the experiment, both with daily
diet and three times a week by catheter in arachidic
oil solution. The surviving experimental animals were
killed after different periods of induction (Table II).
Immediately after killing, their stomachs were processed
according to Kunze et al. (11). A minimum of 50-60
sections (stained with hematoxylin-eosin) per animal
were histologically examined to detect lesions as
reported in Table II. The diagnostic criteria were those
adopted for human stomach (24) because of the great
morphological similarity between the experimental
induced dysplasia and carcinoma types. Pathological
evaluations were done in a blind manner.

MNNG induced gastric carcinomas of intestinal and
diffuse types, both undifferentiated and mucocellular,
were morphologically as in human stomach. They developed

Table II. Appearance of sequential lesions during experimental gastric carcinogenesis by MNNG and
protective effect by BC and CX. Each group
consists of 24 rats ♀ Wistar strain, Nossan,
Milano. (After Santamaria et al., Med. Biol.
Env., 1985).

	Days from initial exposure	polyploid gastritis	gastric atrophy	intestinal metaplasia	mild dysplasia	moderate dysplasia	severe dysplasia	signet ring cell dripping	early cancer	infiltrating carcinoma
MNNG	350		7		8	5	1	3	1	
	400	3	5		6	2		6	2	2
	450	2	1	3	4	5	9	5	7	2
	500		2	1	1	5	3	1	6	3
	550	4	7	5	3	11		2	3	4
Total lesions		9	22	9	22	28	13	17	19	11
MNNG + β-carotene or canthaxanthine	350		8							
	400	3		3	3	9	3		3	
	450	12		6	6					
	500	3	7	7		7	7	14		3
	550	8	8	8	8	13		13	4	
Total lesions		26	23	24	17	29	10	27	7	3

histogenetically from focal atypias or dysplasias of an
otherwise undisturbed mucosa. This process took place
independently of erosions, ulcers, and benign-appearing
proliferative or neoplastic epithelial lesions. They
clearly developed stepwise via several successive stages
of transformation with varying biological potential from
polyploid gastritis, gastric atrophy, intestinal
metaplasia, mild dysplasia, moderate dysplasia, severe
dysplasia including signet ring cell dripping and early
cancer. The multifocal development of gastric cancer was
expressed by the appearance of pre-neoplastic and
neoplastic changes simultaneously in various areas of
the same stomach.

The frequency of carcinogen-induced lesions of the
gastric mucosa in the different experimental groups
induced by limited oral application of MNNG is expressed

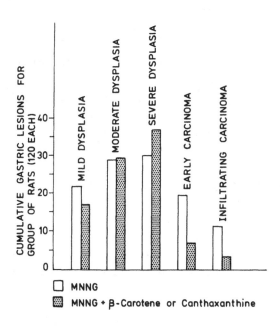

Fig. 3. Inhibition of progression to early and infiltra-
       ting carcinomas by BC and CX. (After Santamaria
       et al., Med. Biol. Env., 1985).

in the upper section of Table II. The same parameter in
animals with supplemental dietary BC or CX, grouped
together because of no significant differences in
results, is expressed in the lower part of Table II. The
cumulative lesions for group of rats with and without
supplemental carotenoids are also expressed by the
histogram in Fig. 3.

From these data it appears that supplemental
carotenoids did not interfere with any pre-neoplastic
lesion arising from glandular mucosa initiated by MNNG
oral application. Somehow, carotenoids might have
increased the severe dysplasias in form of signet ring
cell dripping. Nevertheless, carotenoids clearly

inhibited the progression of dysplasias to early and
infiltrating carcinomas.

In consideration of the multistage carcinogenic
process, one may point out that supplemental carotenoids
did not affect either initiation or promotion, as
expressed by dysplastic lesions, but clearly inhibited
progression to malignant growth. This dramatic
inhibition of progression can be explained giving
support to the hypothesis of oxygen radical involvement
at different stages of the process. Much attention has
been recently paid to the demonstration that reactive
oxygen scavengers and detoxifiers, such as
superoxide-dismutase (SOD), SOD-mimetics, catalase, and
phenolic antioxidants, inhibit biochemical and
biological actions of tumor promoters *in vitro* and *in vi_
vo*,thus providing strong presumptive evidence for oxygen
radical involvement in the later stages of neoplastic
development, that is, progression to infiltrating
malignancy (6,9). Here, carotenoids should exert their
concomitant preventive action. BC can also act like
pro-vitamin A maintaining initiated cells in the dormant
state (4).

These conclusions lead to interesting
considerations on the gastric cancer natural history and
behaviour in animals and humans. Up to now, some
differences have been reported between the
experimentally induced dysplasias in animals, and those
found in human stomach, in spite of their morphological
similarity. Actually, Kunze et al. (11) report the
reversibility of human gastric dysplasias and Ohlert
refers the possible long persistence of this kind of
lesions (21), whereas, these are reported to be
irreversible in animals (11).

Thus, all the above experimental data and related
discussions fit into the theory that the initiation
stage is essentially irreversible, the promotion stage

is reversible at the beginning and subsequently irreversible or blocked, whereas progression allows for the selection of ultimate autonomous malignant cells (6,9). This holds true for an unitarian biological behaviour for both kinds of carcinogenesis.

V. CONCLUSIONS AND PERSPECTIVES IN CANCER PREVENTION PROGRAMS APPLIED TO HUMANS

All the above data demonstrated that carotenoids, when administrated as a daily supplement to diet, to experimental animals starting before cancer initiation and continuing throughout the experiment, exert protection against cancer with a mechanism largely depending on their antioxidant property. In the case of an indirect carcinogen, carotenoids may act at the level of initiation, just scavenging the oxyradical precursor of the ultimate carcinogen, or, in the case of a direct carcinogen, at the level of promotion preventing the progression of dysplasia to infiltrating malignancy.

These clear-cut experimental findings on animals deserve to be critically associated with definite prospective epidemiological investigations in humans. Indeed, the intake of dietary pro-vitamin A (BC) was inversely related to the 19-year incidence of lung cancer in 1,954 middle-aged men (38). Then, new perspectives in cancer prevention programs applied to humans can be advanced.

Carotenoids prevented 8-MOP photoinduction of mammary adenocarcinoma in female mice up to 60%, the same order of magnitude as their protection on 8-MOP photomutagenesis. Further investigations demonstrated the occurrence of a two-step photoreaction, i.e. an anoxic one, followed by an oxygen dependent process controlled by carotenoids. This suggested that PUVA therapy can be carried out cutting down its oncogenic risk, when patients are supplemented with carotenoids.

Actually, the anoxic 8-MOP-DNA photobinding could take
care of the therapeutic effect in clearing chronic
plaque psoriasis, whereas carotenoids could scavenge or
quench the oxyradical and/or $^1O_2$, which should rule the
oxygen dependent second reaction step. This prediction
(29) appeared to be supported by a clinical work on PUVA
therapy carried out with different purposes (13).
Supplemental carotenoids, even if administrated to
patients at high doses, did not help in preventing
burning, but did not affect the PUVA therapeutic action
(13). Nevertheless, in that treatment, most probably,
carotenoids were effective in cutting down the oncogenic
risk. This can be ascertained after several years by a
controlled clinical trial.

Our results may also address to such stimulating
issues as those presented in a review on dietary BC and
human cancer (22), since carotenoids may exert their
antitumorigenic action independently of their
pro-vitamin A activity (29,16). Furthermore, attention
should be given to carotenoids due to their lack of
toxicity in humans, in contrast to retinoids, which may
be harmful to the liver and inactive on skin tumors
(16).

Our previous recommendations (29) to use
supplemental carotenoids, instead of sunscreen
preparations (sun oil), for outdoor workers in order to
prevent skin cancer, appeared to be rational. Presently,
the National Cancer Institute (USA) is funding human
intervention studies on skin cancer prevention by
carotenoids, at least two in USA and one in Africa (in
albino subjects) (37). Accordingly, the primary
prevention of any other epithelial malignancy in humans
by supplemental carotenoids can be also considered
worthwhile.

Furthermore, any post-surgical cancer condition,
when the malignant growth without involvement of

lymphnodes is radically excised, should be treated with supplemental carotenoids to protect the remaining initiated epithelial tissue against promotion and progression to a second malignancy. This type of prevention can be envisaged for any other malignant growth after radical excision in organs like lung, urinary bladder, breast, colon-rectum.

ACKNOWLEDGEMENTS

This work was supported by the Ministero della Sanita', Servizi di Medicina Sociale, Roma, and was enccuraged by the Ministerc della Pubblica Istruzione, Roma. Hoffmann-La Roche Inc., Basel, is acknowledged for providing the carotenoids. Fedegari Autcclavi S.p.A., Albuzzano, Pavia, is acknowledged for providing tecnical facilities. C.N.R., Roma, is acknowledged for partial research contribution no. 83.02606.04.

REFERENCES

1) Blum, H.F. Carcinogenesis by ultraviolet light, pp. 188-191. Princeton, Princeton University Press, 1959.

2) Eungeler, W. Uber die Entstehung von Hautcarcinomen und Hautsarcomen nach Sonnenbestrahlung und Photosensibilisierung. Klin. Wsch., 16: 1012-1013, 1937.

3) Dall' Acqua, F., Marciano, S., Ciavatta, L., and Rodighiero, G. Formation of interstrand cross-linkings in the phctcreaction between furocoumarins and DNA. Z. Naturforsch., 26: 561-569, 1971.

4) De Luca, L.M. Deficiency of vitamin A in hepatccellular carcinoma tissue: considerations on its establishment. Diet, Nutrition, and Cancer: From Basic Research to Policy Implications, pp. 111-115. New York: Alan R. Liss, Inc., 1983.

5) Epstein, J.H. Effects of β-carotene on ultraviolet

induced cancer formation in the hairless mouse skin.
Photochem. Photobiol., 25: 211-213, 1977.

6) Flavin, D.F., and Kolbye, A.C. Nutritional factors
   with the potential to inhibit critical pathways of
   tumor promotion. In: F.L. Meyskens and K.N. Prasad
   (eds.), Modulation and Mediation of Cancer by
   Vitamins, pp. 24-38. Basel: S. Karger, 1983.

7) Ito, T. Cellular and sub-cellular mechanisms of
   photodynamic action: the $^1O_2$ hypothesis as a driving
   force in recent research. Photochem. Photobiol., 28:
   493-508, 1978.

8) Jose, J. Photomutagenesis by chlorinated
   phenothiazines tranquillizers. P.N.A.S., 76 (1):
   469-472, 1979.

9) Kensler, T.W., and Trush, M.A. Role of oxygen
   radicals in tumor promotion. Env. Mutag., 6: 593-616,
   1984.

10) Krinsky , N. Carotenoid protection against
    oxidation. Pure and Applied Chemistry, 51: 649-660,
    1979.

11) Kunze, E., Schauer, A., Eder, M., and Seefeldt, C.
    Early sequential lesions during development of
    experimental gastric cancer with special reference
    to dysplasias. J. Cancer Res. Clin. Oncol., 95:
    247-264, 1979.

12) Lamola, A.A., and Blumberg, W.E. The effectiveness
    of β-carotene and phytoene as systemic sunscreens.
    Proc. Am. Soc. Photobiol, 109, 1976.

13) Macdonald, K., Holti, G., and Marks, J. Is there a
    place for β-carotene/canthaxanthin in
    photochemotherapy for psoriasis ? Dermatologica,
    169: 41-46, 1984.

14) Mathews-Roth, M.M., Pathak, M.A., Parrish, J.A.,
    Fitzpatrick, T.B., Kass, E.H., Toda, K., and
    Clements, W. A clinical trial of the effects of oral
    beta-carotene on the responses of human skin to
    solar radiation. J. Invest. Derm., 59: 349-353,
    1972.

15) Mathews-Roth, M.M., and Pathak, M.A. Phytoene as a

protective agent against sunburn (greater than 280 nm) radiation in guinea pigs. Photochem. Phctobiol., 21: 261-263, 1975.

16) Mathews-Roth, M.M. Carctenoids and skin cancer prevention. Clin. Res., 28: 477, 1980.

17) Mol de, N.J., and Beijersbergen van Henegouwen, G.M.J. Formation of singlet oxygen by 8-methoxypsoralen. Photochem. Photobiol., 30: 331-335, 1979.

18) Mol de, N.J., Beijersbergen van Henegcuwen, C.M.J., Mohn, G.R., Glickman, B.W., and Kleef, P.M.. On the involvement of singlet oxygen in mutation induction by 8-methoxypsoralen and UV-A irradiation in *E. Coli* K 12. Mutat. Res., 82: 23-30, 1981.

19) Musajo, L., Rodighiero, G., and Santamaria, L. Le sostanze fotodinamiche con particolare riguardo alle furocumarine. Atti Soc. Ital. Patol., 5 (1): 1-70, 1957.

20) Oginsky, E.L., Green, G.S., Griffith, D.G., and Fowlks, W.L. Lethal photosensitization of bacteria with 8-methoxypscralen tc long wavelength to UV radiation. J. Bacteriol., 78: 821-833, 1959.

21) Ohlert, W., Henke, M., Strauch, M., and Keller, P. Die Dysplasien der Magenschleimhaut, ihre Pathogenese und ihre Klinische Bedeutung. Therapiewcche, 28: 4966-4975, 1978.

22) Peto, R., Doll, R., Buckley, J.D., and Sporn, M.B. Can dietary beta-carotene materially reduce human cancer rates? Nature, 290: 201-208, 1981.

23) Poppe, W., and Grossweiner, I.I. Photodynamic sensitization by 8-methoxypsoralen via the singlet oxygen mechanism. Photochem. Photobiol., 22: 217-219, 1975.

24) Ravetto, C., and Santamaria, L. Dysplasias and morphogenesis of gastric cancer. Cancer Det. Prev., 4: 369-376, 1981.

25) Rettura, G., Stratford, F., Levenson, S.M., and Seifter, E. Prophylactic and therapeutic action of supplemental β-carotene in mice inoculated with

C3HBA adenocarcinoma cells: lack of therapeutic action of supplemental ascorbic acid. J.N.C.I., 69: 73-77, 1982.

26) Santamaria, L. Problems of energy transfer in photodynamic reactions. Bull. Soc. Chim. Belg., 71: 889-905, 1962.

27) Santamaria, L., Giordano, G.G., Alfisi, M., and Cascione, F. Effects of light on 3,4-benzpyrene carcinogenesis. Nature, 210: 824-825, 1966.

28) Santamaria, L., Bianchi, A., Arnaboldi, A., and Daffara, P. Photocarcinogenesis by methoxypsoralen, neutral red and proflavine. Boll. Chim. Farm., 118: 356-362, 1979.

29) Santamaria, L., Bianchi, A., Arnaboldi, A., and Andreoni, L. Prevention of the benzo(a)pyrene photocarcinogenic effect by β-carotene and canthaxanthine. Preliminary study. Boll. Chim. Farm., 119: 745-748, 1980.

30) Santamaria, L., Bianchi, A., Arnaboldi, A., Andreoni, L., and Bermond, P. Dietary carotenoids block photocarcinogenic enhancement by benzo(a)pyrene and inhibit its carcinogenesis in the dark. Experientia, 39: 1043-1045, 1983.

31) Santamaria, L. Bianchi, A., Arnaboldi, A., Andreoni, L., and Bermond, P. Benzo(a)pyrene carcinogenicity and its prevention by carotenoids. In: F.L. Meyskens and K.N. Prasad (eds.), Modulation and Mediation of Cancer by Vitamins, pp. 81-88. Basel: S. Karger, 1983.

32) Santamaria, L., Bianchi, A, Andreoni, L., Santagati, G., Arnaboldi, A., and Bermond, P. 8-Methoxypsoralen photocarcinogenesis and its preventiom by dietary carotenoids. Preliminary results. Med. Biol. Env., 12 (1): 533-537, 1984.

33) Santamaria, L., Bianchi, L., Bianchi, A., Pizzala, R., Santagati, G., and Bermond, P. Photomutagenicity by 8-methoxypsoralen with and without singlet oxygen involvement and its prevention by beta-carotene. Relevance to the mechanism of 8-MOP

photocarcinogenicity and to PUVA application. Med.
Biol Env., 12: (1), 541-546, 1984.

34) Santamaria, L., Bianchi, A., Ravetto, C., Arnaboldi,
A., Santagati, G., and Andreoni, L. Supplemental
carotenoids prevent gastric cancer in rats induced
by N-methyl-N'-nitro-N-nitrosoguanidine (MNNG).
Communicated at the "Second Int. Conf. on the
Modulation and Mediation of Cancer by Vitamins and
Micronutrients", Tucson, Arizona, Feb. 10-13, 1985;
Med. Biol. Env., 13, 1985. In press.

35) Sayre, R.M., Black, H.S., and Poh Agin, P. Beta
carotene is not an oral sunscreen. Proc. Am. Soc.
Photobiol., 113, 1981.

36) Seifter, E., Rettura, G., Stratford, F., and
Levenson, S.M. C3HBA tumor prevention and treatment
with beta-carotene. Fed. Proc., 40: 652, 1981.

37) Sestili, M.A., (ed.). Chemoprevention Clinical
Trials. Problems and solutions. US Dept. of Health
and Human Services. Publ. no. (NIH) 85: 2715, 1984.

38) Shekelle, R.B., Lepper, M., Liu, S., Maliza, C.,
Raynor, W.J., and Rossof, A.H. Dietary vitamin A and
risk of cancer in the Western Electric Study. The
Lancet, 1185-1190, 1981.

39) Singh, H., and Vadasz, J..A. Singlet oxygen: a major
reactive species in the furocoumarin photosensitized
inactivation of *E. coli* ribosomes. Photochem.
Photobiol., 28: 539-545, 1978.

40) Slater, T.F., and Riley, P.A. Carcinogenicity of
polycyclic hydrocarbons and their interaction with
DNA. Int. J. Quantum Chem., 5: 143-148, 1978.

41) Smith, D.E., Santamaria, L., Smaller, B. Free
radicals in photodyramic systems. In: M.S. Bloys et
al. (eds.), Free Radicals in Biological Systems, pp.
305-310. New York: Academic Press, 1961.

42) Ts' O, P.O.P., Caspary, W.T., Cohen, B.I., Leavit,
J.C., Lesko, S.A., Lorentzen, R.J., Schechtman, L.M.
Basic mechanisms in polycyclic hydrocarbon
carcinogenesis. In P.O.P. Ts'O and J. Di Paolo
(eds.), The Biochemistry of Disease, 4: pp. 113-147.
New York: Dekker, 1974.

RETINOIDS AS CHEMOPREVENTIVE AGENTS: ALONE AND IN COMBINATION

R.C. Moon, D.L. McCormick, and R.G. Mehta

IIT Research Institute

10 West 35th Street, Chicago, IL   60617

The role of retinoids in cancer chemoprevention has been the subject of numerous studies. The rationale for the use of retinoids as chemopreventive agents or inhibitors of carcinogenesis dates back more than 60 years. As early as 1922, Mori (35) observed that a deficiency in vitamin A led to metaplastic changes of the epithelium of the respiratory tract; the normal ciliated columnar epithelium became flattened, lost nuclei, and became cornified while the underlying cells exhibited typical keratohyalin granules. Subsequent studies by Wolbach and Howe (47) extended these observations to epithelia of the gastrointestinal and urinary tracts. These observations of Mori and those of Wolbach and Howe on the development of such retinoid deficient squamous metaplasia indicated a process closely akin to that induced by certain chemical carcinogens (9). A more direct link between retinoids and cancer appeared in 1926 when Fujimaki (5) observed the development of carcinomas of the stomach in rats maintained on a vitamin A deficient diet. More recently, other investigators have shown that animals fed a diet deficient in retinoids and subsequently exposed to chemical carcinogens develop a greater than normal incidence of cancers and putative precursors to these malignancies (37).

In addition to the relationship between retinoid deficiency and neoplasia, other studies have indicated that retinoids can reverse premalignant changes in the epithelium of mouse prostate glands in organ culture (12) and

161

suppress malignant transformation in cells in vitro irre-
spective of whether the transformation is induced by
ionizing radiation (8), chemical carcinogens (27), or
transforming polypeptides (40). Moreover, retinoids have
also been shown to be potent inhibitors of phorbol ester-
induced tumor promotion (42); these studies are detailed
in this volume by Verma. Inasmuch as retinoids inhibit
several aspects of the carcinogenic process (transformation, metaplasia, promotion), several investigators have
extended these studies to show that exogenous retinoids
can inhibit tumor formation in vivo in epithelia at several
different organ sites.

    The majority of primary human cancers arise in epithe-
lial tissues that depend upon retinoids for normal cellular
differentiation and a sustained effort has been directed
towards retinoid modulation of tumorigenesis in these
tissues. Although several reports have appeared relative
to inhibition of carcinogenesis of the respiratory tract,
skin, mammary gland, urinary bladder, intestine, stomach,
esophagus, cervix and pancreas by retinoids, the majority
of studies have dealt with chemoprevention of cancer of the
skin, mammary gland and urinary bladder. Since carcinogenesis of the mammary gland is the only process in which
the chemopreventive activity of retinoids either alone or
in combination with other modifiers has been studied in any
detail, we shall briefly review experiments conducted in
our and other laboratories concerning the influence of
retinoids on carcinogenesis of this structure.

ORGAN AND SPECIES SPECIFICITY

    Modification of the basic structure of the retinoid
molecule (Figure 1) has yielded a range of biologically
active analogs. The majority of these modifications have
occurred at the polar terminal group, but changes in the
aromatic ring and side chain have also led to highly active
compounds, some of which impart less toxicity than the
basic molecule. Not only has toxicity been altered by
changes in the basic retinoid structure, but such alterations can also have dramatic effects upon organ distribution and metabolism and hence, the cancer preventive activity of the retinoid. For instance, the synthetic
retinoid 13-cis retinoic acid is highly effective in the
inhibition of 2 stage tumorigenesis (42) and urinary

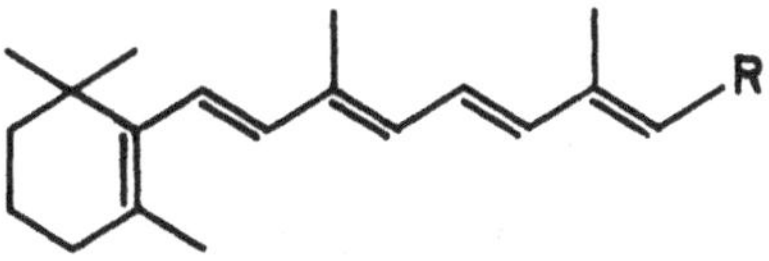

all-*trans*-retinoids

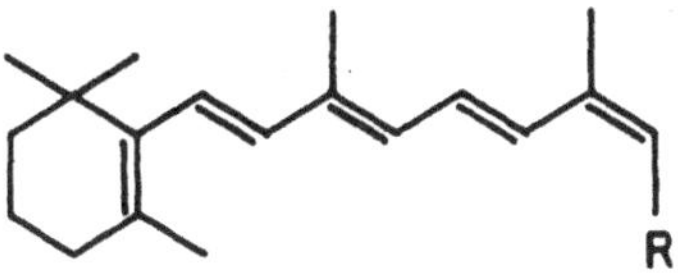

13-*cis*-retinoids

Fig. 1. Retinoid structures, Structure R = COOH, retinoic
acid; CONH-4-C_6H_4OH, N-(4-hydroxyphenyl)retinamide;
CH_2OCOCH_3, retinyl acetate.

bladder cancer induced in rats (6,38) and mice (2) by the
carcinogens N-butyl-N-(4-hydroxybutyl)nitrosamine (OH-BBN)
or N-methyl-N-nitrosourea (MNU). However, by contrast,
the compound has little cancer inhibitory activity in the
rat mammary gland (Table 1). The trimethylmethoxyphenyl
(TMMP) analog of ethyl retinoate is highly effective
against mouse skin carcinogenesis (42), although this compound is ineffective against either bladder carcinogenesis
in mice or mammary cancer in rats. On the other hand,
retinyl acetate is extremely active in the rat mammary
cancer model (31,32), but exhibits little chemopreventive
protection against two stage skin tumorigenesis (42) or
mammary carcinogenesis in mice (13,45).

The relative efficacy of non-toxic doses of several
retinoids in the inhibition of mammary carcinogenesis induced in the rat by MNU is illustrated in Figure 2. Retinyl acetate and 4-hydroxyphenyl retinamide (4-HPR) are
highly effective in reducing mammary cancer incidence and
increasing the latency of induced mammary cancers (34).
In addition, the number of mammary carcinomas are also
significantly reduced by the administration of either of
these retinoids. However, as indicated above, 13-cis
retinoic acid has little effect upon the appearance of MNU
induced mammary carcinomas; retinyl methyl ether is of

Table 1

Target Organ Specificity of Retinoids in
Inhibiting Carcinogenesis

Target Organ	Carcinogen	Effective Retinoid	Noneffective Retinoid
Skin	DMBA	TMMP ethyl retinoate[a]	Retinyl acetate
Mammary Gland	MNU, DMBA	Retinyl acetate	13-cis retinoic acid
Urinary Bladder	OH-BBN	13-cis-retinoic acid	TMMP ethyl retinoate

[a]TMMP ethyl retinoate, 4-methoxy-2,3,6-trimethylphenyl analogue of retinoic acid
ethyl ester; DMBA, 7,12-dimethylbenz(α)anthracene.

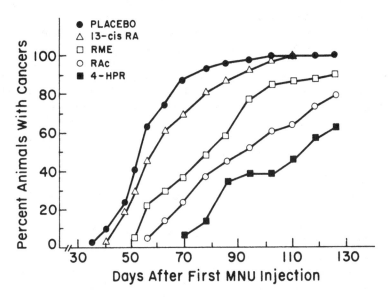

Fig. 2. Composite of several experiments showing the effect of nontoxic levels of retinoids on the incidence and latency of appearance of MNU-induced mammary cancer. In each experiment, virgin female Sprague-Dawley rats received an i.v. injection of 50 mg MNU per kg body weight at 50 and 57 days of age. At age 60 days, animals were placed on diets supplemented with: placebo; 13-cis-retinoic acid (13-cis RA), 1 mmol/kg diet; retinyl methyl ether (RME), 1 mmol/kg diet; retinyl acetate (RAc), 1 mmol/kg diet; 4-HPR, 2 mmol/kg diet. Reprinted from Ref. 29 with permission from Plenum Publishing Corp.

intermediate efficacy, although the latter compound is extremely effective against 7,12-dimethylbenz(α)anthracene induced mammary carcinogenesis. Thus, it is readily apparent that minor alterations in the basic retinoid structure can significantly alter the activity of the molecule with respect to the inhibition of chemical carcinogenesis of the mammary gland.

The toxicity induced by a retinoid is of extreme importance in long term chemoprevention studies. As an example, retinyl acetate and 4-HPR are both effective

inhibitors of chemical carcinogenesis of the rat mammary
gland, but the patterns of metabolism and organ distribution of the two compounds are quite different (34). Chronic
dietary administration of high doses of retinyl acetate
results in an accumulation of retinyl esters in the liver,
a process frequently accompanied by significant hepatic
toxicity (36). On the other hand, dietary administration
of 4-HPR results in a much higher level of retinoid in the
mammary gland, but with relatively little liver accumulation (34). Thus, on the basis of its organ distribution,
it would appear that 4-HPR is preferable to retinyl acetate
for use in the prevention of experimental breast cancer.

CHEMOPREVENTION OF MAMMARY CANCER: RETINOID ALONE

As indicated in Table 2, several retinoids possess
mammary anticarcinogenic activity when administered
chronically in the diet to female rats. Since in these
studies, the retinoid was administered following carcinogen
exposure, it is probable that the retinoid is inhibiting
the promotion or progression of carcinogenesis. However,
evidence exist which suggests that retinoids may also be
effective inhibitors during the initiation phase of the
carcinogenic process (16).

Although retinoids are most effective in inhibiting
mammary carcinogenesis when administered shortly after
carcinogen treatment, they are still effective cancer
chemopreventive agents even if the administration is delayed for some time after the carcinogenic insult (18).
The length of time that retinoid treatment can be delayed
is largely a function of tumor latency. In animals given a
carcinogen dose that induces tumors with a mean induction
time of approximately 60 days (18), retinyl acetate administration begun at one week post-carcinogen is highly effective in cancer inhibition. However, the retinoid treatment is somewhat less effective if initiated 4 weeks after
administration of the carcinogen while beginning the retinoid at 8 weeks after carcinogen treatment has no effect
on tumor induction. By contrast, at a carcinogen dose
inducing mammary cancers with a mean induction time of
approximately 240 days (18), retinyl acetate administration
can be delayed as long as 16 weeks and still retain its
chemopreventive efficacy. Only when the initiation of
retinyl acetate treatment is delayed 20 weeks, does the

Table 2

Effect of Retinoids on Mammary Carcinogenesis of Rats _In Vivo_

Host/Species	Carcinogen	Retinoid[1]	Effect
Rat (S/D)	DMBA	Retinyl Palmitate	No Effect
Rat (S/D)	DMBA	Retinyl Acetate	Inhibition of Carcinogenesis
Rat (Lewis)	DMBA	Retinyl Acetate	
Rat (S/D)	DMBA	N-(4-Hydroxyphenyl)Retinamide	
Rat (S/D)	MNU	Retinyl Acetate	Inhibition of Carcinogenesis
		Retinyl Methyl Ether	
		N-(4-Hydroxyphenyl)Retinamide	
		Axerophthene	
		All-trans-Retinoic Acid	
		N-(4-Hydroxyphenyl)13-cis-Retinamide	
		13-cis Retinoic Acid	No Inhibition
		Retinyl Butyl Ether	
		N-Ethylretinamide	
		Retinylidene Dimedone	
		Retinylidene Acetylacetone	
		TMMP Analog of Retinyl Ethyl Ester	
		TMMP Analog of Retinyl Methyl Ether	
Rat (Lew/Mai)	Benzo(α)pyrene	Retinyl Acetate	Inhibition of Carcinogenesis

[1]For structures, see Newton, et al., Cancer Res., 40: 3413-3425, 1980.

retinoid show a loss of cancer inhibitory activity (Figure 3). The ability of the retinoid to significantly inhibit mammary cancer formation when administered at some time after the carcinogenic insult, is of the utmost clinical importance since the initiation of carcinogenesis in man is largely unknown.

COMBINATION CHEMOPREVENTION: RETINOID AND OTHER MODIFIERS

Although retinoids can inhibit mammary cancer induction, no retinoid has yet been developed which is totally effective, i.e., which reduces mammary cancer incidence to zero. However, significant increases in chemopreventive activity can be achieved when retinoid administration is combined with other modifiers of mammary carcinogenesis. The MNU rat mammary carcinoma model as originally described by Gullino et al (7), and subsequently modified in our laboratory (14) is subject to inhibition both by retinoids

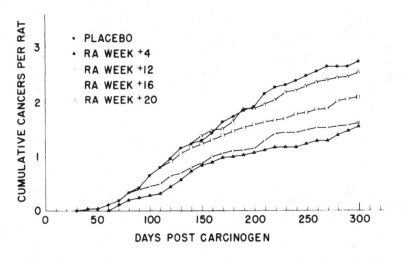

Fig. 3. Influence of delay in retinyl acetate administration on number of mammary carcinomas per rat. Rats received a single i.v. injection of 25 mg MNU per kg body weight at 50 days of age. Retinyl acetate (RA) diet, 1 mmol/kg diet, was begun at either 4, 12, 16, or 20 weeks after (+) injection of MNU. All tumors were histologically confirmed mammary cancers. Reprinted from Ref. 18 with permission from Cancer Research.

and by modification of host hormonal status (17). As indicated in the Figure 4, both retinyl acetate and ovariectomy inhibit mammary cancer induction by MNU; however, the
combination of ovariectomy plus retinyl acetate is significantly more effective in cancer inhibition than is
either treatment regimen alone. A similar combination
effect has been noted using the DMBA rat mammary carcinoma
model (17). That such combined chemoprevention is not
limited to the natural retinoids (retinyl acetate) has been
demonstrated by McCormick et al (17) in which a synthetic
analog (4-HPR) synergistically inhibited mammary carcinogenesis when combined with bilateral ovariectomy. Similar
synergistic responses have also been obtained with use of
the antiestrogen tamoxifen, both in the MNU (Figure 5) and
DMBA tumor models (46). The retinoid-tamoxifen effect,
however, appeared to be additive as contrasted to the
retinoid-ovariectomy effect which was synergistic

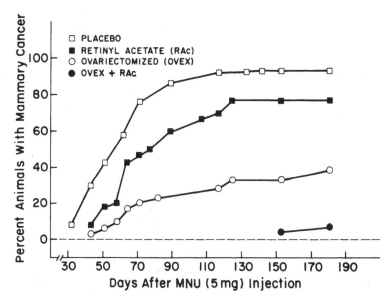

Fig. 4. Influence of ovariectomy and RAc on the multiplicity of mammary adenocarcinoma in rats treated with MNU.
Sprague Dawley female rats were injected i.v. with MNU (50
mg/kg) at 50 days of age. Animals received either placebo
or RAc (1 mmol/kg) supplemented diet at 7 days postcarcinogen, and 2 groups of the animals were bilaterally ovariectomized at 14 days postcarcinogen. Reprinted from Ref. 29,
with permission from Plenum Publishing Corp.

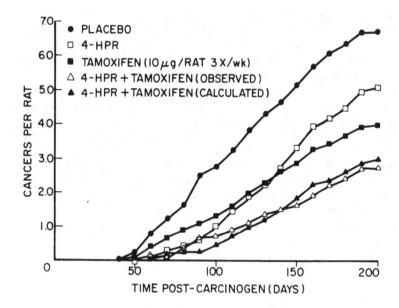

Fig. 5. Influence of HPR and tamoxifen on the multiplicity
of mammary carcinoma in rats treated with MNU. Sprague-
Dawley female rats were injected i.v. with MNU (50 mg/kg)
at 50 days of age. At 7 days postcarcinogen the animals
received either placebo diet or diet supplemented with 2
mmol/kg HPR. Tamoxifen citrate treatment (10 μg, 3 times
each week, s.c.) was also started 7 days postcarcinogen
until the end of the study.

indicating that other hormones may be involved in the interaction with retinoids on mammary carcinogenesis. That
such may be the case has been demonstrated by Welsch et al
(43) who found a synergistic inhibition of MNU induced
mammary carcinogenesis by concomitant administration of
retinyl acetate and 2-bromo-α-ergocryptine, an inhibitor
of pituitary prolactin secretion (Figure 6). Blood prolactin levels of rats treated with retinyl acetate did not
differ from that of control animals, indicating that the
enhanced combination effect was not due to a further suppression of prolactin secretion. The influence of hormones
in the genesis and modulation of experimental mammary carcinogenesis is well established (28), and it is now clear
from the evidence cited above that the retinoids also
effectively modulate tumor development in this structure.

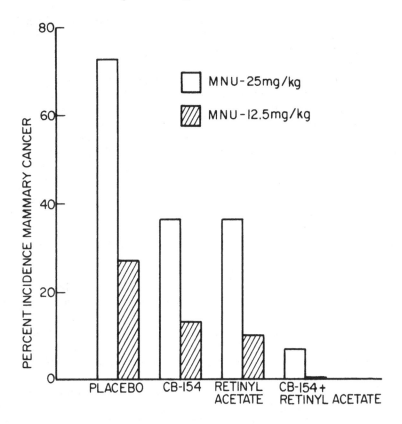

Fig. 6. Effect of retinyl acetate and/or 2-bromo-α-ergocryp-
tine (CB-154) on the incidence of MNU-induced mammary
tumorigenesis. Virgin female Sprague-Dawley rats received
either 12.5 or 25 mg MNU per kg body weight at 50 and 57
days of age. Retinyl acetate diet (1 mmol/kg diet) and/or
2-bromo-α-ergocryptine (4 mg/kg body weight) were initiated
3 days following the second MNU injection. Rats receiving
the high dose of MNU (25 mg/kg) were treated for 129 days,
while those receiving the low dose of MNU (12.5 mg/kg)
were treated for 175 days. All tumors were classified histologically as adenocarcinomas. Reprinted from Ref. 30,
with permission from Cancer Research.

These data suggest the existence of populations of preneoplastic or neoplastic cells with a differential sensitivity to the retinoids and hormones. Thus, the retinoids
might preferentially affect the development of hormone

independent tumors or those that do not regress following
either ovariectomy or treatment with agents that suppress
hormonal function and/or secretion.

Enhanced chemoprevention has also been demonstrated
with retinoids and other agents that inhibit the development of mammary cancer. Thompson et al (39) were the first
to show an enhanced inhibition of MNU rat mammary carcinogenesis with retinyl acetate and selenium. The effect was
confirmed by Ip and Ip (11) using the DMBA induced mammary
tumor model. Although both groups of workers found that
the combined effect of retinyl acetate and selenium was
substantially greater than that of either treatment alone
(Figure 7), both studies were complicated by the significant reduction in food intake and body weight gain in
animals receiving the combination of these chemopreventive
agents.

The use of combined modalities for prevention of mammary cancer have not always been successful. This is particularly true with the combination of retinoids and
immunostimulation. For example, 4-HPR and maleic anhydride-
divinyl ether copolymer (MVE-2), an immunostimulatory agent,
are both effective inhibitors of mammary carcinogenesis
induced in rats by MNU. However, combined administration
of 4-HPR and MVE-2 was no more effective in cancer inhibition than was either agent alone (33). Furthermore, Welsch
and DeHoog (44) have shown that immunostimulation induced
with either methanol extracted residue of the Bacillus
Calmette-Gurein, cell wall skeleton of Nocardia rubra or
mammary tumor cell particulate in Freund's complete adjuvant
and combined with retinyl acetate was no more effective in
inhibiting DMBA induced mammary carcinoma than was retinyl
acetate alone. Furthermore, when retinyl acetate was combined with immunostimulation, tamoxifen and 2-bromo-α-
ergocryptine, the inhibition of carcinoma development was no
greater than that occurring with only retinyl acetate and
hormone inhibition. Thus it would appear, at least in
studies so far reported, that immunostimulation does not
enhance the effect of a retinoid in the inhibition of
mammary carcinogenesis.

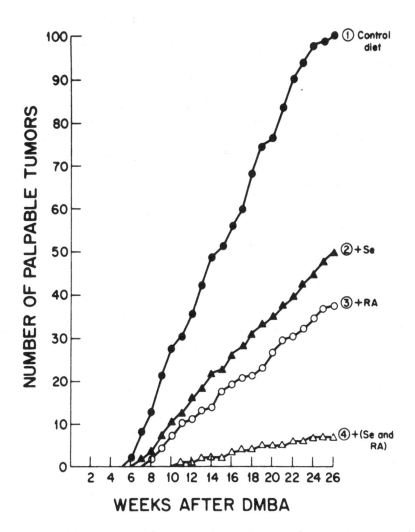

Fig. 7. Effect of Se (selenium) and/or RA (retinyl acetate) supplementation in the diet on the appearance of palpable mammary tumors in rats given a total dose of 15 mg of DMBA. Reprinted from Ref. 11 with permission from Carcinogenesis.

MECHANISM OF CHEMOPREVENTION

The precise mechanism(s) by which retinoids inhibit mammary carcinogenesis is unknown, although some insight into the process has been gained from the effect of retinoids on the mammary gland per se. Both 4-HPR and retinyl acetate exert an antiproliferative effect on the mammary epithelium. This is exemplified by the significant inhibition of ductal branching and end bud proliferation of the glands of rats fed the retinoids chronically in the diet (34). Retinyl acetate has been also shown to inhibit chemical carcinogen-induced increases in mammary gland DNA synthesis (26), and the induction by carcinogens of terminal ductal hyperplasias, a putative precancerous lesion (16). It is interesting to note that the synthetic retinoid, trimethylmethoxyphenyl analog of retinyl methyl ether, which is ineffective in inhibiting carcinogen-induced mammary tumorigenesis, is also ineffective in suppressing mammary DNA synthesis. Furthermore, the addition of 4-HPR or retinoic acid to organ culture of mouse mammary glands (22) inhibits prolactin-induced increases in DNA synthesis, which is reflected in a decreased structural differentiation in such glands. In addition, recent in vivo studies in C$_3$H mice also suggest an antiproliferative effect for 4-HPR in that hyperplastic alveolar nodulogenesis is reduced in animals maintained on a diet supplemented with the retinoid (30). These effects on the mammary gland are probably not mediated via an influence on host hormonal levels, since retinoid administration has little effect upon either circulating prolactin levels (43) or normal ovarian function (31). Moreover, the additive or synergistic effect of the retinoid plus hormonal manipulation in the combination studies cited above would also appear to substantiate this view.

It has been suggested by Bashor et al (1) that the action of retinoids on the cell may be mediated in a manner similar to that of the steroid hormones, in which there is association with a specific cytosolic receptor protein, translocation of steroid-receptor complex to the nucleus, interaction with chromatin, and alteration of the cellular response. Since the report of Bashor et al, several investigators have found both retinol and retinoic acid binding proteins in many normal and neoplastic tissues (3).

Consistent with these studies, Mehta and Moon (25) reported the presence of both retinol and retinoic acid binding proteins in mammary tissue during several physiological states as well as in both animal (19) and human breast cancers (23). Unlabeled all-trans-retinoic acid competes effectively for the binding sites; however, certain retinoids such as 4-HPR and retinyl acetate which are effective against mammary carcinogenesis fail to compete for retinoic acid binding sites. These results suggest that 4-HPR requires metabolism to an active component within the mammary cell which then allows it to effectively bind to cytoplasmic retinoic acid binding protein (CRABP). Although a number of metabolites have been identified in extracts of mammary glands of animals receiving dietary supplements of 4-HPR, the active metabolite of 4-HPR is, however, presently unknown (10).

As indicated above, ovarian hormone independent tumors may be more responsive to retinoid treatment than ovarian hormone dependent tumors. Thus, when tumors appearing in intact animals (both ovarian hormone dependent and independent tumors) as well as those arising in ovariectomized rats (ovarian hormone independent tumors) are analyzed for receptor activity, mammary cancers arising in animals which were ovariectomized (hormone-independent) contained significantly greater concentrations of CRABP than did cancers appearing in intact animals (24). Similar results are also obtained when animals bearing palpable tumors were ovariectomized; the tumors which regressed in size (dependent tumors) contained significantly lower levels of CRABP than the ovarian hormone independent tumors which continued to grow. Thus, it appears that in the rat, a correlation exists between the ability of retinoids to suppress mammary carcinogenesis and the level of CRABP in the cytoplasm of mammary cancers (24).

Recent studies of Mehta et al (20) have also indicated that the formation of a retinoic acid-receptor complex in the mammary tumor cytoplasm is essential for the interaction of retinoic acid with the nucleus; retinoic acid per se does not bind to nuclei or to nuclear components. Although these studies do not explain whether the retinoic acid-receptor complex enters the nucleus or simply delivers retinoic acid to the nucleus, they do provide evidence that the formation of cytoplasmic retinoic acid-receptor complex is essential for the interaction of retinoic acid with the nucleus of mammary cancer cells.

At present, it is speculative to suggest that the
interaction of the retinoid (or a metabolite) with the
nucleus results in altered genomic expression. However,
there are numerous reports which indirectly support such
a view. For example, retinoids inhibit tumor promoter-
induced ornithine decarboxylase activity (41), carcinogen-
induced DNA synthesis (26), and growth factor-induced
transformation (40). Recent studies of RNA polymerase
activity of mammary tumor nuclei are also suggestive of
such an effect: nuclei isolated from mammary cancers pre-
incubated with retinoic acid exhibited reduced RNA polymerase activity compared to tissues incubated under similar
conditions without the retinoid. Furthermore, the nuclei
which were preincubated with mammary cytosol containing
retinoic acid-receptor complex also showed reduced RNA
polymerase activity, as compared with that of nuclei incubated with either buffer or with free retinoic acid.
Activity of both RNA polymerase I and II was reduced as a
result of retinoid treatment (21). These results indicate
that retinoids may be active at the chromatin level, and
that retinoic acid-retinoic acid receptor complexing may
be an important step in the mediation of retinoid action in
the mammary tumor cell.

ACKNOWLEDGMENTS

We greatly appreciate the expert assistance of
Patricia Moser in the preparation of this manuscript.

REFERENCES

1. Bashor, M.M., Toft, D.O., and Chytil, F. In vitro
    binding of retinol to rat tissue components. Proc.
    Natl. Acad. Sci.,70: 3483-3487, 1973.
2. Becci, P.J., Thompson, H.J., Grubbs, C.J., Brown, C.C.,
    and Moon, R.C. Effect of delay in administration of
    13-*cis*-retinoic acid on the inhibition of urinary
    bladder carcinogenesis in the rat. Cancer Res., 39:
    3141-3144, 1979.
3. Chytil, F., and Ong, D.E. Cellular retinoid-binding
    proteins. *In*: Sporn, M.B., Roberts, A.B., and Goodman,

D.S. (eds.), The Retinoids, Vol. 2, Academic Press, Orlando, pp. 97-110.

4. Cohen, S.M., Wittenberg, J.F., and Bryan, G.T. Effect of avitaminosis A and hypervitaminosis A on urinary bladder carcinogenecity of N-[4-(5-nitro-2-furyl)-2-thiazolyl]formamide. Cancer Res., 36: 2334-2339, 1976.

5. Fujimaki, Y. Formation of carcinoma in albino rats fed on deficient diets. J. Cancer Res., 10: 469-477, 1926.

6. Grubbs, C.J., Moon, R.C., Squire, R.A., Farrow, G.M., Stinson, S.F., Goodman, D.G., Brown, C.B., and Sporn, M.B. 13-*cis*-Retinoic acid: Inhibition of bladder carcinogenesis induced in rats by N-butyl-N-(4-hydroxybutyl)nitrosamine. Science, 198: 743-744, 1977.

7. Gullino, P.M., Pettigrew, H.M., and Grantham, F.H. N-nitrosomethylurea as mammary gland carcinogen in rats. J. Natl. Cancer Inst., 54: 401-414, 1975.

8. Harisiadis, L., Miller, R.C., Hall, E.J., and Borek, C. A vitamin A analogue inhibits radiation-induced oncogenic transformation. Nature, 274: 486-487, 1978.

9. Harris, C.C., Sporn, M.B., Kaufman, D.G., Smith, J.M., Jackson, F.E., and Saffiotti, U. Histogenesis of squamous metaplasis in the hamster tracheal epithelium caused by vitamin A deficiency or benzo(α)pyrene-ferric oxide. J. Natl. Cancer Inst., 48: 743-761, 1972.

10. Hultin, T.A., and Moon, R.C. Metabolism of N-(4-hydroxyphenyl)retinamide in female rats and mice. Fed. Proc., 44: 1338, 1985.

11. Ip, C., and Ip, M.M. Chemoprevention of mammary tumorigenesis by a combined regimen of selenium and vitamin A. Carcinogenesis, 2: 915-918, 1981.

12. Lasnitzki, I., and Goodman, D.S. Inhibition of the effects of methylcholanthrene on mouse prostate in organ culture by vitamin A and its analogs. Cancer Res., 34: 1564-1571, 1974.

13. Maiorana, A., and Gullino, P. Effect of retinyl acetate on the incidence of mammary carcinomas and hepatomas in mice. J. Natl. Cancer Inst., 64: 655-663, 1980.

14. McCormick, D.L., Adamowski, C.B., Fiks, A., and Moon, R.C. Lifetime dose-response relationships for mammary tumor induction by a single administration of N-methyl-N-nitrosourea. Cancer Res., 41: 1690-1694, 1981.

15. McCormick, D.L., Becci, P.J., and Moon, R.C. Inhi-
     bition of mammary and urinary bladder carcinogenesis
     by a retinoid and a maleic anhydride-divinyl ether co-
     polymer (MVE-2). Carcinogenesis, 3: 1473-1477, 1982.
16. McCormick, D.L., Burns, F.J., and Albert, R.E. In-
     hibition of benzo(α)pyrene-induced mammary carcino-
     genesis by retinyl acetate. J. Natl. Cancer Inst.,
     66: 559-564, 1981.
17. McCormick, D.L., Mehta, R.G., Thompson, C.A., Dinger,
     N., Caldwell, J.A., and Moon, R.C. Enhanced inhibi-
     tion of mammary carcinogenesis by combination N-(4-
     hydroxyphenyl)retinamide and ovariectomy. Cancer Res.,
     42: 509-512, 1982.
18. McCormick, D.L., and Moon, R.C. Influence of delayed
     administration of retinyl acetate on mammary carcino-
     genesis. Cancer Res., 42: 2639-2643, 1982.
19. Mehta, R.G., Cerny, W.L., and Moon, R.C. Distribution
     of retinoic acid-binding protein in normal and neo-
     plastic mammary tissues. Cancer Res., 40: 47-49, 1980.
20. Mehta, R.G., Cerny, W.L., and Moon, R.C. Nuclear
     interaction of retinoic acid binding protein in chemi-
     cally induced mammary adenocarcinomas. Biochem. J.,
     208: 731-736, 1982.
21. Mehta, R.G., Cerny, W.L., and Moon, R.C. Alteration
     in DNA-dependent RNA polymerase activity by retinoids.
     Proc. Am. Ass. Cancer Res., 23: 21, 1982.
22. Mehta, R.G., Cerny, W.L., and Moon, R.C. Retinoid
     inhibition of prolactin-induced development of the
     mammary gland *in vitro*. Carcinogenesis (Lond.), 4:
     23-26, 1983.
23. Mehta, G.R., Kute, T.E., Hopkins, M., and Moon, R.C.
     Retinoic acid-binding proteins and steroid receptor
     levels in human breast cancer. Eur. J. Cancer Clin.
     Oncol., 18: 221-226, 1982.
24. Mehta, R.G., McCormick, D.L., Cerny, W.L., and Moon,
     R.C. Correlation between retinoid inhibition of N-
     methyl-N-nitrosourea-induced mammary carcinogenesis
     and levels of retinoic acid-binding proteins.
     Carcinogenesis, 3: 89-91, 1982.
25. Mehta, R.G., and Moon, R.C. Hormonal regulation of
     retinoic acid-binding proteins in the mammary gland.
     Biochem. J., 200: 591-595, 1981.
26. Mehta, R.G., and Moon, R.C. Inhibition of DNA synthe-
     sis by retinyl acetate during chemically-induced mam-
     mary carcinogenesis. Cancer Res., 40: 1109-1111, 1981.

27. Merriman, R.L., and Bertram, J.S. Reversible inhibition by retinoids of 3-methyl-cholanthrene-induced neoplastic transformation in C3H/10T1/2 CL8 cells. Cancer Res., 39: 1661-1666, 1979.
28. Moon, R.C. Influence of pregnancy and lactation on experimental mammary carcinogenesis. *In*: Pike, M.C., Siiteri, P.K., and Welsch, C.W. (eds.), Hormones and Breast Cancer, Banbury Report 8, Cold Spring Harbor Laboratory, 1981.
29. Moon, R.C., and Mehta, R.G. Retinoid binding in normal and neoplastic mammary tissue. *In*: W.W. Leavit (ed.), Hormones and Cancer, pp. 231-249. New York: Plenum Publishing Corp., 1982.
30. Moon, R.C., McCormick, D.L., and Mehta, R.G. Inhibition of carcinogenesis by retinoids. Cancer Res., 43, 2469s-2475s, 1983.
31. Moon, R.C., Grubbs, C.J., and Sporn, M.B. Inhibition of 7,12-dimethyl-benz(α)anthracene-induced mammary carcinogenesis by retinyl acetate. Cancer Res., 36: 2626-2630, 1976.
32. Moon, R.C., Grubbs, C.J., Sporn, M.B., and Goodman, D.G. Retinyl acetate inhibits mammary carcinogenesis induced by N-methyl-N-nitrosourea. Nature, 267: 620-621, 1977.
33. Moon, R.C., Mehta, R.G., and McCormick, D.L. Modulation of mammary carcinogenesis by retinoids. *In*: K.N. Prasad (ed.), Vitamins, Nutrition and Cancer, pp. 20-32, Basel, Karger, 1984.
34. Moon, R.C., Thompson, H.J., Becci, P.J., Grubbs, C.J., Gander, R.J., Newton, D.L., Smith, J.M., Phillips, S.R., Henderson, W.R., Mullen, L.T., Brown, C.C., and Sporn, M.B. N-(4-hydroxyphenyl)retinamide, a new retinoid for prevention of breast cancer in the rat. Cancer Res., 39: 1339-1346, 1979.
35. Mori, S. The changes in the para-ocular glands which follow the administration of diets low in fat-soluable A; with notes of the effects of the same diets on the salivary glands and the mucosa of the larynx and trachea. Johns Hopkins Hosp. Bull., 33, 357-359, 1922.
36. Smith, F.R., and Goodman, D.S. Vitamin A transport and human vitamin A toxicity. New Engl. J. Med., 294: 805-808, 1976.
37. Sporn, M.B., Dunlop, N.M., Newton, D.L., and Smith, J.M. Prevention of chemical carcinogenesis by vitamin A and its synthetic analogs (retinoids). Fed. Proc., 35: 1332-1338, 1976.

38. Sporn, M.B., Squire, R.A., Brown, C.C., Smith, J.M., Wenk, M.L., and Springer, S. 13-*cis*-Retinoic acid: Inhibition of bladder carcinogenesis in the rat. Science, 195: 487-489, 1977.

39. Thompson, H.J., Meeker, L.D., and Becci, P.J. Effect of combined selenium and retinyl acetate treatment on mammary carcinogenesis. Cancer Res., 41: 1413-1416, 1981.

40. Todaro, G.J., DeLarco, J.E., and Sporn, M.B. Retinoids block phenotypic cell transformation produced by sarcoma growth factor. Nature, 276: 272, 1978.

41. Verma, A.K., and Boutwell, R.K. Vitamin A acid (retinoic acid), a potent inhibitor of 12-0-tetradecanoyl-phorbol-13-acetate-induced ornithine decarboxylase activity in mouse epidermis. Cancer Res., 37: 2196-2201, 1977.

42. Verma, A.K., Shapas, B.G., Rice, H.M., and Boutwell, R.K. Correlation of the inhibition by retinoids of tumor promoter-induced mouse epidermal ornithine decarboxylase activity and of skin tumor promotion. Cancer Res., 39: 419-425, 1979.

43. Welsch, C.W., Brown, C.K., Goodrich-Smith, M., Chuisano, J., and Moon, R.C. Synergistic effect of chronic prolactin suppression and retinoid treatment in the prophylaxis of N-methyl-N-nitrosourea-induced mammary tumorigenesis in female Sprague-Dawley rats. Cancer Res., 40: 3095-3098, 1980.

44. Welsch, C.W., and DeHoog, J.V. Retinoid feeding, hormone inhibition and/or immune stimulation and the genesis of carcinogen-induced rat mammary carcinomas. Cancer Res., 43: 585-591, 1983.

45. Welsch, C.W., Goodrich-Smith, M., Brown, C.K., and Crowe, N. Enhancement by retinyl acetate of hormone-induced mammary tumorigenesis in female GR/A mice. J. Natl. Cancer Inst., 67: 935-938, 1981.

46. Welsch, C.W., Goodrich-Smith, M., Brown, C.K., Mackie, D., and Johnson, D. 2-Bromo-α-ergocryptine (CB 154 and tamoxifen CICl 46474) induced suppression of the genesis of mammary carcinoma in female rats treated with 7-12-dimethylbenz(α)anthracene (DMBA): a comparison. Oncology, 39: 88-92, 1982.

47. Wolbach, S.D., and Howe, P.R. Tissue changes following deprivation of fat-soluble A vitamin. J. Exp. Med., 42: 753-777, 1925.

DIETARY CHOLESTEROL AND COLON TUMORIGENESIS INDUCED BY 1,2,DIMETHYLHYDRAZINE OR N-METHYL-N-NITROSOUREA IN RATS

Selwyn A. Broitman, Herbert Z. Kupchik and Leonard S. Gottlieb
Departments of Pathology and Microbiology, Boston University School of Medicine, 80 East Concord Street, Boston, MA 02118

INTRODUCTION

The relationship of dietary cholesterol to bowel tumorigenesis is controversial. Lui and associates (1) used food disappearance data and age specific mortality rates for colon cancer in a descriptive epidemiologic study. By cross classification of data they observed that dietary cholesterol independently exhibited a significant direct effect with colon cancer mortality but fat and fiber did not. In a case control study of colo-rectal cancer by Jain, et al (2) multivariate analysis, with major nutrients controlled, revealed a dose responsive direct relationship for each sex between dietary cholesterol intake and colorectal cancer.

In experimental studies, Cruse (3) suggested that dietary cholesterol was co-carcinogenic when fed to female Wistar rats given the colon carcinogen 1,2 dimethylhydrazine (DMH). They observed that rats fed Vivonex (a commercial human food supplement) with 0.1% added cholesterol and given DMH, exhibited a greater incidence and numbers of bowel tumors and higher frequency of metastases than rats fed Vivonex alone. While the validity of such a dietary regimen in experimental animals is subject to question, these studies raised

concern on the relationship of dietary cholesterol to bowel tumorigenesis.

Hiramatsu and colleagues (4) fed a 1% cholesterol
supplemented low fat commercial analyzed chow
diet to male Donryu rats injected with azoxymethane. Cholesterol supplementation resulted in
increased numbers of tumors and distant metastases compared to controls. Klurfeld, et al (5)
using DMH for bowel tumor induction, noted that
the addition of dietary cholesterol to a semi-
synthetic diet was associated with a significantly higher percentage of invasive tumors.

Effects of alterations of serum cholesterol levels on DMH induced bowel tumors was studied in
rats (6). Rats were fed atherogenic isocaloric
cholesterol containing diets with either 20%
coconut oil to promote hypercholesterolemia and
vascular lipidosis or 20% safflower oil to maintain lower serum cholesterol levels and, presumably shunt cholesterol through the bowel. Rats
fed the polyunsaturated fat diet had lower serum
cholesterol levels and experienced less vascular
lipidosis but developed more bowel tumors than
those fed the saturated fat diet. The possibility
that polyunsaturated fat contributed to large
bowel tumorigenesis in a greater extent than the
saturated fat could not be discounted.

The current studies were undertaken to evaluate
the role of dietary cholesterol in large bowel
tumorigenesis induced by a direct or indirect
dietary carcinogen. Diets high in fat (20%) were
utilized to ascertain if the effects of dietary
cholesterol on bowel tumorigenesis could be demonstrated in a system in which the promotional
effects of dietary fat were near a practical
maximum. Semi-synthetic diets containing either a
polyunsaturated or a saturated fat (with attention to essential fatty acid requirement) were
chosen. These were evaluated to ascertain if
either were more effective alone or in combination with cholesterol on bowel tumorigenesis. In
a second series of studies, dietary cholesterol
was fed during the initiation or promotion stage

of bowel tumorigenesis to determine the stage in which dietary cholesterol exerted an effect.

MATERIALS AND METHODS

Two model systems were utilized to evaluate the effects of dietary cholesterol on large bowel tumorigenesis in which an indirect carcinogen 1,2 dimethylhydrazine (DMH) or a direct acting carcinogen N-methyl-N-nitrosourea (MNU) was used. With the latter, studies were directed at determining if the effects of cholesterol on bowel tumorigenesis could be discerned during the initiation or promotion phase of two step carcinogenesis.

Sprague Dawley CD weanling rats (Charles River Breeding Labs) were randomized into groups and each group fed a modified AIN-76 (7) diet as follows: Group 1 – a basal diet containing 20% safflower oil, Group 2 – a basal diet containing 18.86 g safflower oil (hydrogenated) and 1.14 g safflower oil (to supply 1.75% of calories as essential fatty acids), Group 3 – the safflower oil basal diet with 1.0% cholesterol, Group 4 – the coconut oil basal diet with 1.0% cholesterol, Group 5 – the coconut oil basal diet with 0.3% cholic acid and Group 6 – the coconut oil basal diet with 1.0% cholesterol and 0.3% cholic acid. Each group initially contained 12 rats except Group 1, which had 21 and which were also utilized for another study run simultaneously. After one week on diet, each rat was given 10 mg/kg of DMH injected intramuscularly once each week for 20 weeks.

In the second series, 3 groups of 15 rats each were fed according to the following schedule: Group B were fed the basal coconut oil diet for 40 weeks. Group BC were fed the basal coconut diet for the first 10 weeks (during which time MNU was given). After the last dose of MNU, the diet was switched to the basal coconut oil diet with 1% cholesterol. Group C were fed the basal coconut oil diet with 1% cholesterol for 40 weeks. MNU, kept frozen and prepared immediately prior to use, was dissolved in saline (5 mg/ml). 0.2 ml was given intrarectally twice weekly for 8 weeks - from week 2 through 10.

Control rats, 6 in each dietary group, were given saline intramuscularly for the first study and intrarectally for the second.

Rats were housed in individual cages at 70° ± 1° F and weighed twice weekly. Diets were prepared fresh each week and stored frozen in evacuated bags until utilized. As diet cups were filled on alternate days, they were weighed to estimate food consumption. At the termination of each study, animals were killed, and autopsied. Tumors in the bowel were counted and lesions at distal sites evaluated. All lesions in the gross were verified by routine histologic techniques.

RESULTS

The first series of studies were undertaken to determine if the addition of cholesterol to a diet high in saturated or polyunsaturated fat influenced large bowel tumorigenesis. Tumor incidence in DMH treated animals (Group 1 to 4) is illustrated in Figure 1. Addition of cholesterol to either the safflower oil or coconut oil diet significantly increased the incidence of small bowel tumors ($p < 0.001$)* but had no significant effect on large bowel or total tumor incidence. Average number of tumors, however, as depicted in Figure 2, was significantly increased by the addition of cholesterol to either fat diet in the small bowel ($p < 0.001$)*; the large bowel ($p < 0.001$)*; and for the total number of bowel tumors ($p < 0.001$)*. Safflower oil in combination with cholesterol was more effective than coconut oil and cholesterol in augmenting the numbers of small bowel tumors but there were no differences in the average numbers of large bowel and total tumors between the two dietary fats alone or in combination with cholesterol.

*Wilson distribution free ANOVA

FIGURE 1

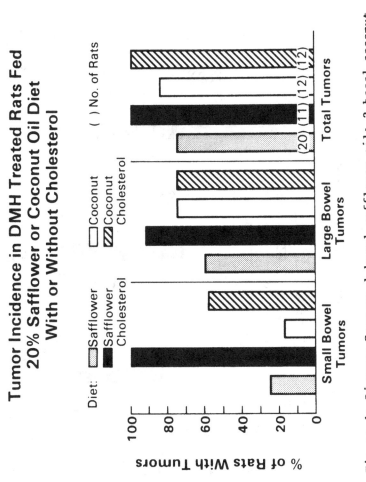

Figure 1: Dietary Groups: 1 basal safflower oil; 2 basal coconut oil; 3 basal safflower oil + 1% cholesterol; and 4 basal coconut oil + 1% cholesterol.

FIGURE 2

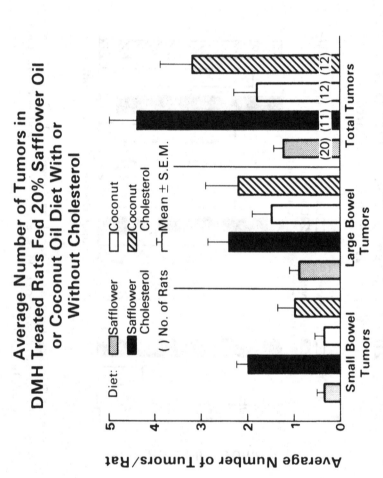

Figure 2: Dietary Groups: 1 basal safflower oil; 2 basal coconut oil; 3 basal safflower oil + 1% cholesterol; and 4 basal coconut oil + 1% cholesterol.

To ascertain if bile acids played a contributing role in augmenting bowel tumorigenesis when cholesterol was added to diets high in fat, cholic acid was incorporated. Tumor incidence induced by DMH in these animals is shown in Figure 3. Feeding of cholesterol, cholic acid or both in a basal coconut oil diet moderately increased the incidence of small bowel tumors compared to rats fed the basal coconut oil diet alone. No significant differences were noted in the incidence of large bowel or total tumors.

The average number of small, large bowel and total tumors (Figure 4) was uneffected by the addition of cholic acid to the diet compared to rats fed the basal coconut oil diet. Dietary cholic acid and cholesterol together were no more effective in augmenting bowel tumorigenesis than cholesterol alone.

It was observed that the growth rates of rats fed safflower oil or coconut oil with or without cholesterol were not significantly different. However, addition of cholic acid to the coconut oil basal diet retarded weight gain in this group; it became apparent at the 16th week of the study and continued throughout the duration of the study (Figure 5). Since DMH was administered on a weight basis, it was of interest to determine how weight variations could effect the total amount of carcinogen given and if this was a factor in the results observed.

Figure 6 depicts the total quantities of DMH administered to rats fed the various diets. Rats fed the basal coconut oil diet with cholesterol received about 13% less DMH ($p < 0.01$)* than those fed the basal diet, and those fed the basal with cholic acid received 23% less ($p < 0.01$)*. Rats fed the basal diet with cholesterol and cholic acid received the same quantity of DMH as those fed the basal coconut diet with cholesterol. It is possible that the failure to see an increase in average numbers or bowel tumors with cholic acid

*Analysis of variance

FIGURE 3

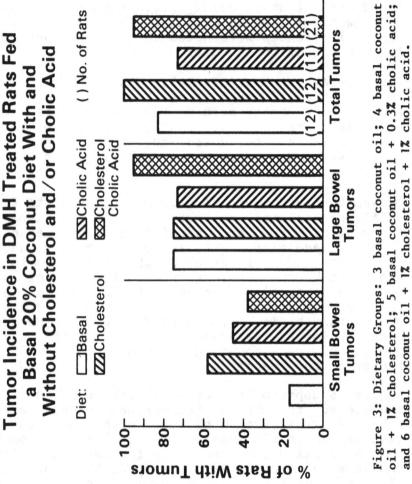

Figure 3: Dietary Groups: 3 basal coconut oil; 4 basal coconut oil + 1% cholesterol; 5 basal coconut oil + 0.3% cholic acid; and 6 basal coconut oil + 1% cholesterol + 1% cholic acid.

FIGURE 4

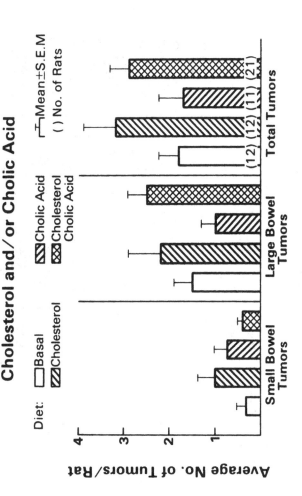

Figure 4: Dietary Groups: 3 basal coconut oil; 4 basal coconut oil + 1% cholesterol; 5 basal coconut oil + 0.3% cholic acid; and 6 basal coconut oil + 1% cholesterol + 1% cholic acid.

FIGURE 5

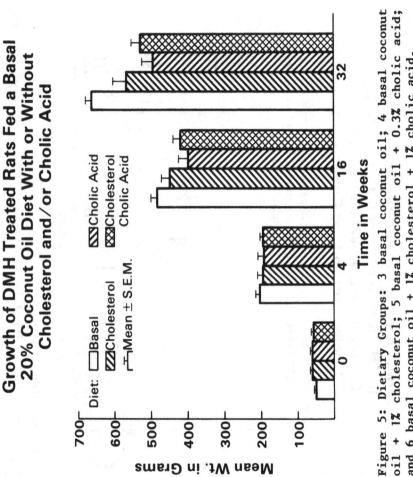

Figure 5: Dietary Groups: 3 basal coconut oil; 4 basal coconut oil + 1% cholesterol; 5 basal coconut oil + 0.3% cholic acid; and 6 basal coconut oil + 1% cholesterol + 1% cholic acid.

FIGURE 6

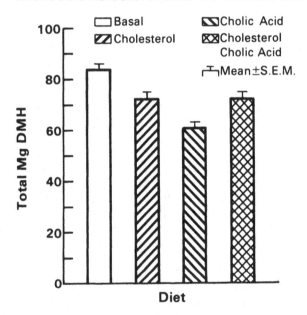

**Mean Cummulative Quantities of DMH
Administered To Groups of Rats Fed a
20% Basal Coconut Oil Diet With and
Without Cholesterol and/or Cholic Acid**

Figure 6: Dietary Groups: 3 basal coconut oil; 4 basal coconut oil + 1% cholesterol; 5 basal coconut oil + 0.3% cholic acid; and 6 basal coconut oil + 1% cholesterol + 1% cholic acid.

feeding could result from the reduced total
quantity of carcinogen administered to this group
compared to controls. However, rats fed cholesterol also received less total carcinogen, but
exhibited an increased average number of tumors
compared to controls.

No tumors were detected in any animals given
saline in lieu of DMH. Growth rates of these
animals were comparable to experimental animals
in each respective dietary group.

In the second series of studies (Table 1) rats
were fed the basal coconut diet, dietary group B,
or the basal coconut diet with 1% cholesterol,
group C, throughout the 40 weeks of the study. In
dietary group BC, rats were fed the basal coconut
diet throughout the administration of MNU and
following the last dose switched to the basal
coconut diet with cholesterol. Premature deaths
accounted for 1 rat in group BC and two in group
C and were not included in the calculations.
Weight gains and food consumption were similar in
all groups. The incidence of large bowel tumors
was slightly but not significantly greater in
group BC and C. However, the average numbers of
large bowel tumors was slightly increased in
group BC (p<0.01). The greatest difference was a
97% (p<0.01) increase in the number of large
bowel tumors in rats fed the cholesterol containing diet (group C) over those fed the basal diet
(group B). The studies indicate that the enhancing effects of dietary cholesterol on the multiplicity of tumors occurs primarily during the
initiation phase of two step carcinogenesis with
a very slight effect during the promotion phase.

No bowel lesions were detected in animals given
intrarectal saline in lieu of MNU.

DISCUSSION

These studies indicate that dietary cholesterol
plays a role in experimental bowel tumorigenesis
using either an indirect (DMH) or direct acting
carcinogen (MNU). Dietary fat levels of 20% are

TABLE 1

EFFECT OF DIETARY CHOLESTEROL ON LARGE BOWEL TUMORIGENESIS
INDUCED BY MULTIPLE INTRARECTAL ADMINISTRATIONS OF MNU

DIETARY GROUP	NO OF RATS	LARGE BOWEL TUMORS INCIDENCE[1]	AVERAGE NO. OF TUMORS[2]
B	15	86.7%	1.87 ± 0.32[3]
BC	14	78.6%	2.07 ± 0.46
C	13	100.0%	3.69 ± 0.36

[1] By Fisher's Exact:
  B vs. BC N.S.
  B vs. C N.S.
  BC vs. C N.S.

[2] By ANOVA, Newman-Keuls
  groups differ
  B vs BC $p < 0.01$
  B vs C $p < 0.01$
  BC vs C $p < 0.01$

[3] Mean $\pm$ SEM

known to enhance carcinogen induced bowel tumorigenesis in the rat over that seen with low dietary fat levels (8). In these studies, cholesterol
was added to a 20% fat diet to ascertain if
augmentation of bowel tumorigenesis occurred in
a model system in which the promotional effects
of dietary fat were at a practical maximum. The
finding of enhanced tumorigenesis by cholesterol
under these conditions implies that the effects
of dietary cholesterol of tumorigenesis are at
least additive to the effects of dietary fats.
Whether synergistic effects occur between these
dietary nutrients in bowel tumorigenesis, or
whether these act in similar or different fashion
in carcinogenesis is not fully established. These
results are consistent with previous experimental
reports (3-5). They differ from a study in which
0.2% cholesterol added to commercial laboratory
chow (cholesterol and plant sterol content unknown) resulted in decreased tumorigenesis compared to controls (9). A comparison of these
findings with the current study in which a semi-
synthetic diet was utilized may be misleading.

It has been suggested that polyunsaturated fats
may augment experimental bowel tumorigenesis to a
greater degree than saturated fats (10) in a manner initially reported for breast tumorigenesis
(11). However, it is now appreciated that the
addition of essential fatty acids to diets high
in saturated fat results in essentially the same
yields of breast tumors as a diet high in polyunsaturated fat (12). An analogous finding is
reported here in which a high saturated fat diet
with essential fatty acids provided the same
incidence and yield of bowel tumors as a high
polyunsaturated fat diet. This supports an earlier report by Reddy, et al (8).

The participation of dietary bile acids in the
enhancing effects of cholesterol on tumorigenesis
could not be demonstrated in these studies. Cholic acid feeding did not increase the yield and
incidence of bowel tumors as reported previously
in studies utilizing chow diets (13).

Two possibilities are apparent. The first is that feeding bile acids under the conditions of these experiments simply has no effects on bowel tumorigenesis. Or second, the impaired weight gain in bile acid fed animals associated with significantly less DMH administered does not permit a valid comparison with those not fed cholic acid.

In the second series of studies, when MNU was administered to rats fed a high saturated fat diet with cholesterol, a greater tumor yield was noted compared to rats fed the basal saturated fat diet only. Thus the enhancing effects of dietary cholesterol on bowel tumorigenesis was essentially the same whether a direct or indirect acting carcinogen was used. This finding minimizes, but does not exclude, the possibility that high fat diets with cholesterol could conceivably enhance the hepatic activation of DMH (1st series of studies) resulting in increased active carcinogen delivered to the bowel in cholesterol fed animals. When dietary cholesterol was fed after the last administered dose of MNU (during the promotion phase), a minimal effect of cholesterol on tumor yield was seen compared to rats not fed cholesterol. However, increased tumor yields resulted when cholesterol was fed during both the initiation and promotion phases of carcinogenesis. These findings imply that the effects of cholesterol of bowel tumorigenesis are manifest during the initiation phase or very early promotion phase . In rats fed cholesterol throughout the experiment, MNU was administered in multiple doses during a period of 8 weeks. Thus the possibility cannot be discounted that cholesterol could have acted in the early promotion phase after the first few doses of MNU. This problem has been resolved in ongoing studies in which a single dose of MNU has been utilized for tumor induction.

Nevertheless, the findings that cholesterol exerts its effects during initiation or possibly early promotion phase of bowel tumorigenesis is clearly different from the purported promotional effects of bile acids (14). Furthermore, these

effects appear to differ also from the promotional effects of high levels of dietary fat, and is
likely to account for the suggestion that the
effects of dietary cholesterol in enhancing bowel
tumorigenesis are at least additive to those of
high levels of dietary fat.

The mode of action of dietary cholesterol in
bowel tumorigenesis is speculative at this time
but could involve a) enhanced diffusion of carcinogen across mucosal cells; b) increased formation or persistence of DNA-adducts; c) diminished
capacity of DNA repair; d) participation as a
tumor growth factor; or e) enhanced proliferation
rate of bowel mucosa mediated by increased fecal
excretion of bile acids modulated by alterations
in enzymatic activity of the bowel microflora.

SUMMARY

Addition of 1% dietary cholesterol to a 20% safflower or coconut oil diet increased the tumor
yield of DMH induced bowel tumors in rats. No
differences in bowel tumor yield or incidence was
detected between animals fed a polyunsaturated
fat or saturated fat diet. Bowel tumorigenesis
was enhanced by dietary cholesterol with both an
indirect (DMH) or direct (MNU) acting carcinogen.
Using MNU for bowel tumor induction, dietary cholesterol was found to act during the initiation
or early promotion phase in two stage carcinogenesis. This action of cholesterol appears to be
different from promotional effects of bile acids
or dietary fat. Thus the effects of dietary cholesterol appear to be at least additive to the
effects of high levels of dietary fat in bowel
carcinogenesis in these models.

REFERENCES

1. Liu K, Moss D, Persky V, et al: Dietary chol-
    esterol, fat, and fibre, and colon-cancer
    mortality. An analysis of international data.
    Lancet 2:782-785, 1979.

(α) anthracene. Lipids 6:415-420, 1971.
12. Carroll KK, Hopkins GH: Dietary polyunsaturated fat versus saturated fat in relation to mammary carcinogenesis. Lipids 14:155-158, 1979.
13. Cohen BI, Raicht RF, Deschner EG, et al: Effect of cholic acid feeding on N-methyl-N-nitrosourea induced colon tumors and cell kinetics in rats. J Natl Cancer Inst 64:573-578, 1980.
14. Narisawa T, Magadia NE, Weisburger JH, et al: Promoting effect of bile acids on colon carcinogenesis after intrarectal instillation of N-methyl-N'-nitrosoguandine in rats. J Natl Cancer Inst 53: 1093-1097, 1974.

ACKNOWLEDGEMENTS

The authors would like to acknowledge the excellent technical assistance of Mr. Paul L. Colon and Ms. Maureen Kelly.

This work was supported in part by grants CA 16750 from the National Large Bowel Cancer Project and T32-CA 09423, National Cancer Institute, National Institutes of Health.

EFFECTS OF VITAMIN E ON THE IMMUNE SYSTEM

Mary P. Carpenter

Biomembrane Research Program
Oklahoma Medical Research Foundation
and
Department of Biochemistry and Molecular Biology
University of Oklahoma Health Sciences Center
Oklahoma City, Oklahoma

Vitamin E, tocopherol, a methylated derivative of 6-hydroxychromonal with a phytyl side chain, is an essential nutrient. In cells, this hydrophobic molecule is intercalated into the membrane bilayer. Studies with structural models (1) and of vitamin E in phospholipid monolayers (2) indicate that it is associated primarily with arachidonic acid. As a membrane component, vitamin E has the potential to affect the functional biology of cells of the immune system.

The regulation of immune function is very complex and involves membrane-mediated interactions between cells and humoral factors. Cellular components of the immune system include: 1) phagocytes--monocytes, macrophages and neutrophils and, 2) lymphocytes--T-lymphocytes which do not produce circulating antibody, but affect the responses of the B lymphocytes which do produce antibody. Cooperativity between these cells is required to produce a response. Phagocytic cells are required for lymphocytes to proliferate and make antibody. The macrophage is a critical regulatory cell which concentrates, processes and presents antigen to lymphocytes. Macrophages ingest, phagocytize and process microbial antigen, which is then displayed on the cell surface. Helper T-lymphocytes recognize the antigen and bind to the macrophage. This activates the

T-lymphocyte and elicits a number of responses, including
proliferation of a clone of that particular lymphocyte. B-
lymphocytes also recognize the antigen and bind to the same
macrophage. The B-lymphocyte is not activated until it
receives a signal from the activated T-lymphocyte. Activated B-lymphocytes then proliferate to expand their clone
and differentiate into antibody-producing cells, plasma-
cytes. The activated T-lymphocyte also causes the activation of cytotoic lymphocytes to killer lymphocytes and
stimulates suppressor lymphocytes. Secretory products
mediated by these cell-cell interactions include enzymes,
kinins, activated oxygen species and oxygenated metabolites
of arachidonic acid-prostaglandins, thromboxane, leukotrienes and other lipoxygenase products. As membrane-bound
antioxidant, vitamin E has the potential to regulate immune
cell function by affecting the physical/chemical properties
of membranes, serving as a chain-breaking free radical
scavenger, and/or some other yet unknown effect.

VITAMIN E EFFECTS ON THE IMMUNE SYSTEM

       Available evidence indicates that vitamin E affects
both humoral and cell-mediated immune response. There is
heterogeneity in these studies reflecting the use of
different animal species and strains as well as gender.
Moreover, there has been considerable variation in the
nutritional design of the work. Some studies have included
in vitro addition of vitamin E to preparations of immune
cells. When used as a dietary supplement, vitamin E has
been added to commercial, stock diets containing adequate
vitamin E. Other studies have utilized semipurified diets
with and without vitamin E. The amount and type of dietary
lipid in the diets has also varied. Consideration of the
experimental design is important in the interpretation and
comparison of the results of work on the effect of vitamin
E on immune function. In a number of the studies, immune
function has been evaluated using polyclonal mitogens--
conconavalin A (con A), phytohemmagglutinin (PHA), which
induce proliferation of T-lymphocytes, or bacterial lipo-
polysaccharides (LPS), which stimulates the proliferation
of B-cells.

Both humoral and cellular immune response appears to be enhanced in chicks fed excess vitamin E (3). Chicks fed a commercial, stock diet containing 43 mg of vitamin E/kg diet, supplemented with 150-300 mg/kg of α-tocopherol acetate showed increased survival against the lethal effects of E coli infection (4), increase in hemaggluntinating antibody (5), and clearance of E coli from blood. In chicks immunized against sheep red blood cells, plaque-forming cells were 4-fold increased. To evaluate whether these effects of vitamin E reflected modulation of prostaglandin synthesis, aspirin, which inhibits prostaglandin synthase at the cyclooxygenase step, was incorporated into the diet (6). Although there was improved survival to E coli infection when both excess vitamin E and aspirin were fed, concurrent radioimmunoassay analyses of several prostaglandins produced by spleen and bursa homogenates gave equivocal results, which did not correlate with the results on survival.

Results of studies from several different laboratories using both different mouse strains and protocols also suggest a correlation between enhanced function and excess vitamin E. Culture of normal spleen cells with vitamin E in vitro for 5 days resulted in a small increase in plaque-forming cells (7). Although the number of plaque-forming cells was lower, a more pronounced effect of vitamin E was observed when adherent cells were removed. The same laboratory also assessed vitamin E as well as the addition of the antioxidant, DPPD, to chow diets in CF-1 mice challenged with either sheep red blood cells (SRBC) or tetanus toxoid (8). Increased plaque-forming cells were found with either challenge, but the response was stronger with SRBC suggesting a selective affect of vitamin E on IgG-producing cells. DPPD was ineffective, suggesting the effect of vitamin E is not that of a simple antioxidant effect. The effect of feeding a stock diet containing adequate vitamin E supplemented with additional tocopherol (as either the nicotinamide or acetate) has been tested on helper T-cell function in two inbred strains of female mice (9). Excess vitamin E resulted in an increase in haemagglutin titers to hamster red blood cells and an increased carrier effect on antibody immunization. The vitamin E enhanced humoral immunity was postulated to reflect stimulation by vitamin E of cooperation between T- and B-cells in antibody production, perhaps by a specific effect on helper T-cells and/or by stimulating cell proliferation.

Both dietary and in vitro additions of vitamin E have been evaluated on the immune response of male CBA/J mice. Addition of α-tocopherol to mixed spleen preparations of chow-fed mice stimulated mitogenesis (10). Similar effects were observed when 2-mercaptoethanol was added. Both vitamin E and 2-mercaptoethanol stimulated spleen cell response to low concentrations of con A (0.125 μg/0.2 ml), but had no effect at higher doses of mitogen. Further studies with the same mouse strain fed a semipurified diet containing 4% lard and either 5 or 50 mg/kg of α-tocopherol acetate, confirmed the vitamin E effect using low doses of con A, and also demonstrated stimulation of cell proliferation with PHA and LPS at the higher level of dietary vitamin E (10). The effects of feeding the mice semipurified diets containing unsaturated fat (8% corn oil) or saturated fat (8% coconut oil) in the presence and absence of dietary vitamin E (10) suggest that dietary fat may modulate the vitamin E effect. Although con A, PHA and LPS were more effective in spleen preparations from vitamin E-fed mice than those from vitamin E-deficient mice on the corn oil diet, differences in mitogen response were observed only for low doses of con A on the more saturated diet. In vitro of α-tocopherol (1 μM) to spleenocytes of deficient animals gave a response similar to that seen with dietary vitamin E treatment. The effect of vitamin E on stimulation of mitogenic response to low levels of con A appears not to be that of a simple antioxidant effect. Addition of the synthetic antioxidant, DPPD, to mixed spleen cells of mice fed the corn oil diet stimulated the response to suboptimal concentrations of con A and to PHA as well as the B cell mitogen, LPS, suggesting an antioxidant effect (11). A similar study carried out with mice fed the hydrogenated coconut oil diet revealed that DPPD was less effective on the preparations from vitamin E-fed mice than above, but there were good responses to low con A, PHA and LPS in those from vitamin E-deficient animals. BHT, a very good antioxidant, added in vitro, was not effective in any of the dietary groups. Trolox, a synthetic vitamin E which does not have an isoprene side chain, but which is a very effective antioxidant, also did not enhance mitogenesis. Furthermore, tocopherol quinone, which does not function as an antioxidant, was as effective as α-tocopherol. The effects of vitamin E on spleen cell proliferation appear not to be correlated with prostaglandin synthesis, as the addition of indomethacin, an inhibitor of prostaglandin cyclooxygenase activity, had no effect on vitamin E stimulation.

The same group of investigators also performed studies on fractionation of the murine spleen cells to determine which populations were vitamin E responders (12). After removal of Ia^+ cells on plastic and/or removal of spleen cells which were Ia^+ by treatment with Ia^+ antiserum, vitamin E was still effective in stimulating mitogenesis. As the adherent cells are macrophages which are Ia^+ cells, the results were interpreted to indicate that vitamin E stimulates an Ia^- cell population in the absence of macrophages. However, unless the removal of macrophages was quantitative, this conclusion may not be valid as current evidence shows that the presence of only a small number of macrophages is adequate to activate T-cell responses. Subsequent studies revealed that when the spleen cells were washed, the response to low concentrations of con A was stimulated and vitamin E no longer enhanced mitogenesis. The factor in the medium which acts as a suppressor was identified as spermine (13). The results of these studies on the CBA/J mouse strain clearly implicate a role for vitamin E in stimulating T-cell mitogenesis.

Effects of vitamin E dietary on immune function have also been documented in the rat. Examination of spleenocyte mitogenesis in the spontaneously hypertensive (SHR) and normotensive (WKY) rat strains showed that con A, PHA and LPS-induced blastogenesis was depressed in the vitamin E-deficient as compared to vitamin E supplemented animals (14). Similar blastogenic responses to T- and B-cell mitogens of mixed spleen cells were observed for vitamin E-deficient compared to vitamin E-fed guinea pigs (15). In addition to these effects of vitamin E on the proliferation of both T- and B-lymphocytes, vitamin E has also been shown to affect other responses of cells of the immune system. When the phagocytic and oxidative functions of peritoneal polymorpholeukocytes (PMNs) of male Sprague-Dawley rats fed purified diets with and without vitamin E were assessed, no differences reflecting dietary vitamin E were observed on adherence of the cells, lysosomal release of B-glucuronidase, or phagocytosis (16). Recovery of PMNs was 40% less from vitamin E-deficient than vitamin E-fed rats. Chemotaxis of the cells and ingestion of albumin and C_3b or IgG-coated paraffin oil droplets, but not ingestion and killing

of Staph aureus, were impaired in the cells of vitamin E-
deficient, compared to those of supplemented rats. Additionally, both O_2 consumption and H_2O_2 release were elevated in the deficient compared to control cells. Impaired
paraffin oil ingestion was reversed 5 hours after vitamin E
treatment (i.m.) and chemotaxis within 18 hours.

Vitamin E has also been shown to affect phagocyte
function in human subjects. In an infant with a congenital
deficiency of glutathione synthetase activity and abnormal
PMN function, vitamin E treatment corrected the overproduc-
tion of H_2O_2 and decreased ability to iodinate protein and
to kill bacteria (17). In a study with 25 diabetics compared to 25 controls, phagocyte function was found to be
defective. Monocytes from diabetics had depressed chemotaxis to zymosan-activated serum as well as decreased
random motility (18). In vivo therapy of diabetics (25
IU/kg/day) with α-tocopherol for 2-3 weeks restored these
activities to normal levels. On the otherhand, treatment
of normal male, human subjects for 3 weeks with 300 mg/day
of α-tocopherol acetate depressed PMN bactericidal activity
and PHA-induced lymphocyte proliferation (19).

POTENTIAL MECHANISMS OF VITAMIN E ACTION ON THE IMMUNE
SYSTEM

Although there are differences both in regard to the
animal species and the experimental protocol used, the
results of the above studies clearly implicate a role for
vitamin E in modulating the immune response (Table 1). The
immune functions which are enhanced by vitamin E include
protection against infection, increase in the number of
plaque-forming cells, increased antibody production,
increased proliferative response to T-and B-cell mitogens,
enhanced chemotaxis and particle ingestion, and a decrease
in oxygen uptake and H_2O_2 production. These effects
reflect modulation of function of both phagocytes and lymphocytes. Phagocytes are essential for lymphoid function;
lymphocytes modulate phagocyte function. On the basis of
the information that is presently available, the complex
interactions between cells of the immune systems, and the
vast array of products which are secreted, as well as
potential feed-back loops, identification of a specific

TABLE 1

Immune Functions Affected by Vitamin E

Species	Function
Chicken	Protection against infection Plaque-forming Cells antibody production
Mouse	Plaque-forming cells Antibody production Helper cell activity Mitogenesis of T and B lymphocytes
Rat	Mitogenesis of T and B lymphocytes Chemotaxis Ingestion O_2 and H_2O_2 production
Guinea pig	Mitogenesis of T and B lymphocytes
Human	PMN killing ability O_2 and H_2O_2 production Lymphocyte proliferation Chemotaxis and random motility of monocytes

lesion in a specific cell is not possible. Vitamin E appears to have an effect on neutrophils, monocytes, macrophages, and T- and B-lymphocytes.

Effects are observed when moderate levels of vitamin E are added to diets in the mouse, rat and guinea pig. However, in some of the models, effects were apparent only with high, pharmacological doses of vitamin E. The basis for the latter responses is not clear. In some models, it may represent an enhanced need for vitamin E in antigen-challenged animals. In others it may represent depletion of vitamin E during culture of immune cells. This point needs to be clarified. Modulation of lipoxygenation of arachidonic acid by human leukocytes has been shown to be bidirectional. Addition of vitamin E at concentrations equivalent to normal plasma levels enhanced conversion of both endogenous and exogenous arachidonic acid to hydroperoxy and hydroxy arachidonate derivatives, whereas higher concentrations suppressed lipoxygenation (20). In several species, vitamin E has an effect on the proliferation of both T- and B- lymphocytes. Interactions between these cells and adherent spleen cells, macrophages, are functionally important and are extremely complex. Responses to different amounts of con A have been interpreted to indicate that vitamin E selectively stimulates certain populations of T-cells in a macrophage-independent manner. Differences in response to PHA are also reported for spleen cell preparations of vitamin E-deficient compared to supplemented animals. Information on these cells as individual as well as mixed populations would clarify considerably which cells are vitamin E responsive. The macrophage plays a central role in the activation of both T- and B-lymphocytes. Vitamin E effects on this phagocyte could result in changes in the activation of both T- and B-lymphocytes. Further studies on the effect of vitamin E on this target cell would be of interest.

The effects of vitamin E on the immune system do not appear to reflect simple antioxidant action. Few studies have been done with other antioxidants as additions to the diet; however, DPPD appears not to replace vitamin E. Addition of vitamin E to immune cells in culture results in responses apparently analogous to those resulting from dietary vitamin E treatment. Studies on the in vitro addition of DPPD, BHT and trolox, which are very effective antioxidants, and of tocopherol quinone and menadione, which are not antioxidants, suggest that the effects of tocopherol may be specific.

Results of studies on several mouse strains have been interpreted to indicate that vitamin E selectively stimulates certain populations of T-cells. Immature thymocytes are not as responsive to PHA as are mature T-cells. The vitamin E-dependent PHA response may indicate an effect of vitamin E on the maturation of T-cells. Differentiation of precursor cells in the bone marrow is an important source of cells of the immune system. Abnormalities in bone marrow haemotopoiesis have been correlated with vitamin E deficiency-induced anemias in the pig (21) and monkey (22). In ongoing studies on the role of vitamin E on the function of blood platelets in my laboratory, we have confirmed that blood platelet content is increased in the vitamin E-deficient male Sprague-Dawley rat and extended this effect to include the female (Table 2). Dietary addition of the antioxidant, propyl gallate, did not substitute for vitamin E in regard to platelet number. Transfer of vitamin E-deficient male or female rats to a vitamin E diet restores platelet number to the vitamin E supplemented values within 9-14 days. Pilot studies on bone marrow suggest that megakarycytes increase in number in vitamin E-deficiency. Alterations in the differentiation of precursor cells of the immune system and/or effects of vitamin E on the proliferation of cells of the immune system could have a role in the immune function effects observed.

Cell-cell contact between macrophages and T and B lymphocytes is essential for cooperativity between these cells and the expression of immune function. The presence of vitamin E in the membrane bilayer has the potential to affect the physical properties of the membrane and membrane function. The phytyl side chain of vitamin E is proposed to form a helix with the cis double bonds of arachidonic acid, restrict the movement of the membrane, and decrease fluidity. Using fluoresence depolarization techniques, we have observed that rat platelets containing vitamin E are less fluid than those which do not contain vitamin E: microviscosity at 37°C for male platelets from vitamin E

TABLE 2

PLATELET CONTENT OF WHOLE BLOOD

	Platelets x 10^6/ml blood	
Diet	Male	Female
+ Vitamin E	533 ± 93	570 ± 49
− Vitamin E	805 ± 109	922 ± 94

Data are expressed and the mean S.D., n=15. Platelet number was determined on whole blood by laser hematology using the Ortho ELT-8 instrument. Differences between +vitamin E and −vitamin E are significant by the paired Student t test, p<0.01.

supplemented rats = 0.92 ± 0.04 poise and for those from
vitamin E-deficient animals = 0.75 ± 0.02 poise. Changes
in membrane fluidity effected by vitamin E of cells of the
immune system could affect cell-cell interactions as well
as antigenic recognition.

As a membrane component and antioxidant, vitamin E may
affect arachidonate oxygenation. Oxygenated metabolites of
arachidonic acid have an important role in modulating the
immune system. Macrophage-lectin response involves the
release of secretory products including enzymes, complement
proteins, growth factors, and eicosanoids--both prostaglandins and lipoxygenase products. Major prostanoids produced
by macrophages are PGE_2 and TXA_2 (23). In general, the
effects of prostaglandins on the immune system are suppressive. Inhibitors of prostaglandin synthesis, such as indomethacin and aspirin, improve the proliferative response to
lectins. Recent studies show that lipoxygenase products
have an important role in the immune system (24). Phagocytes have very active lipoxygenases. Lipoxygenase products inhibit spleen lymphocyte responses to con A and PHA
(25,26). Of particular interest is the leukotriene pathway, which is initiated by the introduction of O_2 at C-5 of
arachidonic acid, followed by formation of an epoxide.
Hydrolysis of the epoxide, LTA_4, results in LTB_4, which is
an extremely potent chemotactic agent (27), stimulates PMN
leukocyte enzyme release and superoxide generation and
induces degranulation. LTB_4 enhances generation of T-sup-
pressor lymphyocytes (26). Alternatively, addition of
glutathione to the epoxide results in a series of peptidyl
leukotrienes, LTC_4, LTD_4 and LTE_4, which are the slow
reacting substances of anaphylaxis.

Other lipoxygenase products of arachidonic acid are
also involved in the mitogenic responses of lymphocytes to
plant lectins and tumor promoters. 15-HPETE, a product of
15-lipoxygenase activity in monocytes, induces T-cells to
become suppressor cells. Addition of HPETEs to mouse
spleenocytes inhibits the proliferative response to PHA and
con A, and also suppresses the development of killer cells.
There is considerable evidence that lipoxygenase products
have important modulating effects on lymphocyte function.
Some of the HETEs are incorporated into the membrane and,
as a result, affect the fluidity of the membrane.

Vitamin E may affect immune function by modulating the release of arachidonic acid from membrane phosphatide and/ or affecting PG synthesis and lipoxygenase activity. Both biosynthetic pathways proceed via free radical mechanisms. Eicosanoid synthesis is modulated by vitamin E in rat platelets. Platelets from vitamin E-deficient rats pre-labeled with (^{14}C) arachidonate and activated by thrombin produce more thromboxane and 12-lipoxygenase product than platelets from rats fed vitamin E (Table 3). Indomethacin blocks TXA$_2$ but stimulates 12-HETE synthesis. There is evidence for modulation of lipoxygenase activity by vitamin E in human leukocytes (20). Critical studies on the effects of vitamin E on arachidonate turnover and oxygenation will be necessary to determine whether these pathways are affected in cells of the immune system.

In summary, vitamin E clearly has regulatory effects on the immune system. The specific site and mechanism by which these effects are exerted are not presently known. Future studies using new information and currently available immunological tools should clarify the role of vitamin E on the immune system.

TABLE 3

Oxygenation of Arachidonate by Prelabeled Platelets

Diet	Product	Thrombin	Thrombin + Indomethacin
		% cpm	
Vitamin E-sufficient	TXB$_2$	1.5	0.6
	12-HETE	10.6	25.3
Vitamin E-deficient	TXB$_2$	3.8	1.4
	12-HETE	34.8	32.6

Platelets were prelabeled with 1-(^{14}C)20:4, for 30 min at 37°C. After 5 min preincubation at 37° in the presence or absence of indocin (10 μg/ml), 1 unit human thrombin was added and the incubation continued for 5 min. Supernates of inactivated platelets were extracted with ethylacetate, partitioned by Silica gel TLC, scraped and the radioactivity counted. Data are expressed as % cpm in the supernate.

REFERENCES

1. Diplock, A.T. and Lucy, J.A. (1976) FEBS Lett. 29, 205-212.
2. Maggio, B., Diplock, A.T. and Lucy, J.A. (1977) Biochem. J. 161, 111-121
3. Tengerdy, R.P. (1980) Vitamin E: A Comprehensive Treatise, Basic and Clinical Nurition, Vol. 1, 429-444.
4. Tengerdy, R.P., Mathias, M.M. and Nockels, C.F. (1981) Adv. Exp. Med. Biol. 135, 27-41.
5. Heinserling, R.H., Nockels, C.F., Quarles, C.L. and Tengerdy, R.P. (1974) Proc. Soc. Exp. Biol. Med. 146, 279-283.
6. Likoff, R.O., Guptill, D.R., Lawrence, L.M., McKay, C.C., Mathias, M.M., Nocketls, C.F. and Tengerdy, R.P. (1981) Am. J. Clin. Nutr. 34, 245-251.
7. Campbell, P.A., Cooper, H.R., Heinzerling, R.H. and Tengerdy, R.P. (1974) Proc. Soc. Exp. Biol. Med. 146, 465-369.
8. Tengerdy, R.P., Heinzerling, R.H., Brown, G.L. and Mathias, M.M. (1973) Int. Arch. Allergy 44, 221-232.
9. Tanaka, J., Fujiwara, H. and Torisu, M. (1979) Immunology 38, 727-734.
10. Corwin, L.M. and Shloss, J. (1980) J. Nutr. 110, 916-923.
11. Corwin, L.M. and Shloss, J. (1980) J. Nutr. 110, 2497-2505.
12. Corwin, L.M., Gordon, R.K. and Shloss, J. (1981) Scand. J. Immunol. 14, 565-571.
13. Corwin, L.M. and Gordon, R.K. (1982) Vitamin E: Biochemical, Hematological and Clinical Aspects, Annals of the New York Academy of Sciences, Vol. 393, 437-451.
14. Bendich, A. Gabriel, E. and Machlin, L.J. (1983) J. Nutr. 113, 1920-1926.
15. Bendich, A., D'Apolito, P., Gabriel, E. and Machlin, L.J. (1984) J. Nutr. 114, 1588-1593.
16. Harris, R.E., Boxer, L.A. and Baehner, R.L. (1980) Blood 55, 338-343.
17. Boxer, L.A., Oliver, J.M., Spielberg, S.P., Allen, J.M. and Schulman, J.D. (1979) N. Engl. J. Med. 301, 901-905.

18. Hill, H.R., Augustine, N.H., Rallison, M.L. and Santos, J.I. (1983) J. Clin. Immunol. 3, 70-77.
19. Prasad, J.S. (1980) Am. J. Clin. Nutr. 33, 606-608.
20. Goetzl, E.J. (1980) Nature 288, 183-185.
21. Lynch, R.E., Hammer, S.P., Lee, G.R. and Cartwright, G.E. (1977) Am. J. Hematol. 2, 145-162.
22. Fitch, C.D., Brown, G.O., Chou, A.C. and Gallagher, N.I. (1980) Am. J. Clin. Nutr. 33, 1251-1259.
23. Humes, J.L., Sadowski, S., Galavage, M., Goldenberg. M., Subers, E., Bonney, R.J. and Kuehl, F.A. Jr., (1982) J. Biol. Chem. 257, 1591-1594.
24. Vanderhock, J.Y., Bryant, R.W. and Barley, J.M. (1980) J. Biol. Chem. 255, 10064-10066.
25. Gualde, N., Chable-Rabinovitch, H., Mott, O.C, Durand, J., Benneytout, J.L. and Rigand, M. (1983) Biochim. Biophys. Acta 750, 429-437.
26. Low, C.I., Pupillo, M.B., Bryant, R.W. and Bailey, J.M. (1984) J. Lipid Res. 25, 1090-1095.
27. Samuelsson, B. (1983) Science 220, 568-575.
28. Bailey, J.M., Bryant, R.W., Low, C.E., Pupillo, M.B. and Vanderhoek, J.Y. (1982) Cell. Immunol. 67, 112-120.

MECHANISM AND PREVENTION OF ANTICANCER AGENT-INDUCED

CANCER: Interactions of Vitamin E and Daunorubicin

Yeu-Ming Wang
Department of Experimental Pediatrics The University of
Texas M.D. Anderson Hospital and Tumor Institute
6723 Bertner Street
Houston, Texas 77030

INTRODUCTION

The investigations of vitamin E and cancer have been stimulated by an unreproducible finding of Rowntree et al. (1) that crude wheat germ oil induced sarcomas in rats. Wheat germ oil is naturally enriched with vitamin E. To date, more than 20 reports have appeared in the literature demonstrating that animals fed with vitamin E, mostly in ester form, have a reduced incidence or a delayed appearance of tumor after the administration of a carcinogen or UV radiation. There are also a few reports against the efficacy of vitamin E as a cancer preventive agent (2-4).

Along with the animal experimentations, the effect of α-tocopherol or α-tocopheryl quinone in the differentiation and growth of tumor cell or cell lines in culture has been investigated (5-7). For instance, Takenaga et al. (5) observed that α-tocopherol inhibited the differentiation of mouse myeloid leukemia cells. Prasad and Prasad (6) reported that α-tocopheryl succinate induced growth inhibition of melanoma cells in culture. Furthermore, the efficacy of dietary vitamin E on the reduction of human fecal mutagenicity has also been suggested (8,9).

213

THE BIOCHEMICAL FUNCTION OF VITAMIN E

Vitamin E or α-tocopherol has three major biochemical functions relevant to this discussion. The mechanism and action of the vitamin have been extensively reviewed in recent years (10-12).

1. α-Tocopherol is a physiologic antioxidant that not only protects the cellular membrane from oxidation, it also maintains some cellular enzyme and protein in a reduced active state. These include cyto-chrome-P-450 and phosphoenolpyruvate carboxykinase (13). α-Tocopherol appears to have a specific effect on the architecture of the membrane phospholipids by maintaining the profiles of membrane unsaturated fatty acid components (14). It also can directly interact with nitrosating agents and neutralize its toxicity.

    Recently, Burton et al. (15) reported that α-tocopherol is the major, and probably the only, lipid soluble, chain-breaking antioxidant in human plasma as well as erythrocyte ghost membrane. They also theorized that α-tocopherol functions as a far more efficient inhibitor of lipid peroxidation in vivo than in vitro because of a stereo electronic mechanism (16).

2. α-Tocopherol maintains the integrity of the macromolecular structure of the cell and can effectively reduce the binding of a number of carcinogens to cellular DNA (17-19).

3. α-Tocopherol may act as a regulator of gene activity. There is sufficient evidence to indicate that α-tocopherol suppresses the cellular biosynthesis of xanthine oxidase and, likely, creatinine kinase (20).

THERAPY-INDUCED CANCER

Antineoplastic agents have been known as carcinogens for a number of years, (21) and second malignancies in cancer patients treated with single-drug or multidrug chemotherapeutic agents have also been documented (22,23). The multimodal therapy mainly due to irradiation has been found to induce second malignancies in 4-16% of the survivors (24,25). Recently, Frei (26) estimated that current cancer chemotherapy can result in about 30,000 to 40,000 long-term survivors per year. Therefore, second malignancies induced by antineoplastic agents particularly in children will soon become an acute problem.

Anthracycline-Induced Tumors and Mechanisms of Toxicity

The anthracycline antibiotics daunorubicin and doxorubicin (14-hydroxydaunorubicin) have been used extensively since 1970 for the treatment of human cancers. The major toxicities of the anthracycline antibiotics are cardiotoxicity and, likely, carcinogenic activities. The anthracycline antibiotics are mutagenic according to the Ames test. They induce chromosomal breakage in human cells. Bertazzoli et al. (27) reported a high incidence of mammary tumors in a relatively small group of Sprague-Dawley rats treated with single doses of doxorubicin or daunorubicin. These results were later confirmed by us and other (28). Both drugs induce cancer in rat mammary gland exclusively. Sieber et al. (29) reported that one of ten healthy monkeys studied died of acute myeloblastic leukemia after treatment with doxorubicin at a cumulative dose of 324 mg/m^2. The induction time for cancer development was 29 months.

The mechanisms by which the anthracycline antibiotics exert their cytotoxicity and carcinogenicity are not clearly established. It is known, however, that:

1. Daunorubicin intercalates into DNA, thus affecting DNA and RNA synthesis.

2. Daunorubicin generates free radicals during its metabolic process, thereby damaging cellular components including DNA.

3. Daunorubicin chelates metal ions and binds to membrane and cellular proteins. Tewey, et al. (30) reported the involvement of DNA topoisomerase II in the mechanism of action of doxorubicin. Tökes et

al. (31) and Tritton and Yee (32) suggested that anthracycline antibiotics exert their cytotoxicity by interaction at the cell membrane level.

Metabolism of Daunorubicin

Daunorubicin is metabolized in liver by three pathways: (a) free-radical generation by one-electron oxidation-reduction, (b) a carbonyl reduction process, (33) and (c) the involvement of a two-electron transfer enzyme, quinone reductase.

Microsomal and nuclear NADPH cytochrome (P-450) reductase, NADH oxidoreductase, and xanthine oxidase, one-electron transfer enzymes, can catalyze the reduction of the anthracyclines to a semiquinone free-radical intermediate. This radical, in turn, reacts with a cellular oxygen to produce superoxide anions. The superoxide radical formed will subsequently convert to hydrogen peroxide and hydroxyl radical that induce lipid peroxidation and DNA breaks. In the absence of cellular oxygen, the semiquinone radical can also rearrange slowly to form an aglycone free radical, which can alkylate DNA. The end product of this metabolic route is 7-deoxydaunorubicin aglycone.

Carbonyl reduction is another metabolic pathway of daunorubicin. It is apparently a detoxification process. This metabolic process forms daunorubicinol and 7-deoxydaunorubicinol aglycone and is mediated by NADPH requiring cytoplasmic reductases (33).

The third and the other potential metabolic route is the involvement of DT-diaphorase [NAD(P)H-quinone reductase] in the metabolism or detoxification of daunorubicin. It reduces quinone to a rather stable hydroquinone. Therefore, it has been suggested recently that quinone reductase is a cellular control device against semiquinone and superoxide radicals formation (34). Further, Butylhydroxylated anisole, a dietary antitoxidant at very high doses of 7 g/kg diet has been found to substantially increase the NAD(P)H quinone reductase activity in liver, kidney, and a number of other rat tissues (35).

We have investigated and compared the metabolism of daunorubicin in isolated single mammary epithelial cells and hepatocytes. The results of daunorubicin metabolism showed that mammary cells either do not metabolize daunorubicin or they metabolize daunorubicin very slowly. However, more than 70% of daunorubicin was metabolized when incubated with hepatocytes for a 90-minute period (Table 1). A substantial quantity of 7-deoxydaunorubicinol aglycone and daunorubicinol (the major metabolites of carbonyl reduction of daunorubicin) and a small percentage of 7-deoxydaunorubicin aglycone (the end product of the free-radical reaction and likely the end product of the proposed quinone reductase metabolic route) were found. Cytochrome P-450 reductase inhibitors SKF-525 ($1x10^{-3}$M) and α-naphthoflavone ($2x10^{-4}$M) modify significantly the metabolic patterns of the drug (Table 1).

Furthermore, the presence of dicumarol ($3x10^{-4}$M), a competitive inhibitor of the quinone reductase, completely inhibits the metabolism of 2,6-dichloro-indophenol as well as daunorubicin in liver cytosol. Our preliminary results indicate that there could be an NADH-dependent reductase as well as an NADPH-dependent reductase in rat hepatocytes as reported by Koli et al. (36) in hog liver.

The presence of a rat liver microsomal or a rat liver postmitochondrial preparation reduced the noncovalent interaction between the anthracycline antibiotics and DNA. The addition of rat liver post-mitochondrial preparations to a bacterial mutagen assay or the induction of microsomal enzymic activities in mouse M_2 fibroblasts decreased the capacity of doxorubicin-induced mutagenesis and malignant transformation. By contrast, inhibitors of microsomal enzyme activity increased the yield of the drug-induced transformants (37).

The activities of two metabolic enzymes of daunorubicin, xanthine oxidase and NAD(P)H quinone reductase, were determined in rat hepatocytes and isolated mammary epithelial cells. The results are shown in Table 2. Furthermore, the uptake of dauno-rubicin by these two types of cells was similar when quantitated per DNA content. These results suggested

Table 1: EFFECTS OF MICROSOMAL INHIBITORS ON THE METABOLISM OF DAUNORUBICIN IN RAT HEPATOCYTE HOMOGENATES

EXPERIMENT	PERCENT AFTER 90 MIN INCUBATION			
	DAUNORUBICIN	DAUNORUBICINOL	7-DEOXYDAUNO-RUBICINOL AGLYCONE	7-DEOXYDAUNO-RUBICIN AGLYCONE
CONTROL[a]	17	4.8	66.0	11
+SKF-525	65	24.0	4.5	6
+NAPHTHOFLAVONE	35	7.3	45.0	13
+2-METHYLPROPANONE	25	5.8	56.0	13

a. Incubation conditions: Protein concentration, 4.0 mg/ml; daunorubicin concentration, 8.0×10^{-5}M; NADPH concentration, 8.3×10^{-4}M; Tris, 0.05M, pH 7.4; temperature 37°.

TABLE 2: ENZYME ACTIVITIES IN NORMAL AND VITAMIN E DEFICIENT RAT CELLS[a]

($nmol\ min^{-1}\ mg\ protein^{-1}$)

CELLS	VITAMIN E STATUS	α-TOCOPHEROL ($\mu g/10^7$ cells)	GLUTATHIONE REDUCTASE	γ-GLUTAMYL TRANSPEPTIDASE	NADPH:QUINONE REDUCTASE	XANTHINE OXIDASE
HEPATOCYTES	Normal (3)	N.D.[b]	21 ± 5.7	0.43 ± 0.32	215 ± 28.6	1.6 ± 0.2
	Deficient (3)	N.D.	21 ± 5.5	0.27 ± 0.15	357 ± 276	1.6 ± 0.7
MAMMARY CELLS	Normal (3)	<0.13	239 ± 67	21.4 ± 10.0	40 ± 25.7	3.8 ± 1.1
	Deficient (3)	0.57 ± 0.07	150 ± 101	37.5 ± 22.6	65 ± 30.6	3.6 ± 1.1

[a] The cells were isolated after feeding weanling rats with normal (100 mg α-tocopherylacetate/kg diet) or deficient (0 mg α-tocopherolacetate/kg diet) AIN-76 diet for 6 weeks. Diets were purchased from Dyets, Inc., Bethlehem, Penn, 18017.

[b] N.D. — Not determined.

that mammary cells might generate more semiquinone radicals by xanthine oxidase per mg protein than hepatocytes. In addition, mammary cells are less able to detoxify daunorubicin by the enzymatic action of the quinone reductase. Therefore, rat mammary cell in the presence of oxygen may continuously generate superoxide anions through the reversible reaction.

The Difference of Daunorubicin-Induced DNA Breaks Between Mammary Cells and Hepatocytes

Alkaline elution techniques (38) were used to compare the frequencies and type of DNA lesions in mammary cells and hepatocytes. Daunorubicin concentrations that gave a dose-response curve were utilized first in mammary epithelial cells and then in hepatocytes. Mammary cells, at 10^6 cells per ml, were incubated with the 1.5, 4.0, and 10.0 μg drug for one hour. After incubation, the cells were pelleted at 200 x g for 4 minutes, washed once with HBSS, and resuspended in PBS. DNA single-strand breaks (SSB) were assessed in the absence and the presence of proteinase K. Analyses of experiments with mammary epithelial cells revealed DNA protein-associated SSB were induced in DNA at all drug dose levels. SSB were also detected without proteinase K treatment, but at a diminished level when compared with proteinase-K-treated assays. Proteinase-K-treated assays showed a small number of SSB at the lowest drug concentration (1.5 μg/ml) in hepatocytes. Negligible amounts of SSB were seen at the other drug concentrations in both treatments. Similar results were obtained in proteinase-K-untreated assays (38). In general, the quantity of SSB seen in liver cells was statistically significantly lower than that in comparably treated mammary epithelial cells.

Further analyses of differences in carcinogen-DNA interaction between the two cell types were undertaken. The type and degree of cross-linking were studied using experiments involving treatment of cells with 10 μg/ml of daunorubicin for 1 hour followed by 300 rad of irradiation. Preliminary results suggest that the total number of cross-linking lesions show no statistical difference between isolated mammary cells and hepatocytes. The metabolite, 7-deoxydaunorubicinol aglycone at a concentration of 5 μg/ml, showed that mammary cells might generate more semiquinone radicals by xanthine oxidase per mg protein than hepatocytes. In addition, mammary cells are less able to detoxify daunorubicin by the enzymatic action of the quinone reductase. Therefore, rat mammary cell in the presence of oxygen may continuously generate superoxide anions through the reversible reaction.

The Difference of Daunorubicin-Induced DNA Breaks Between Mammary Cells and Hepatocytes

Alkaline elution techniques (38) were used to compare the frequencies and type of DNA lesions in mammary cells and hepatocytes. Daunorubicin concentrations that gave a dose-response curve were utilized first in mammary epithelial cells and then in hepatocytes. Mammary cells, at 10^6 cells per ml, were incubated with the 1.5, 4.0, and 10.0 µg drug for one hour. After incubation, the cells were pelleted at 200 x g for 4 minutes, washed once with HBSS, and resuspended in PBS. DNA single-strand breaks (SSB) were assessed in the absence and the presence of proteinase K. Analyses of experiments with mammary epithelial cells revealed DNA protein-associated SSB were induced in DNA at all drug dose levels. SSB were also detected without proteinase K treatment, but at a diminished level when compared with proteinase-K-treated assays. Proteinase-K-treated assays showed a small number of SSB at the lowest drug concentration (1.5 µg/ml) in hepatocytes. Negligible amounts of SSB were seen at the other drug concentrations in both treatments. Similar results were obtained in proteinase-K-untreated assays (38). In general, the quantity of SSB seen in liver cells was statistically significantly lower than that in comparably treated mammary epithelial cells.

Further analyses of differences in carcinogen-DNA interaction between the two cell types were undertaken. The type and degree of cross-linking were studied using experiments involving treatment of cells with 10 µg/ml of daunorubicin for 1 hour followed by 300 rad of irradiation. Preliminary results suggest that the total number of cross-linking lesions show no statistical difference between isolated mammary cells and hepatocytes. The metabolite, 7-deoxydaunorubicinol aglycone at a concentration of 5 µg/ml, showed

negligible SSB in proteinase-K-treated DNA. The
combination of this dose of metabolite with daunorubicin
did not change the frequency of SSB produced by daunorubicin alone. Five μg/ml of 7-deoxydaunorubicinol
aglycone alone did not show any ability to produce
cross-links in mammary cells. The combination of
various mixtures of the two compounds did not produce a
change in the cross-linking profile of daunorubicin.

Since daunorubicin alone does not induce strand
breaks in liver cells, we were not able to investigate
DNA repair capabilities of the two cell types after drug
incubation. However, we have studied DNA repair after
both cell types were irradiated with 300 rad of ionizing
radiation (cesium 137). This experiment showed that in
this specific type of damage, both cells types exhibited
similar functional capabilities (Wang, unpublished).

VITAMIN E AS A CANCER PREVENTIVE AGENT

Based upon a hypothesis that the free radicals or
superoxide anions generated through the cellular
activity and the metabolism of daunorubicin might be the
causes of the tumorigenesis in animals, α-tocopherylacetate (1.8 g/m^2) was given intraperitoneally daily for
four days prior to a single injection of daunorubicin
through a tail vein. The 60 mg/m^2 of daunorubicin is
usually a single dose given to humans. The frequency of
tumor formation was compared with those animals treated
with doxorubicin alone. The animals treated with α-
tocopherylacetate had a significantly lower incidence
($p < 0.05$) of tumor induction than those treated with
daunorubicin alone. In animals injected with daunorubicin only, 24/54 animals had histologically proven
mammary tumor; in animals treated with both α-
tocopherylacetate and daunomycin, 9/38 animals had
mammary cancer (Wang et al., unpublished).

In this study, we observed the following:

1. Level of α-tocopherol was significantly higher in
   the spleen and heart of animals not receiving
   daunorubicin;

2. Mammary gland and mammary fat along with plasma and

erythrocyte had significant increases of α-tocopherol radioactivities in animals treated with
daunorubicin;

3. Liver, spleen, kidney, and lung tissues had the
   highest daunorubicin concentration. Mammary tissue
   areas and surrounding fat had the lowest drug
   concentration;

4. Drug clearance was significantly faster in liver
   than in mammary tissue area;

5. The increase of α-tocopherol was less than 100% in
   mammary gland and mammary fat after four intra-
   peritoneal injections of α-tocopherylacetate.

The increase of α-tocopherol was less than 100% in
mammary gland and fat areas 24 hours after four
injections of high doses of α-tocopherol. Therefore, to
investigate whether the effect of α-tocopherol is in the
early stage of tumor development, weanling female SD
rats were fed with α-tocopherylacetate and α-
tocopherylacetate-supplemented diet (containing 100 and
1,000 mg α-tocopherol per kg diet) for 5 weeks. Single
mammary epithelial cells were isolated from these rats
and biochemical studies were performed. Mammary
epithelial cells had cellular α-tocopherol concentrations of less than 0.13 μg/10^7 cells isolated from rats
fed with the deficient diet for 5 weeks as compared with
2.1 μg/10^7 cells isolated from the animals fed with the
1000 mg/kg diet. Alkaline elution assays of these cells
after incubation with various quantities of daunorubicin
were performed. It is apparent that vitamin-E-
supplemented cells can resist the oxidation induced by
daunorubicin. The results also indicated that α-
tocopherol can, to a degree, modify the effect of
daunorubicin-induced, single-strand DNA breaks.
Normally, cells isolated from rats fed a normal diet can
retain 40-60% of their DNA in double-strand format. In
cells isolated from an animal fed with a vitamin-E-
deficient diet, these cells can only retain about 20% of
their DNA after incubation with 10 μg daunorubicin in
the presence of proteinase K. On the other hand, to
those cells isolated from an animal fed with vitamin-E-
supplemented diet, about 80% of their DNA was in an
intact form. However, our preliminary results indicated

that the adequacy of α-tocopherol does not alter the
activities of xanthine oxidase or quinone reductase in
rats fed with either vitamin-E-deficient diet (0 mg/kg)
or supplemented diet (100 mg/kg). Experiments with
animals fed an even higher vitamin E diets (1,000 or
10,000 mg/kg) are ongoing.

In the last few years there have been a few reports
dealing with the involvement of α-tocopherol as to the
protection of DNA integrity. For instance, Summerfield
and Tapple (39) reported that with minimal dietary
supplement of α-tocopherol, up to 10 mg/kg diet, the
increased α-tocopherol supplementation can reduce rat
brain DNA-protein and DNA-DNA-interstrand cross-linking
induced by the injection of methylethyl ketone
peroxide. Kappen and Goldberg (40) reported that the
presence of α-tocopherol succinate reduced the breakage
of ^{3}H-labeled-λ-DNA induced by neocarcinostatin in
vitro.

THE DILEMMA OF RESEARCH IN NUTRIPREVENTION

Epidemiologic studies have suggested that dietary
practice is one of the contributing factors in cancer
risk and incidence. These investigations correlated
cancer causation and dietary factors, such as food
contaminants, additives, and meat consumption, and also
correlated cancer prevention and dietary factors such as
fiber contents and fruit/vegetable and cereal consumption (41). There are many interactions in tumor-bearing
hosts having an impact on the utilization of macro- or
micronutrients. A mutual interrelation exists among
nutrition, immunity, cancer, therapy, and prevention.
It is, therefore, difficult to simplify these
interactions. However, it is feasible to examine the
mechanisms by which a defined nutrient affects the
multifactorial interactions, and thus to examine their
interactions in causation and prevention of cancer.
There is ample evidence, for instance, to suggest the
cause and effect of vitamin E as an anticarcinogen in
model systems. However, the lack of demonstrated
quantitative relation at a basic level becomes
obvious. The understanding of the fundamental
properties and biochemical actions of carcinogen and
anticarcinogen becomes essential and necessary. This
kind of investigation may suggest or preclude the need

for vitamin supplements that already prevail in our society (42).

REFERENCES

1. Rowntree, L.G., Steinberg, A., Dorrance, G.M., and Criccone, E.F.: Sarcoma in rats from the ingestion of a crude wheat germ oil made by ether extraction. Am. J. Cancer 31:359-372, 1937.

2. Wattenberg, L.W.: Inhibition of carcinogenic and toxic effects of polycyclic hydrocarbon by phenolic antioxidants and ethoxyquin. J. Natl. Cancer Inst. 48:1425-1430, 1972.

3. Newmark, H.L., and Mergens, W.J.: α-Tocopherol (Vitamin E) and its relationship to tumor induction, in "Inhibition of Tumor Induction and Development." Zedeck, M.S., and Lipkin, M. (eds.); Plenum Publishing Co., New York, p. 127-168, 1981.

4. Newborne, P.M., and Suphakarn, V.: Nutrition and cancer: A review with emphasis on the role of vitamin C and E and selenium. Nutri. Cancer 5:107-119, 1983.

5. Takenaga, K.: Inhibition of differentiation of mouse myeloid leukemic cells by phenolic antioxidants and α-tocopherol. Gann 72:104-112, 1981.

6. Prasad, K.N., and Edwards-Prasad, J.: Effects of tocopherol (vitamin E) and growth inhibition in melanoma cells in culture. Cancer Res. 42:550-555, 1982.

7. Liepkalns, V.A., Icard-Liepkalns, C., and Cornwell, D.G.: Regulation of cell division in human glioma cell clone by arachidonic acid and α-tocopherol-quinone. Cancer Lett. 15:173-178, 1982.

8. Dion, P.W., Bright-See, E.G., Smith, C.C., and Bruce, W.R.: The effects of dietary ascorbic acid and α-tocopherol on fecal mutagenicity. Mutation Res. 102:27-37, 1982.

9. Wilkins, T.D., Lederman, M., and van Tassell, R.L.: Isolation of a mutagen produced in the human colon by bacterial action. Banburg Rep. 7:205-214, 1981.

10. Machlin, L.J. (eds.). "Vitamin E, A Comprehensive Treatise," Marcel Dekker, Inc., New York, pp. 660, 1980.

11. Lubin, B., and Machlin, L.J. (eds.). Vitamin E: Biochemical, Hematological, and Clinical Aspects. Ann. N. Y. Acad. Sci. 393:1-506, 1982.

12. Porter, R., and Whelan, J. (eds.). Biology of Vitamin E, Liba Fnd. Symposium, 101, The Pitaman Press, Bath, pp. 260, 1983.

13. MacDonald, M.J.: Rapid inactivation of rat liver phosphoenolpyruvate carboxykinase and reversal by reductants. Biochim. Biophys. Acta. 615:223-236, 1980.

14. Giasuddin, A.S.M., and Diplock, A.J.: The influence of vitamin E on membrane lipids of mouse fibroblasts in culture. Arch. Biochem. Biophys. 210:348-362, 1981.

15. Burton, G.W., Joyce, A., and Ingold, K.U.: First proof that vitamin E is a major lipid soluble, chainbreaking antioxidant in human blood plasma. Lancet 2:327, 1982.

16. Burton, G.W., Page, Y.L., Gabe, E.J., and Ingold, K.U.: Antioxidant activity of vitamin E and related phenols. Importance of stereoelectronic factors. J. Am. Chem. Soc. 102:7792-7794, 1980.

17. Harris, C.C., Autrup, H., van Haaflen, C., Connor, R., Frank, A.L., Barrett, L.A., McDowell, E.M., and Trump, B.F.: Inhibition of benzo(a)pyrene to DNA in cultured human bronchi. In: "Prevention and Detection of Cancer," vol. 2, (part 1), Nieburgs, H.E., eds., Marcel Dekker, New York, pp. 1359-1364, 1978.

18. Sakai, S., Rienhold, C.E., Wirth, P.J., and Thorgeirsson, S.S.: Mechanism of in vitro mutagenic activation and covalent binding of N-hydroxy-2-acetylaminofluorene in isolated liver cell nuclei from rat and mouse. Cancer Res. 38:2058-2067, 1978.

19. Matsura, T., Ueyama, H., Nomi, S., and Veda, K.: Effect of α-tocopherol on the binding of benzo(a)pyrene to nuclear macromolecules. J. Nutr. Sci. Vitaminol. 25:495-504, 1979.

20. Catignani, G.L.: Vitamin E: Role in nucleic acid and protein metabolism. In: "Vitamin E, A Comprehensive Treatise," (ed.), Machlin, L.J., Marcel Dekker, Inc., New York, pp. 318-331, 1980.

21. Hoover, R., and Fraumeni, J.H., Jr.: Drug-induced cancer. Cancer 47:1071, 1080, 1981.

22. Youness, E., Dosik, G., Benjamin, R.S., and Trujillo, J.M.: Acute myelomonocytic leukemia following a chemotherapeutic regimen. Cancer Treat. Rep. 62:1513-1516, 1978.

23. Bersagel, D.E., Bailey, A.J., and Langley, G.R.: The chemotherapy of plasma cell myeloma and the

incidence of acute leukemia. N. Engl. J. Med. 301:743-748, 1979.

24. Sullivan, M.P., Ramirez, I., and Ried, H.L.: Second malignancies following Hodgkin's disease in children differ from those of adults: Incidence occurring among 228 pediatric Hodgkin's disease patients. Proc. AACR 24:160, 1983 (Abstract).

25. Li, F.P.: Second malignant tumors after cancer in childhood. Cancer 40(4 Suppl):1899-1902, 1977.

26. Frei, E. III: The national cancer program. Science (U.S.A.) 217:600-606, 1982.

27. Bertazzolli, C., Chieli, T., and Solcia, E.: Different incidence of breast carcinomas or fibroadenomas in daunorubicin or Adriamycin treated rats. Experimentia 27:1209-1210, 1971.

28. Wang, Y.M., Howell, S.K., Kimball, J.C., Tsai, C.C., Sato, J., and Gleiser, C.A.: Alpha-tocopherol as a potential modifier of daunomycin carcinogenicity in Sprague-Dawley rats. In: "Molecular Interrelations of Nutrition and Cancer." Arnott, M.S., van Eys, J., and Wang, Y.M. (eds.), Raven Press, New York, pp., 369-379, 1982.

29. Sieber, S.M., Correa, P., Young, D.M., Dalgard, D.W., and Adamson, R.H.: Cardiotoxic and possible leukemogenic effects of Adriamycin in non-human primates. Pharmacology 20:9-14, 1980.

30. Tewey, K.M., Rowe, T.C., Yang, L., Halligan, B.D., And Liu, L.F.: Adriamycin-induced DNA damage mediated by mammalian DNA topoisomerase II. Science 226:446-468, 1984.

31. Tökes, Z.A., Rogers, K.E., and Rombaum, A.: Synthesis of Adriamycin-coupled polygutaraldehyde microspheres and evaluation of their cytostatic activity. Proc. Natl. Acad. Sci. (U.S.A.) 79:2026-2030, 1982.

32. Tritton, T.R., and Yee, G.: The anticancer agent Adriamycin can be actively cytotoxic without entering cells. Science 217:248-250, 1982.

33. Myers, C.E.: Anthracyclines. In: "Principles of Cancer Treatment", Chabner, B. (ed.), W. B. Saunders Co., Philadelphia, pp. 416-434, 1982.

34. Lind, C., Hochstein, P., and Ernsten, L.: DT-diaphorase as a quinone reductase: A cellular control device against seminquinone and superoxide radical formation. Arch. Biochem. Biophys. 216:178-185, 1982.

35. Benson, A.M., Hunkeler, M.J., and Tolalay, P.: Increase of NAD(P)H:quinone reductase by dietary antioxidants: Possible role in protection against carcinogenesis and toxicity. Proc. Natl. Acad. Sci. (U.S.A.) 77:5216-5220, 1980.

36. Koli, A.K., Yearby, C., Scott, W., and Donaldson, K.O.: Purification and properties of three separate medione reductases from hog liver. J. Biol. Chem. 244:621-629, 1969.

37. Wang, Y.M., and Howell, S.K.: α-Tocopherol as a potential modifier of daunorubicin-induced mammary tumors in rats. Ann. N.Y. Acad. Sci. 393:186-189, 1982.

38. Howell, S.K.: Daunorubicin-Induced DNA Lesions in Mammalian Somatic Cells. M.S. Thesis. The University of Texas at Houston, Texas, pp. 81, 1983.

39. Summerfield, F.W., and Tapple, A.L.: Vitamin E protects against methylethyl ketone peroxide-induced peroxitative damage to rat brain DNA. Mutation Res. 126:113-120, 1984.

40. Kappen, L.S., and Goldberg, I.H.: Activation and inactivation of neocarcinostatin-induced cleavage of DNA. Nucleic Acids Res. 5:2959-2967, 1978.

41. Ames, B.N.:   Dietary carcinogens and anticarcinogens. Oxygen radical and degenerative diseases. Science 221:1256-1264, 1983.

42. Read, M.H., Bhalla, V., Harill, I., Bendel, R., Monagle, J.E., Schultz, H.G., Sheehan, E.T., and Standal, B.R.:   Potentially toxic vitamin supplementation practices among adults in seven Western states. Nutr. Reps. International 24:133-1138, 1981.

CHEMOPREVENTION (HUMAN)

Methodological Issues

A NEW HPLC METHOD FOR THE SIMULTANEOUS ANALYSIS OF PLASMA RETINOL, TOCOPHEROLS, AND CAROTENOIDS AND ITS APPLICATION IN CANCER EPIDEMIOLOGY

Chung S. Yang, Kenneth W. Miller and Mao-Jung Lee
Department of Biochemistry, UMDNJ-New Jersey Medical School, Newark, NJ 07103 USA

ABSTRACT

An isocratic high-performance liquid chromatography (HPLC) method for the simultaneous determination of various fat-soluble vitamins and carotenoids has been developed. The method utilizes a Radial-Pak C18, 8 mm i.d. x 10 cm, 5-μm column and an elution solvent composed of methanol, acetonitrile, and chloroform. Retinol, α-tocopherol, α-carotene, β-carotene, lycopene, zeaxanthin, and two other unidentified carotenoids can be clearly separated and quantified in one HPLC run using α-tocopheryl acetate or tocol as the internal standard. The eluted peaks are quantified by either a photodiode-array detector at preprogrammed wavelengths at the absorption maxima of the compounds or by a dual-wavelength detector at 280 and 436 nm. The total run time is 16 min. With an automatic injector and a programmable detector the system allows unattended operation. The within-run and day-to-day coefficients of variation range from 1 to 8%. In addition, the system can monitor the absorption spectra of the eluent during the HPLC run; this allows the spectral identification of various compounds separated in the same run. The application of this new method in cancer epidemiology was demonstrated in a joint U.S.-China cooperative study on nutrition and esophageal cancer.

INTRODUCTION

The possible roles of vitamin A, vitamin E, and β-carotene in cancer prevention have received a great deal of attention in recent years (1-3). As an adjunct to dietary surveys, biochemical assessment of tissue nutrient levels is of great importance in epidemilogical studies on nutrition and cancer. Concerning the methodology for these determinations, conventional methods for the spectrophotometric determination of retinol, α-tocopherol, and β-carotene are either insensitive, nonspecific, or time consuming (4-6), and high-performance liquid chromatography (HPLC) methods are considered superior (6). Among the existing HPLC methods, some can determine vitamins A and E (7-9) and others can separate lycopene, β-carotene, α-carotene and other carotenoids, (11). A recent paper reported that three HPLC systems have to be used simultaneously for the determination of retinol, α-tocopherol, and α-carotene (12). A system for the simultaneous quantitation of plasma fat-soluble vitamins and other compounds in one HPLC run is highly desirable because it decreases sample size, increases the efficiency of HPLC utilization, and saves technical manpower.

In this communication we shall discuss a new isocratic HPLC method for the simultaneous quantitation of retinol, α-tocopherol, β-carotene, α-carotene, lycopene, and other compounds in plasma samples in one HPLC run. This system, which quantifies each compound at pre-programed wavelengths, is automated to allow unattended operation. The application of this method in epidemiological study will also be discussed.

MATERIALS AND METHODS

Sample preparation and HPLC: The fat-soluble compounds were extracted from human plasma samples using a procedure described previously (13). In brief, an internal standard, α-tocopheryl acetate or tocol, and 100 μl of ethanol were added to 100 μl of plasma and mixed. Then 230 μl hexane was added and the mixture was vortexed for 2 min. The samples were centrifuged for 5 min at 1000 rpm in a benchtop centrifuge to aid the solvent layer separation. The hexane layer (150 μl) was removed into a vial (usable in a Waters Model 710B WISP^{TM} automatic injector), dried in a centrifugal evaporator, and the residue was dissolved in 100 μl of the elution solvent. The sample vials were loaded onto the automatic injector. A 80 μl sample was injected into the HPLC and the column was eluted isocratically with methanol:acetonitrile:chloroform (25:60:15) at a flow rate of 1.5 ml/min. A pump (Waters Model 6000A), a Radial Compression Module (Waters Model RCM-100), and a Waters Radial-Pak C18, 8 mm i.d. x 10 cm, 5-μm column, were used. For monitoring the peaks and quantifying the compounds, a Hewlett-Packard multiwavelength detection system consisting of a 1040A photodiode-array HPLC detector, a HP-85B computer, a HP-9121 dual mini disc drive, 7470A graphics plotter, and a 3392A integrator were employed. Alternatively, a Waters Model 440 absorbance detector with 280 nm and 436 nm filters together with a Model 730 data module was used.

Standards: Standards for retinol, α-tocopheryl acetate, α-tocopherol, lycopene, α-carotene, and β-carotene were obtained from Sigma Chemical Company (St. Louis, MO). Tocol was a gift from Hoffmann-La Roche Inc. (Nutley, NJ). Solutions of α-carotene, β-carotene, and lycopene were prepared in chloroform. Retinol, α-tocopheryl acetate, and α-tocopherol standards were prepared in 100% ethanol. Concentrations of the standard solutions were determined using the following extinction coefficients (E 1%/cm): α-carotene, 2800 at 444 nm; β-carotene, 2396 at 465 nm; lycopene, 3450 at 472nm; retinol, 1780 at 325 nm; and α-tocopherol, 75.8 at 292 nm (8,10). The standards were not stable and were prepared fresh (within two days of their use). Standard curves were prepared by the addition, singly or in combination, of the standards to plasma samples or a solution of bovine serum albumin (7 g/100 ml saline). Results were calculated using the ratio of the peak area of the compound over the peak area of the internal standard. Recovery and linearity of the standard curves were determined and are presented in a subsequent section.

RESULTS AND DISCUSSION

Separation and Quantitation: Typical HPLC separations of fat-soluble vitamins and carotenes in a human plasma sample are shown in Figure 1. It presents overlapping profiles obtained in the same chromatography run by a preprogramed multiwavelength detection system and by

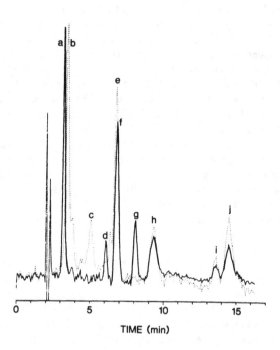

Figure 1. Chromatographs of human plasma extract. Results were obtained by the HP-1040A system. Peak identification: a, retinol; b, zeaxanthin; c–e unknowns; f, α-tocopherol; g, α-tocopheryl acetate; h, lycopene; i, α-carotene; and j, β-carotene. The solid line was obtained by monitoring peaks a, d and f, g, h, and i and j at 325, 290, 284, 470, and 450 nm, respectively. The dotted line was obtained by monitoring at 450 nm at a lower attenuation.

monitoring at 450 nm. The HP-1040A detection system scans the absorption spectra of the eluent every 10 ms and allows the HPLC peaks to be plotted and integrated at preprogramed wavelengths at or near the absorption maxima of the compounds. Comparisons of the respective retention times and absorption spectra with those of pure standards indicated that peaks a, f, h, i, and j were retinol, α-tocopherol, lycopene α-carotene, and β-carotene, respectively. Peak b was tentatively identified as zeaxanthin. Peak d was presumed to be β- or γ-tocopherol and peaks c and e to be carotenoids based on their absorption spectra, but the identification of these peaks and several minor components has not been completed. For quantitative analysis, peaks a and b did not significantly interfere with each other because they were each quantified at their respective absorption maxima. For spectral analysis, pure spectra of retinol and zeaxanthin were obtained from the upslope of peak a and the down slope of peak b, respectively. A retinyl palmitate standard was eluted at 16.5 min, slightly behind the β-carotene peak (result not shown). By monitoring the absorbance at 325 nm, therefore, it is possible to quantify this retinyl ester if present in nanogram quantities. When the system is programed for the integration of the β-carotene peak (at 450 nm), the absorbance at 325 nm can be recorded in the HP-85B computer and replotted after the HPLC run.

Figure 2 shows that excellent quantitation was also obtained using a Waters 440 dual wavelength detector. Absorbance at 280 nm was plotted and integrated for the

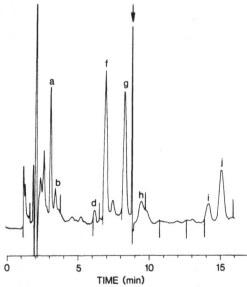

Figure 2. Chromatograph of human plasma extract. Results were obtained by a Waters model 440 detector. Peak identification is the same as for Figure 1. The first 8.8 min were monitored at 280 nm and then (after the arrow) at 436 nm.

first 8.8 min of the run for the determination of retinol
and tocopherols; then the monitoring wavelength was
switched manually to 436 nm for carotenoids (Figure 2).
A second pen can record the absorbance at either 280 or
436 nm to provide additional information. When the
determination of α-tocopherol is not important, the
retinol peak can be quantified by absorbance at 313 nm
(with a 313 nm filter) to increase the specificity and
sensitivity of the determination.

Standard curves and variability: For quantitative
analysis, standard curves were constructed and the
efficiency of the extraction procedure was examined as
described previously (13). The extraction efficiencies
of retinol, α-tocopherol, α-tocopheryl acetate, tocol,
and carotenes from the plasma sample were between 92 and
98%. Standard curves were established by adding known

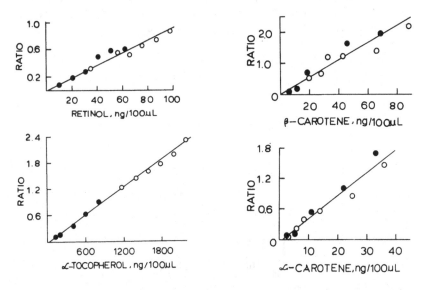

Figure 3. Standard curves for retinol (upper left),
α-tocopherol (lower left), β-carotene (upper right), and
α-carotene (lower right). Known amounts of standards
were added to either bovine serum albumin solution (•) or
human plasma (0) and the peak area is expressed as a
ratio to that of the internal standard (α-tocopherol
acetate) determined by the Waters Model 440 detector.
Each point represents the mean of duplicate determinations.

quantities of standards to plasma samples and bovine serum albumin solutions (Figure 3). Linearity of these standard curves was established with correlation coefficients of 0.938, 0.995, 0.990, and 0.958 for retinol, α-tocopherol, α-carotene, and β-carotene, respectively. It was estimated on the basis of the peak area that the lower limits of determination with both detecting systems were 2, 40, and 2 ng for retinol, α-tocopherol, and β-cartene (and α-carotene), respectively.

The within-run and day-to-day variations obtained with a reference plasma sample were presented in Table 1. Reproducible results were observed using either α-tocopheryl acetate or tocol (retention time 5 min) as the internal standard. Coefficients of variation of the determinations ranged from 1.5 to 8.2% with the highest variation seen for carotenes. Careful adjustment of integration parameters should further improve the quantitation of the broader carotene peaks.

TABLE 1. Within-run and day-to-day variations[a]

	Retinol	α-toco-pherol	β-caro-tene	α-caro-tene	Internal Standard
Exp. 1					
Mean	0.476	0.613	0.260	0.083	549
CV (%)	1.5	3.6	8.0	3.6	2.6
Exp. 2					
Mean	0.411	1.313	1.102	0.220	336
CV (%)	7.1	5.4	6.8	6.4	5.7
Exp. 3					
Mean	0.406	1.248	1.237	0.271	355
CV (%)	6.2	4.0	8.2	8.1	6.5

[a] Experiment 1: within-run variation (n=7) with HP-1040A detector; Experiment 2: within-run variation (n=9) with Waters 440 detector; and Experiment 3: day-to-day variation (n=19) with Waters 440 detector. The mean is expressed in peak area ratios to the internal standard (tocol in Experiment 1; α-tocopheryl acetate in Experiments 2 and 3) which is expressed in peak area units. Coefficient of variation (CV = standard deviation/mean) is expressed as a percentage.

Applications and possible problems: The advantages of
the present method are short analysis time and small
sample size. Furthermore, sensitivity and specificity
are greater than with previously published methods. The
method is also suitable for the analysis of serum
samples. By modifying the extraction procedure, this
method can be readily used for the analyses of vitamins
and carotenoids in animal tissues and food products. The
ability of the HP-1040A system to monitor up to 8
wavelengths simultaneously also allows the identification
and quantitation of other compounds in tissues and body
fluids. We found that a 8 mm i.d. x 10 cm, 5-μm Radial-
Pak C18 column gave the best separation. A 5 mm i.d. x
10 cm, 10-μm C18 column, which was used in our gradient
method (13), also provided a good separation with an
isocratic solvent mixture of methanol:acetonitrile:-
chloroform (75:20:5) at a flow rate of 1 ml/min. The run
time under these conditions was 13 to 14 min. Minor
adjustments of the solvent ratio and flow rate should
adapt this method to similar columns of other
manufacturers.

As is the case with many analytical procedures,
several possible problems may affect the accuracy and
reproducibility of the present HPLC method. One is water
contamination in the elution solvent which increases the
retention of α- and β-carotenes in the column. This problem can be overcome by drying the solvent with molecular
sieve. A second problem is the high lipid content of
some of the plasma or serum samples. The lipids are
extracted into the hexane layer and, on occassion, not
readily dissolved in the elution solvent (methanol:ace-
tonitrile:chloroform). The lipid may be trapped onto the
guard column or the C18 separation column of the HPLC
system and may affect the separation. A possible solution of this problem involving the hydrolysis of plasma
lipid by saponification or lipase digestion is currently
being tested in this laboratory.

Automation: With an automatic injector and a programmable multiwavelength detector such as the HP-1040A system, the system allows unattended operation. In this
case the spectra are not stored with our current data
system and only one wavelength can be monitored at a
time. However up to three wavelengths can be monitored
with a multi-channel integrator. The Waters Model 440

dual wavelength detector is not designed for automation.
If such operation is desired, it may be possible to use
both pens (channels) 1 and 2 simultaneously. Pen 1
monitors the absorbance at 280 nm for the quantification
of retinol and α-tocopherol with α-tocopheryl acetate or
tocol and the internal standard. Pen 2 monitors the
absorbance at 450 nm for carotenoids and the inclusion of
a second internal standard for this wavelength may be
necessary. With the Waters Model 730 data module, only
one pen is integrated and the peaks recorded by the other
pen can be integrated manually. The new Waters 490
multi-wavelength detector affords higher sensitivity and
reproducibility and is suitable for automated analysis.

Application in Cancer Epidemiology: The applicability of
this method in epidemiology was recently demonstrated in
a collaborative study on the effects of nutrition on
esophageal carcinogenesis. During a feasibility study
of a joint U.S.-China nutritional intervention study on
esophageal cancer in Linxian, China, plasma samples were
collected from individuals (ages 40-69) in April 1983
before supplementation with daily multiple vitamin pills
("One A Day" brand from Miles Laboratories, Inc.) and
again in August 1983 after a 16-week supplementation. The
samples were frozen and shipped to New Jersey for
analysis. The results were published in detail elsewhere
(16,17). Some representative data on vitamin A nutrition
are shown in Fig. 4. In April about 33-37% of the
individuals had plasma retinol levels of less than 20
μg/dl, a level considered to be "low or deficient" in
nutritional surveys. Differences between the general
population (Groups I and III) and individuals with
esophageal epithelial dysplasia (Groups II) were not
observed. After a 16-week supplementation, the plasma
retinol levels were significantly increased in Groups I
and II and almost all the individuals had levels above 20
μg/dl. The individuals in Group III who did not receive
the vitamin supplement did not show an increased mean
plasma retinol level (Table 2), even though fewer of them
(13.3%) were in the "low or deficient" category. A
summary of the results on retinol, α-tocopherol, α-carotene, and β-carotene is shown in Table 2. Lower nutritional status in α-tocopherol was also observed. In
April, about half of the individuals surveyed had plasma
α-tocopherol levels of less than 100 μg/dl, a level

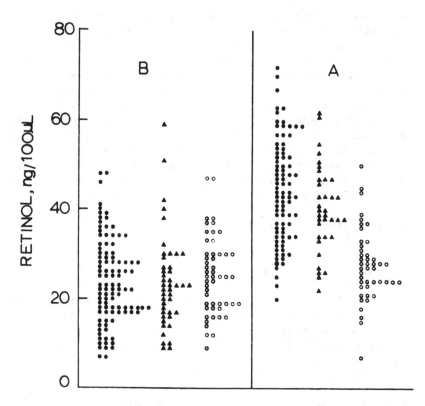

Figure 4. Plasma retinol levels of the population in
Linxian. Blood samples were collected in April (B) and
August (A). Samples were from the general population,
Group I (•) who received vitamin supplement and Group III
(o) who did not, and individuals with esophageal
dysplasia, Group II (▲) who also received the vitamin
supplement.

considered to be "deficient or low" in nutritional
surveys. In August, the percentage was reduced to 24–
29%. Significant increases in the mean plasma α–
tocopherol levels, however, were observed in Groups I and
II (supplemented) but not in Group III (not
supplemented). The plasma β–carotene levels were lower
in April than August in Groups I and II, but not in Group
III. The observed values of β–carotene, of course, are
much lower than the "total carotenes" determined
spectrophotometrically for this population (14). In

TABLE 2. Human Plasma Fat-Soluble Vitamin Levels Obtained in a Pilot Study in Linxian in 1983[a]

	GROUP I		GROUP II		GROUP III	
	April (n=100)	August (n=90)	April (n=45)	August (n=39)	April (n=51)	August (n=45)
Retinol	23.8 ± 9.5	44.6* ±11.4	23.5 ±10.5	40.3* ±11.4	26.7 ±12.8	27.7 ± 8.1
α-tocopherol	700 ±229	931* ±208	723 ±274	867[+] ±224	737 ±219	793 ±159
β-carotene	10.7 ± 8.1	15.9* ±12.6	8.3 ± 6.0	13.1[+] ± 8.1	11.8 ± 7.3	11.1 ± 6.5
α-carotene	2.0 ± 2.2	3.8* ± 3.2	1.2 ± 1.4	4.0* ± 5.0	1.5 ± 2.1	2.8[+] ± 1.8

[a]Populations in the age group of 40 to 69 were studied. Groups I and III were normal populations and Group II consisted of individuals with esophageal dysplasia. Groups I and II but not Group III received a daily supplement of retinol, α-tocopherol, and other vitamins in a tablet for 16 weeks. Samples were taken before (April) and after (August) the supplementation. The mean ± standard deviation (μg/dl) of each nutrients are shown.

*Significantly different from the corresponding April sample ($P < 0.001$).

+Significantly different from the corresponding April sample ($P < 0.05$).

Linxian, corn is an important staple food and xeazanthin is a major contributor in the spectrophotometric assay of carotenes. It was estimated that in the plasma samples from Linxian, β-carotene accounted for only 10-20% of the "total carotenes" assayed spectrophotometrically. The plasma α-carotene levels were low (and higher in August), but the significance of this compound, at these levels, in vitamin A nutrition or cancer prevention is not known.

This study demonstrates the usefulness of the new HPLC method in the analysis of fat-soluble vitamins and carotenes in cancer epidemiology. These results together with the data on other micro-nutrients (16,17) form the biochemical background for the presently ongoing nutritional intervention study on esophageal cancer in Linxian.

REFERENCES

1.   Sporn, M. B. and Roberts, A. B. (1983) <u>Cancer Res.</u> 43, 3034-3040.

2.   Peto, R., Doll, R., Buckley, J.D., and Sporn, M.B. (1981) <u>Nature</u> 290, 201-208.

3.   Willett, W.C., Polk, F., Underwood, B.A., Stampfer, M.J., Pressel, S., Rosner, B., Taylor, J.O., Schneider, K., and Hames, C.G. (1984) <u>New Engl. J. Med.</u> 310, 430-434.

4.   Suberlich, H.E., Dowdy, R.P., and Skala, J.H. (1974) Laboratory tests for the Assessement of Nutrional Status, p. 6, 7 and 76, CRC Press, Boca Raton, FL.

5.   Linhares, E.D.R. (1971) <u>Microchem.</u> 16, 467-471.

6.   Arroyave, G., Chichester, C.O., Flores, H., Glover, J., Mejia, L. A., Olson, J. A., Simpson, K. L., and Underwood, B. A. (1982) Biochemical Methodology for the Assessment of Vitamin A Status pp. 60-64. The Nutrition Foundation, Washington, D. C.

7.   De Leenheer, A.P., De Bevere, V.O.R.C., De Ruyter, M.G.M., and Claeys, A.E. (1979) <u>J. Chromatogr.</u> 162. 408-413.

8.   Bieri, J.G., Tolliver, T.J., and Catignani, G.L. (1979) <u>Am J. Clin. Nutr.</u> 32, 2143-2149.

9.   Driskell, W.J., Neese, J.W., Bryant, C.C., and Bashor, M.M. (1982) <u>J. Chromatogr.</u> 231, 439-444.

10. Broich, C.R., Gerber, L.E., and Erdman, J.W. Jr. (1983) <u>Lipids</u> 18, 253-258.

11. Nelis, H.J.C.F. and De Leenheer, A.P. (1983) <u>Anal Chem.</u> 55, 270-275.

12. Vuilleumier, J.-P., Keller, H.E., Gysel, D., and Hunziker, F. (1983) <u>Int. J. Vit. Nutri. Res.</u> 53, 265-272.

13. Miller, K. W., Lorr, N. A., and Yang, C. S. (1984) <u>Anal. Biochem.</u> 138, 340-345.

14. Yang, C. S., Miao, J., Yang, W., Huang, M., Wang, T., Xue, H. You, S., Lu, J., and Wu, J. (1982) <u>Nutr. Cancer</u> 4, 154-164.

15. Willet, W. C., Stampfer, M., Underwood, B. A., Taylor, J., and Hennekens, C. H. (1983) <u>Am J. Clin. Nutri.</u> 38, 559-566.

16. Yang, C.S., Sun, Y., Yang, Q., Miller, K.W., Li, G., Zheng, S.-F., Ershow, A.G., Blot, W.J., and Li, J. (1984) <u>J. Natl. Cancer Inst.</u> 73, 1449-1453.

17. Ershow, A.G., Zheng, S.-F., Li, G., Li, J., Yang, C.S., and Blot, W.J. (1984) <u>J. Natl. Cancer Inst.</u> 73, 1477-1481.

CLINICAL TOXICOLOGY PHARMACOKINETICS OF 13-CIS-RETINOIC ACID ADMINISTERED CHRONICALLY AT LOW DOSES EXPECTED FOR CANCER CHEMOPREVENTION TRIALS

David S. Alberts, Libby Edwards, Yei-Mei Peng,
Ruth Serokman, Thomas P. Davis, and
Frank L. Meyskens, Jr.
Sections of Hematology and Oncology and Dermatology,
Department of Medicine, Department of Pharmacology,
and the Cancer Center
Arizona Health Sciences Center
Tucson, Arizona 85724

This work was supported by research grants CA-27502 and
CA-17094 from the National Institutes of Health,
Department of Health and Human Services, Bethesda, MD
20205. We would like to thank Dr. Thomas Moon for his
excellent scientific advice and Susan Leigh for her
outstanding dedication in the coordination of collection
of biological samples.

INTRODUCTION

The synthetic vitamin A analog 13-cis-retinoic acid
(13-CRA) has proven a clinically useful drug in the
treatment of both neoplastic and preneoplastic diseases
(1-6). Because of this activity against established
benign and malignant lesions, the ease of its oral
administration and its relatively low incidence of
significant side effects, the clinical role of 13-CRA has
been expanded to include its use in cancer chemoprevention
trials. While the clinical pharmacology of this drug has
been well described in patients receiving 1-5 mg/kg per
day (7-10), little data exists concerning the toxicology
and pharmacokinetics of 13-CRA following the chronic daily
administration of the lower doses anticipated to be used
in cancer chemoprevention trials.

245

We and others have reported previously the human toxicology and pharmacokinetics of 13-CRA when used in high dose (i.e. 1-5 mg/kg/day) in normal subjects and cancer patients (4,7-10). Before initiating large chemoprevention trials with this agent, we decided to evaluate the toxicity and pharmacokinetics of 13-CRA in normal subjects administered daily oral doses of 0.11-0.14 mg/kg for a period of nine months. This report presents the results of our trial in ten normal subjects and establishes guidelines for the use of low dose 13-CRA in future chemoprevention trials.

METHODS

Subjects and Pre-Study Evaluation

Ten healthy volunteers (5 males and 5 females) with no history of acute or chronic illness were enrolled in this study over a period of 4 months. Subject age ranged between 21 and 50 and subject weight ranged between 65.5 and 90 kg. Women of childbearing potential were required to institute contraceptive protection and the subjects were asked to discontinue all vitamin supplements at least 2 weeks prior to the start of the trial.

Pre-study evaluations included a complete history and physical examination, CBC with differential and platelet counts and serum determinations for SGOT, LDH, alkaline phosphatase, fasting cholesterol, HDL, triglycerides, total protein, and albumin. History and physical examinations were performed monthly throughout the trial and all laboratory tests were repeated at 3, 6, and 9 months.

13-CRA Dosing and Pharmacokinetic Study Design

All subjects were administered 13-CRA in a dose of 10 mg daily to be taken at 8 a.m. in the fasting state. Since the daily dose of the drug was fixed for all subjects, the actual dose of drug on a per kilogram basis ranged between 0.11-0.14 mg/kg/day.

Pharmacokinetic studies of 13-CRA and its major

metabolite, 4-OXO-13-CRA were performed on the first day and at 3, 6, and 9 months of the trial. In addition at monthly intervals blood samples were obtained just prior to the 8 a.m. dose and 4 hours later. During the pharmacokinetic studies, 10 ml blood samples were collected in foil-wrapped vacutainers containing 200 units of sodium heparin at varying intervals up to 72 hours after drug administration. During this time, no further doses of 13-CRA were administered. Blood samples were stored on ice in the dark prior to centrifugation at 2000 X g for 10 minutes at 4°C. The plasma layer was then removed, placed in polypropylene freezer tubes (Vangard International, Inc. Neptune, NJ), and stored in the dark at -25°C until analysis. Patients were allowed to resume normal p.o. intake 3 hours after drug administration.

Toxicity Evaluation

Clinical toxicities related to 13-CRA administration were judged to be present when either the subject or the examiner noted a change from the pretreatment status. The level of toxicity was graded according to a clinical toxicity scale developed at our institution during previous investigations (Table 1).

TABLE 1

Clinical Toxicity Scale for Patients Receiving 13-Cis-Retinoic-Acid

Level I Toxicity

Dry skin, mucous membranes, mild, controlled with
  emollients
Cheilitis, mild, controlled with emollients
Epistaxis, mild, $\leq$2 episodes per week
Peeling of palms and soles, mild, controlled with
  emollients
Headache, mild, $\leq$2 per week over pretreatment incidence
Increased sunburn susceptibility
Conjunctivitis, mild, controlled with artificial tears
Menstrual changes, mild

TABLE 1 (cont.)

Level II Toxicity

Dry skin, mucous membranes, moderate, partially controlled
  with emollients
Cheilitis, moderate, partially controlled with emollients
Epistaxis, mild >2 per week, or significant epistaxis
  (>10cc) >1 episode per week
Peeling of palms and soles, moderate, partially controlled
  with emollients
Headache, mild >2 per week over pretreatment incidence
Conjunctivitis, moderate, partially controlled with
  artificial tears
Alopecia of scalp, mild
Musculoskeletal symptoms (pain, stiffness), mild
Chronic fatigue, mild (able to perform normal functions)
Dysuria (uretheral irritation), $\leq$3 episodes per week
Skin infections, $\leq$2 episodes per month
Menstrual changes, hypomenorrhea

Level III Toxicity

Dry skin, mucous membranes, severe, poorly controlled with
  emollients
Cheilitis, severe, poorly controlled with emollients
Epistaxis with significant blood loss (>10cc) >3 times per
  week
Peeling of palms and soles controlled with analgesics, >5
  per week over pretreatment incidence
Alopecia of scalp (clinically obvious) with moderate hair
  loss
Musculoskeletal symptoms (pain, stiffness), moderate,
  requiring awnalgesics for relief of symptoms
Chronic fatigue, moderate, difficulty in performing normal
  functions (working, driving)
Menstrual changes, amenorrhea

Adapted from Meyskens, FL, Goodman, GE, Alberts, DS:
13-Cis-Retinoic Acid: Pharmacology, toxicology, and
clinical applications for the prevention and treatment of
human cancer. Critical Reviews in Hematology and
Oncology, in press, 1985.

13-CRA Assay Procedure

At the time of analysis, the plasma samples were allowed to thaw in the dark at room temperature and 13-CRA plasma extraction and high performance liquid chromatography were carried out as described previously (7,11). The assay for the 4-OXO-13-CRA was carried out by a minor modification of the HPLC methodology developed by Vane and Bugge (12). The recovery of 13-CRA from plasma was linear from 10-1000 ng/ml and averaged 90% $\pm$ 6% (S.D.). The assay had a detection limit of 10 ng/ml determined on the basis of a signal equal to twice the noise level. The precision of the assay for 13-CRA was 8%.

Plasma concentration of 13-CRA versus time data were obtained from each patient and fitted to a multi-exponential equation using a non-linear regression computer program (13). Preliminary parameter estimates were obtained with the aid of a previously published computer method (14). Equations used in analysis are identical to those previously published (15).

RESULTS

Clinical Toxicity of 13-CRA

All ten of the normal subjects experienced at least level I toxicity during the 9 month trial. The toxicity was severe enough in two of the subjects to require discontinuation of the 13-CRA. Shown in Table 2 are the types and levels of toxicity experienced by the 10 volunteers. Note that the most commonly experienced toxicities were xerosis (70%) and cheilitis (80%). In general these two toxicities were well tolerated and at least partly controlled by emollients. Headaches were another common side effect of 13-CRA, but were only of grade III severity in one subject. Perhaps the most troublesome problem was musculoskeletal toxicity which was severe in two of the volunteers. One of these subjects requested discontinuation of 13-CRA after 6 months because of musculoskeletal discomfort. The other subject who requested early termination of 13-CRA experienced a large variety of symptoms, only a few of which could be directly related to 13-CRA administration. These complaints included nausea, metallic dysgeusia, increased appetite, decreased alcohol tolerance, mouth sores, swelling and bleeding of the gums, and increased irritability as well as several of the more common adverse reactions.

All five female subjects noted changes in their menstrual cycle. Four of the subjects reported hypomenorrhea. Two reported mid-cycle spotting. The fifth subject noted more frequent, longer and heavier menses, as well as post-coital bleeding.

There were no significant routine laboratory abnormalities observed during the 9 month study. One subject did have a minor elevation of serum triglycerides to 319 mg/dl (normal 50-200 mg/dl) on one occasion.

All of the toxicities related to 13-CRA administration resolved quickly and completely following termination of drug dosing. The onset of xerosis, cheilitis, eye discomfort, sensitivity to sunlight and menstrual changes were experienced during the first weeks of treatment. The more serious complaints of headaches and musculoskeletal pain or discomfort had a later onset during the trial.

TABLE 2

LOW DOSE 13-CRA IN NORMAL SUBJECTS

| | TOXICITY LEVEL* | | |
TOXICITY TYPE	I (MILD) %	II (MODERATE) %	III (SEVERE) %
Xerosis	50	20	0
Cheilitis	40	30	10
Headaches	50	10	10
Menstrual	0	100	0
Musculoskeletal	10	0	20[+]
Sensitivity to Sunlight	20	0	0
Eye Discomfort	40	0	0
Epistaxis	20	0	0
Palmar-Plantar Peeling	20	0	0

*Refer to Table 1 for Toxicity Levels
[+]Discontinued 13 CRA

Pharmacokinetics of Low Dose 13-CRA

The median interval to the achievement of peak plasma concentrations of 13-CRA and 4-OXO-13-CRA was 2 hours (range 1-4+ hours) and 7+ hours (range 1-25 hours), respectively. Shown in Table 3 are the plasma peak and trough concentrations of 13-CRA as determined at 1, 90, 180 and 270 days of administration. Note that the peak plasma concentrations of 13-CRA averaged greater than 90 ng/ml. Plasma trough concentrations of 13-CRA were observed in more than 80% of samples and averaged greater than 25 ng/ml.

Peak plasma concentrations of 4-OXO-13-CRA averaged greater than 100 ng/ml. Trough plasma concentrations of this metabolite were observed in more than 60% of blood samples and proved quite variable. There was no evidence of a rising peak or trough plasma concentration of either 13-CRA or 4-OXO-13-CRA during the 270 day trial.

The composite plasma initial phase half-life ($t^{\alpha}1/2$) of 13-CRA in the 10 subjects calculated over the 270 day trial duration was 1.6 ± 1.1 hours. The plasma terminal phase half-life ($t^{\beta}1/2$) was 28 ± 24 hours. There was a significant trend for an increasing plasma terminal phase half-life, an increasing plasma concentration . time product and a decreasing total body elimination rate for both 13-CRA and its 4-OXO metabolite between the first and last trial days. The plasma concentration . time products increased significantly (p = .018, comparing CxTs at 1 and 90 days versus 180 and 270 days) and progressively from day 1 to day 270 in 80% of the normal subjects.

A careful evaluation was performed to relate plasma peak, trough and CxT concentrations of 13 CRA and 4-OXO-13-CRA to the documented clinical toxicities. There was no obvious evidence of a relationship between any of these pharmacokinetic parameters and side effects of 13-CRA administration.

TABLE 3

PLASMA PEAK AND TROUGH CONCENTRATIONS OF LOW DOSE 13 CRA
IN NORMAL SUBJECTS

DAY ON-STUDY	NO. SUBJECTS	MEAN PEAK CONCENTRATION (NG/ML)	MEAN TROUGH* CONCENTRATION (NG/ML)
1	10	64	12
90	8	99	24
180	9	96	29+
270	7	92	29

*Trough Values Measured at 24 Hours After Last Dose
+Two Subjects Had No Measurable 13 CRA in Plasma on Day
   180 of Trial

DISCUSSION

There are plans to incorporate low daily doses of
13-CRA into several chemoprevention trials in the United
States. Although a large pool of toxicity data exist for
the use of high dose 13-CRA (i.e. doses of 1-5 mg/kg/day)
in patients with cancer and dermatological disorders
(3-5), little data has been published concerning the
toxicities of this vitamin A analog when used in
significantly lower doses for longer periods of time. The
subjects in this trial experienced a relatively high
incidence of moderate (40%) or severe (30%) toxicities
following administration of a daily dose of 10 mg.
Unfortunately, the trial design was dictated by the
availability of only 10 mg tablets of 13-CRA. Thus, daily
administration required a dose of at least .11-.14 mg/kg.
The more recent availability of 5 mg size tablets will
allow a halving of the daily dose used in this trial.
Although we could expect a lower incidence of significant
toxicities related to a 13-CRA dose of .055-.07 mg/kg/day,
further clinical pharmacology trials in normal subjects
will be required to determine the tolerance of these lower
doses. Nevertheless, on the basis of the present trial
results, we cannot recommend chronic daily dosing with the
10 mg tablets in the relatively normal subjects entered
into chemoprevention trials.

It is of considerable interest that the relatively low .11-.14 mg/kg dose of 13-CRA was associated with detectable concentrations of the parent compound and its major metabolite (i.e., 4-OXO-13-CRA) in blood samples obtained 24 hours after the last drug dose. Thus, 13-CRA dosing compliance can be monitored using HPLC assay methodology. On the basis of the mean plasma trough concentrations of 13-CRA (i.e. approximately 25 ng/ml at 24 hours after the last dose) it is not likely that the parent compound will be detectable in the majority of subjects entered into chemoprevention trials at lower doses. However, the plasma trough concentrations of the 4-OXO-13-CRA metabolites could prove useful for monitoring dosing compliance of 13-CRA in future chemoprevention trials which use even lower doses of the drug.

It is unfortunate that the clinical toxicities associated with 13-CRA administration could not be predicted by plasma concentrations of either the parent compound or its major metabolite. Thus, future chemoprevention trials with this agent cannot rely on plasma monitoring of the parent compound or metabolite in order to anticipate serious toxicities.

REFERENCES

1.   Bollag W: Vitamin A and vitamin A acid in the
      prophylaxis and therapy of epithelial tumors. Int J
      Vit Res 40:299-314, 1976.

2.   Bollag W: Vitamin A and retinoids: from nutrition
      to pharmacotherapy in dermatology and oncology.
      Lancet 1:860-863, 1983.

3.   Haydey RP, Reed ML, Dzubow LM et al.: Treatment of
      keratoacanthormas with oral 13-cis-retinoic acid. N
      Engl J Med 303:560-562, 1980.

4.   Meyskens FL Jr, Gilmartin E, Alberts DS, Levine NS,
      Brooks R, Salmon SE, and Surwit EA: Activity of
      isotretinoin against squamous cell cancers and
      preneoplastic lesions. Cancer Treat Rep
      66:1315-1319, 1982.

5.   Levine N, Miller RC, and Meyskens FL Jr: Oral
      13-cis-retinoic acid therapy for multiple cutaneous
      squamous cell carcinomas and keratoacanthomas. Arch
      Derm 120:1215-1217, 1984.

6.   Kessler JF, Meyskens FL Jr, Levine N, Lynch PJ, and
      Jones SE: Treatment of cutaneous T-cell lymphoma
      (mycosis fungoides) with 13-cis-retinoid acid.
      Lancet 1:1345-1347, 1983.

7.   Goodman GE, Einspahr JG, Alberts DS, Davis TP, Leigh,
      SA, Chen HSG, and Meyskens, FL Jr: Pharmacokinetics
      of 13-cis-retinoic acid in patients with advanced
      cancer. Cancer Res 42:2087-2091, 1982.

8.   Brazzell RK and Colburn WA: Pharmacology and
      toxicology of oral retinoids: Pharmacokinetics of
      the retinoids isotretinoin and etretinate: a
      comparative review. Am Acad Dermatol 6:643-651, 1982.

9.   Khoo K-C, Reik D, and Colburn, WA: Pharmacokinetics
      of isotretinoin following a single oral dose. J Clin
      Pharmacol 22:395-402, 1982.

10. Kerr IG, Lippman ME, Jenkins J, and Myers CE:
    Pharmacology of 13-cis-retinoic acid in humans.
    Cancer Res 42:2069-2073, 1982.

11. Davis TP, Peng Y-M, Goodman GE, and Alberts DS:
    HPLC, MS, and pharmacokinetics of melphalan,
    bisantrene and 13-cis retinoic acid. J of
    Chromatographic Science 20:511-516, 1982.

12. Vane FJ and Bugge CJL: Identification of
    4-oxo-13-cis-retinoic acid as the major metabolite of
    13-cis-retinoic acid in human blood. Fed Proc
    39:757, 1980.

13. Metzler CM: Nonlin: a computer program for parameter
    estimation in non-linear situations. Technical
    Report 7292/69/7272/005. Kalamazoo, Mich.: UpJohn
    Co., 1969.

14. Sedman AJ and Wagner JG: CSTRIP: a Fortran IV
    Computer program for obtaining initial
    polyexponential parameter estimates. J Pharm Sci
    65:1006-1010, 1976.

15. Alberts DS, Chang SY, Chen HSG, Evans TL, and Moon
    TE: Oral melphalan kinetics. Clin Pharmacol Ther
    26:737-745, 1979.

CHANGING THE PUBLIC'S HEALTH BEHAVIORS BY

DIET AND CHEMOPREVENTIVE INTERVENTIONS

Curtis Mettlin   Ph.D.

Roswell Park Memorial Institute

Buffalo, New York   14263

INTRODUCTION

In the last decade, cancer prevention has
witnessed a great increase in the importance
attached to diet and related chemopreventive
interventions. There are several apparent
stimuli for this. Firstly, the positive health
value of nutrition in general and of some specific nutrients may be an outgrowth of developments
in basic laboratory studies of carcinogenesis.
As the number of substances examined in laboratory models grew, it was perhaps inevitable that
some test substances would prove to have inhibitory, rather than carcinogenic, effects. Indeed,
the application of basic carcinogenesis research
methodology has proved as capable of identifying
inhibitors as carcinogens.

A second underlying force stimulating
interest in diet and cancer prevention has been
the work of epidemiologists who, in multiple
investigations have demonstrated that it is possible to assess, even if only in a crude fashion,
exposures to dietary phenomenon which may be
associated with cancer risk. Thirdly, clinicians
treating cancer patients have shown that nutritional variables may affect significantly the

257

course of treatment and recovery and this work
indirectly may have supported the work of others
in the field of disease etiology and cancer prevention.

As these multiple threads of research begin
to form a fabric of understanding of the role of
diet and nutrition in cancer causation, the time
is approaching when another group, the public
health practitioner, takes interest in the subject. Herein, we examine some of the concepts
and principles involved in the translation of
basic knowledge of cause and prevention into
interventions which may be effective in reducing
risk to the population and rates of disease
occurrence and mortality.

This topic is deserving of scrutiny in its
own right because past experience has shown that
a considerable gap may occur between the discovery of the scientific leads to cancer prevention,
the confirmation of these leads to sufficient
satisfaction of reasonable observers, and the
application of the knowledge in a manner that
actually leads to risk reduction. Nearly twenty
years passed between the early identification of
the risk of cigarette smoking and the documenta-
tion of an official scientific consensus. Even
three decades after the early epidemiologic dis-
coveries, one third of the US population continues to smoke. Similarly, the basic discovery
essential to the pap smear occurred nearly four
decades before the truly widescale implementation
of this early detection tool was achieved. Any
expectation that present-day novel research
results regarding the modulation of cancer by
micronutrients, vitamins, or even macro
nutrients, will ipso facto prevent cancer, is not
realistic given the track record of implementation of chronic disease prevention measures.

REQUIREMENTS FOR PUBLIC HEALTH INTERVENTIONS

The conditions for successful intervention
are relatively well understood and have been

discussed   elsewhere   at some   length   (1).   The
essential   requirements for successful   intervention are believed to include: 1) the presence of
a significant health risk,   2) credible and   compelling scientific evidence of the factors   that
lead   to that risk,   3) a behavior change in response   to   the risk that is compatible   with   the
attitudinal   and   behavioral   complexion   of   the
individual, and 4) a social and cultural environment   that is supportive of the desired   behavior
change.   Each of these elements may independently
retard or accelerate the pace of change toward   a
desired public health response.

The   perception of serious health risk   with
respect   to   nutrient intervention and cancer   is
perhaps the easiest condition to   satisfy.   Conventional   public wisdom is that cancer is   among
the   most serious health risks that one can   face
and   this has been documented in well   conducted
public surveys (2).   The reports of the National
Cancer Institute SEER program annually   reinforce
this perception,   documenting as they do the fact
that   cancer   continues to be the second   leading
cause of death in the nation.

The   establishment of the second   condition,
convincing scientific evidence,   is proving   more
difficult.   The   need   strong evidence has   been
expressed well by Ahrens (3) who points out   that
the   current state of our diet is presumed to   be
the   result   of   a sum of forces   that   represent
progress and that proponents of change must   bear
the burden of proof.   While our knowledge of the
cancer-related   roles of vitamins and other   nutrients   has   expanded immensely in recent   years,
the   nature of the research tools that have   been
applied   thus   far reasonably invite   public   and
professional skepticism.

Laboratory   and   animal   models   inevitably
suffer from the fact that an inferential leap   of
uncertain   validity   must be made to apply   those
results to human health.   International correlations   of dietary practices and disease risk   are
potentially fallacious because they fail to   take

into account the numerous other differences in populations that may contribute to differences in disease risk.

Some have argued, correctly, that epidemiologic studies of the diets of persons with cancer, compared to those without, are superior for testing hypotheses about diet and cancer risk. However, where populations are generally exposed to risk enhancing factors, insufficient contrast between cases and controls may be present to assess risk. Thus, while numerous case control studies have shown effects for vitamin A and cancer risk, the fact that the U.S. population generally ingests a high fat diet makes this study design of limited value for this aspect of diet.

To establish convincingly the association of a dietary factor to cancer risk it appears necessary that the hypotheses which appear most important and promising be tested by the most rigorous and convincing means. At present, the most convincing research tool we have is the randomized, controlled clinical trial and several such trials of nutritional factors and cancer are underway or are being planned. A good example of this is the so-called Physicians' Health Study which is investigating the prophylactic potential of beta-carotene among over 20,000 U.S. physicians. Other important examples of such trials are those studying retinoids and skin cancer, and antioxidants and colorectal polyps.

Particularly when applied to study of the diet, as opposed to chemopreventive supplementation, such trials have major inherent difficulties that are not experienced when one studies the efficacy of a medication or treatment. These problems include:

    1. achieving compliance to the dietary intervention,

    2. the infeasibility of providing placebos to control subjects,

3. the inspecificity of the intervention (eg. one dietary change brings about many other changes, thusly confounding interpretation of results),

4. the control group can not be isolated from general dietary trends affecting the population,

5. the effects of dietary intervention may not be evident until long after the intervention, and

6. the trial participants may be an unrepresentative subset of the population.

In spite of these difficulties, dietary intervention trials have been conducted successfully. The experience of researchers of heart disease risk offers some guidance in this regard. However, the several cholesterol lowering trials differ significantly from cancer prevention trials in that the intervention typically is not on some serum measure that may be manipulated by a variety of dietary interventions or by pharmacologic means, but rather, on a particular dietary exposure which may be affected only by affecting that exposure. Thus, the cholesterol lowering strategy of altering multiple aspects of the diet to achieve a desired biochemical change will not be suitable for cancer prevention trials because the multiplicity of changes may confound the identification of the responsible factor, should an effect be observed.

The third requirement for life-style change to promote public health is that the behavior change desired be compatible with the attitudinal and behavioral make-up of the individual. This concept of cultural compatibility is derived from anthropological and communications research on the diffusion of innovations in a population. This work shows that the most compatible changes tend to be those that require change in the least

number of aspects of the individual. This concept would suggest that change in diet may be
most successful when the focus is narrowed.
Attention to individual nutrients may yield more
evident benefit than will general prescriptions
for dietary change such as are incorporated in
the concept of the "prudent diet."

Finally, behavior is, in large part, a social
product and behavior change may be expected also
to be largely a social product. Dietary habits
are influenced during childhood socialization,
modified by the forces of economics and food
marketing and, supported and altered by the
influences of family and other companions. Risk
factor intervention studies previously have shown
that involvement of a spouse in the process of
change may be an important determinant of compliance to the intervention and the ability to
maintain long-term adherence to a clinical trial
protocol (4,5).

FEASIBILITY OF ALTERNATIVE APPROACHES

Considering the factors that effect the
capability to affect changes in lifestyle to promote public health, we may differentiate types of
dietary interventions with respect to their prospects as public health tools. Dietary changes
and interventions by means of micronutrients or
comparable synthetic inhibitors such as beta-
carotene or retinoids, as opposed to macro nutrients such as fat or fiber, generally have not
been differentiated with respect to their potentials for implementation. Yet, given their
different natures, it is reasonable to expect
that that different nutritional interventions
will have distinct advantages and disadvantages.

The tables below list advantages of interventions through chemopreventive means as opposed
to dietary changes. By chemopreventive we refer
to those interventions which may be accomplished
by supplementation of foods or potables with
inhibitors of carcinogenesis or by individual

prescription of substances to individuals at specific levels of cancer risk. Dietary change on, the other hand, refers to modification of general practices of food purchase, preparation, and consumption.

Table 1
Advantages of Chemopreventive
Interventions

1. Compatibility of intervention

2. Specificity of effects

3. Celerity of impact

Table 2
Advantages of Dietary Intervention

1. Self-sustaining

2. Multiplicity of effects

3. Diffusiveness of impact

The potential advantages of chemopreventive interventions include the possibilities that they be accomplished with little active response on the part of the target population in much the same manner as ordinary foodstuffs are supplemented with vitamins or water is fluoridated. Assuming that our understanding achieves such a level, specific agents may be prescribed to specific populations at risk of given cancers, eg. a lung protective agent for heavy smokers, a breast protective agent for women at high risk of breast cancer etc. Finally given the specificity with which they agents may be applied and their potential potency, effects may be achieved more quickly than would be possible with interventions that require more generalized social and behavioral change.

Dietary interventions, in contrast, have the potential advantages of being sustained by social habit once achieved, of yielding multiple effects such as the prevention of cancer as well as coronary heart disease, and of generally affecting the population rather than specific target groups. A major drawback of dietary interventions intended for an entire population may be the length of time that will be required to achieve them.

Figure 1 illustrates the increasing, calorie standardized, levels of fat consumption reflected by U.S. food expenditure data between 1915 and 1983 (6). These five-year moving averages show a 25% increase with the recent data suggesting a leveling of the trend. One projected line indicates the time that would be required to achieve a 25% reduction in fat consumption if we were to sustain a rate of decrease comparable to the rate of increase previously observed. The steeper line reflects the rate of change that must be sustained if we are to reduce fat intake by 25% by the end of the century. The latter is probably a pace of change that is not possible to achieve in light of present-day food habits and food marketing practices.

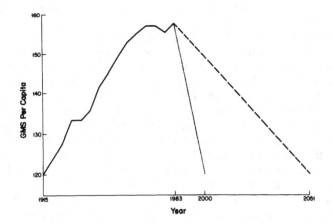

Fig. 1 Past and Projected Fat Consumption Trends (US expenditures, calorie-adj, 5-yr moving avg)

This illustration may suggest, however, that any clinical trials which attempt significant reductions in fat consumption may be protected, in the short term, from secular trends in the population. It may be reasonable to expect that a group of control subjects would change their fat consumption relatively little over the next decade if not intervened upon.

SUMMARY

The concept of cancer prevention by means of nutritional or chemopreventive manipulation offers interesting potential as a means of public health control of cancer. The gaps in our knowledge remain great and it is important that, whenever possible, the scientific community move beyond laboratory and observational studies to research designs which offer the greatest rigor and which will have the greatest impact on public perception. Controlled clinical trials are perhaps the most powerful tool we have to study potential public health interventions. This approach, however, has many limitations when applied to human populations.

It also is important to consider the behavioral determinants of acceptance of dietary and chemopreventive interventions. Little research on this subject currently is available but relevant models may be derived from previous research on the diffusion of innovations and on the acceptance of dietary interventions for other chronic diseases.

Finally, little consideration has been given to the differing potentials of different types of dietary and nutritional interventions. Selection of research and intervention approaches may affect significantly the future level of effort and time-frames required for meaningful progress.

REFERENCES

1. Mettlin C, Prerequisites to successful life-
   style intervention. Social Science and Medicine, 13A:559, 1979.

2. James WG, Lieberman S, What the American public knows and does about cancer and cancer
   tests. UICC Technical Series Report 45:66,
   1978.

3. Ahrens EH, Diet and heart disease: shaping
   public perception when proof is lacking.
   Arteriosclerosis. 2:85, 1982.

4. Streja DA, Boyko E, Rabkin SW, Predictor of
   outcome in a risk factor intervention
   trial using behavior modification. Preventive
   Medicine, 11:291, 1982.

5. Witschi JC, Singer M, Wu-Lee M, Stare FJ, Family cooperation and effectiveness in a
   cholesterol lowering diet. Journal of the
   American Dietetic Association, 72:384, 1978.

6. United States Department of Agriculture Eco-
   nomic Research Service, Food Consumption,
   Prices and Expenditures. USDA-ERS Statistical
   Bulletin, Number 713, 1984.

DESIGN AND COMPLIANCE CONSIDERATIONS

OF DIETARY INTERVENTION TRIALS

THOMAS E. MOON, PhD
RESEARCH PROFESSOR OF MEDICINE
ASSISTANT DIRECTOR, CANCER CENTER
DIRECTOR OF BIOMETRY, COMPUTING & EPIDEMIOLOGY

STEVEN ROSS RODNEY, B.S.
RESEARCH ASSISTANT
BIOMETRY, COMPUTING & EPIDEMIOLOGY

YEI-MEI PENG, PhD
RESEARCH ASSISTANT
PROFESSOR OF INTERNAL MEDICINE

DAVID S. ALBERTS, M.D.
PROFESSOR OF MEDICINE AND PHARMACOLOGY

FRANK MEYSKENS, M.D.
PROFESSOR OF MEDICINE
DIRECTOR OF CANCER PREVENTION AND CONTROL

ARIZONA CANCER CENTER AT THE
UNIVERSITY OF ARIZONA
TUCSON, ARIZONA 85724

Supported in part by National Cancer
Institute Grants CA 34256, CA27502
and CA27504

INTRODUCTION

Clinical trials are widely used and accepted as the best method to evaluate the effect of therapy or prophylactic interventions. The design of cancer prevention trials are based on the same principles as cancer therapy trials (Peto, et al, 1976). However, there are a number of important differences in the methodology, logistics and costs of prevention trials as contrasted to therapy trials. A clear recognition and careful consideration of such differences provide a better study design resulting in improved evaluation of cancer prophylactic interventions.

The Chemoprevention of Skin Cancer by Retinoids Trial will be used for illustration. The trial is currently being carried out by investigators at the Arizona Cancer Center in collaboration with community dermatologists. Persons eligible for enrollment in the study have a history of ten or more actinic keratoses as diagnosed by one of the dermatologists in the Tucson, Arizona area. Participants in the trial are randomly assigned to either retinol (25,000 IU/day) or placebo in a double blinded design. The objectives of the trial include the comparison of newly diagnosed skin cancer.

CLINICAL TRIALS

Items for consideration during the design of a clinical trial are numerous (Table 1). The design of a clinical trial substantially impacts its conduct, analysis and scientific impact. Principles common to all clinical trials include a design that is efficient and provides integrity to the results (Staquet, 1984). Ethical considerations also apply to all clinical trials but have an increased emphasis because the intervention is commonly applied to currently healthy people. Methods, logistics and costs are of major importance in the design of all clinical trials. However, methods and logistics are more complex and costs are greater in prophylactic trials and thus deserve added consideration (Magnus and Miller, 1980).

Evaluation of Interventions

Evaluation of a prophylactic intervention follows the same general developmental steps as commonly used for the evaluation of a new therapy.
These steps include preclinical evaluation and a hierarchy of clinical trials commonly called Phase I-IV. Sequential evaluation of an intervention through the preclinical and clinical phases provides increasing information as to biologic efficacy of the intervention, safety and applicability to a population at risk of cancer. The preclinical evaluation can be used to screen different dietary interventions in a panel of animal models using different animals species, and different carcinogens acting at different tumor sites. Different intervention schedules and doses should also be evaluated. The primary objective of a Phase I clinical trial is the definition of a safe range of doses and schedules that are applicable to a human population. Generally, only acute toxicities would be identified during a Phase I trial. The primary objective of a Phase II clinical trial is to evaluate the effectiveness of an intervention dose and schedule identified during the Phase I trial. It is hoped that ineffective or toxic interventions will be identified during a Phase II trial and that additional clinical evaluation will not be carried out using that same intervention dose and schedule.

A Phase II trial of a dietary intervention can evaluate the feasibility of identifying, recruiting and following study participants. Recruitment and follow-up procedures include the motivation and evaluation of subject compliance. There appears to be methodologic limitations in the use of Phase II clinical trials for evaluating dietary interventions.

The number of subjects enrolled in a Phase II trial of a dietary intervention need be substantially greater than for the evaluation of a cancer therapy. This is a result of the low annual incidence of cancer and the necessity to evaluate not only accute life threatening toxicities but also toxicities that would reduce participant compliance to the intervention. The annual incidence of even the most common type of cancer is very low. Subjects with 10 or more prior actinic keratoses have an estimated annual incidence of basal or squamous skin cancers of approximately 3.5 %. However, women with a high risk of breast cancer due to family history of breast cancer and men with an extensive 40+ pack-year history of cigarette smoking have approximately a 1% per year annual incidence of the respective cancers of the breast and lung. The incidence of other cancers is substantially lower. The perception of the study participant versus the perception of the trial coordinators may differ in their interpretation of severity and acceptability of non-life threatening toxicity associated with the intervention. For example, study participants may tolerate some degree of skin toxicity associated with some synthetic retinoids. A Phase II trial can estimate the compliance and the associated toxicity using the selected dose and schedule. The sample size of a Phase II trial of a dietary intervention must be in direct proportion to the incidence of cancer and the incidence of toxicity to be evaluated. A working procedure is to evauate approximately the same number of study participants as the reciprocal of the incidence of toxicity. For example, 500 study participants need to be evaluated in order to have slightly better than a 50-50 chance of identifying a toxicity with an incidence of 1 in 500. However, even this large number of study participants would be inadequate to expect to observe one or more cases of a toxicity with an incidence of 1 in 1,000. In addition, the low frequency of cancer incidence and the heterogenous distribution of persons at high risk to cancer in a population severely limits the traditional Phase II trial's ability to evaluate efficacy of a cancer prophylactic intervention.

The importance of a careful hierarchical evaluation of a dietary intervention must be maintained. Information obtained from epidemiological studies has been of value in the choice of retinoids and carotenoids for several ongoing chemoprevention trials. However, epidemiological studies will have more limited value as synthetic analogs of nutrients are developed and evaluated. Results of animal studies with tumors induced by carcinogens permit laboratory evaluation of doses and schedules of dietary interventions. However, substantially more research is required in order to correctly identify which animal species, which carcinogenic initiators and promoters and which animal tumor sites are best predictive for the evaluation of cancer prevention agents in humans.

Thus, a Phase II trial of a dietary intervention for the prevention of cancer has as its achievable objectives the estimation of study feasibility and intervention safety. The ability to estimate intervention efficacy appears to have to be deferred to the Phase III comparative trial, thus requiring substantially large numbers of participants. Such a deferral of the evalution of efficacy implies that dietary interventions will be determined feasible but later found to lack efficacy during the Phase III trial. This will result in increased costs not only due to the larger number of participants required during the evaluation of a dietary intervention, but also because interventions will be passed on to a Phase III trial that may lack efficacy. This emphasizes the importance of reducing the cost associated with Phase III trials of cancer prevention interventions.

Sample Size and Compliance:

Calculation of sample size of a clinical trial is related to the phase of the clinical evaluation, underlying incidence of cancer and toxicity in the study population and the statistical uncertainty. For a Phase III or IV trial, the reduction of incidence of cancer due to the active intervention must also be specified. The resulting sample size often is larger for prevention trials as contrasted to therapy trials.

Investigators planning a dietary intervention study must keep in mind that the calculated sample size is the minimum number of subjects needed and assumes that participants are 100% compliant to the prescribed intervention. The actual sample size required for a dietary intervention study must be greater than the calculated sample size. The impact of low compliance has an inverse relationship on sample size. Thus, participant compliance must be considered in the design of a dietary intervention trial. The understanding of medication compliance and methods to motivate high compliance has greatly expanded during the past few years (Haynes, et al, 1980).

All subjects randomly allocated during a Phase III or IV trial to active or control intervention must be included in the comparison to assure the basis for statistical inferences. The use of a placebo run-in period during which all participants enrolled on study are assigned to placebo permits an evaluation of compliance prior to random allocation. This permits the identification of subjects unable or unwilling to comply with a prescribed intervention schedule and thus their elimination prior to the random assignment procedure. If the dietary intervention can be formulated as a capsule, then the participant need not be aware (blinded) of the placebo run-in procedure. Even if blinding is not possible, the use of such a placebo run-in period may be of value. For example, in our ongoing Skin Cancer Prevention Trial amongst persons with 10 or more actinic keratoses, a five month placebo run-in period is utilized. Preliminary data based upon the first 226 persons entered on trial indicates that persons wishing to drop out of the study do so during the first two months after enrollment.

A number of methods have been suggested for the evaluation of participant compliance to the prescribed intervention. Methods currently being used in our ongoing Skin Cancer Prevention Trial include both subjective as well as objective measures of compliance. Subjective methods include the participants self reporting of their level of compliance, use of a pill calendar in which the participant is asked to fill out the time each day they take their capsule or to indicate they did not take their capsule, and the (pill count) number of capsules returned at each follow-up visit to the Skin Cancer Prevention Clinic. Data based upon the first 80 subjects completing the five month run-in period indicates that all subjects reported that they had missed no more than 20% of their capsules. Based upon pill count, 95% of the participants had taken at least 80% of their capsules.

The use of a pharmacologic assessment of blood or urine levels of the dietary intervention, its metabolite or a marker compound would provide information that could be used to objectively evaluate and, if needed, improve participant compliance. A pilot study evaluating feasibility for use of riboflavin to objectively monitor medication compliance was carried out in 33 consecutive particpants enrolled on the ongoing Skin Cancer Prevention Trial. The protocol for this pilot study included the addition of 10 milligrams of riboflavin per day to the participants' capsules. Similar packaging and labeling was used for all capsules. Following the same enrollment procedures participants on this pilot study were sent requests through the U. S. Mail during each of their first four months on-study. The mail procedure requested each pilot study participant to obtain a urine specimen, place it in the mailable container provided and send it back to the Skin Cancer Prevention Clinic using a self addressed, stamped envelope. Participants were informed that urine specimens were required to monitor safety. The mail requests were sent to each pilot study participant during a randomly selected Friday each month. Upon receiving the returned urine specimens at the Skin Cancer Prevention Clinic, they were stored under refrigeration and analyzed for riboflavin content using a highly sensitive and specific HPLC assay.

Results of the riboflavin ancillary study were based upon 27 participants who returned a urine specimen for at least one of the four requests. Six study subjects were not evaluable. Four subjects were not included in this evaluation, as they terminated their study participation during the first month on trial, and two subjects reported supplementing their dietary intake with B Vitamins. Of the 27 evaluable subjects, Table 2 illustrates that 24 returned a urine specimen following the first mail request. Similarly, 25 subjects returned a urine specimen following the second, third and fourth mail request. Assay of urine specimens indicated that 100% of subjects returning urine specimens had substantial increases in urinary riboflavin content over their on study (pre-dosing) urinary levels. Ninety-two percent (23/25) of the subjects returning a urine specimen following the fourth mail request indicated high levels of riboflavin in their urine. The preliminary analysis and results of this pilot study suggests that use of riboflavin as a marker for patient compliance is feasible. It is interesting to note that the objective riboflavin assay results were consistent with the subjective reports provided by the participants in the form of self reporting compliance as well as returning unused capsules.

Limitations in the use of riboflavin or analysis of blood or urine levels for the intervention or its metabolite are important to point out. Both riboflavin and several of the retinoids have a plasma disappearance half-life of a few hours. This suggests that the ability to monitor compliance to the prescribed intervention is limited to a valuation of whether or not the participant took a capsule during the previous day. Use of riboflavin to

evaluate compliance prior to the previous day is not
currently evaluable with any reliability.

Table 3 shows the impact of non-compliance on the
statistical power and thus ability of the trial to
correctly identify a significant reduction in cancer
incidence for an efficacious intervention. Assuming that
the background incidence of cancer is 3% per year and the
intervention is anticipated to have a 1.5% per year
incidence (50% reduction in incidence) then Table 3
illustrates three different hypothetical levels of
compliance. Lack of compliance is assumed in this
illustration to mean that the participant stops all
consumption of the intervention but continues under
follow-up with ascertainment of endpoints (diagnosis of
cancer). When study subjects have a 100% compliance and
the trial was designed to have a power of 0.80, then the
observed statistical power assuming complete follow-up of
participants would also be 0.80. A compliance of 50%
meaning that half of the persons regularly allocated to
the active intervention would in fact not be compliant
with the intervention, thus having the same cancer
incidence as placebo controls would have an observed
annual cancer incidence of 2.3%. In addition,
participants with a 50% compliance would have a reduction
in their statistical power to 0.29. Similarly, if all
subjects allocated to the active intervention in fact did
not take the intervention (resulting in 0% compliance)
then both subjects assigned to the active as well as
subjects assigned to the placebo intervention would have
the same 3% per year cancer incidence rate and a
resulting statistical power would be 0.0.

Delayed Effect of Intervention

A dietary intervention trial should not be terminated too
early. The duration of an intervention trial should be
carefully planned to include considerations of the total
number of participants but also the desired number of
events. The number and rate of cancers diagnosed during
the first few months of a trial should be carefully
monitored not only for the ongoing evaluation of
intervention efficacy, but also for the determination of
a possible delayed effect of the intervention. The
occurence of cancers during the first few months of the
trial may not reflect an effective intervention but may
only reflect participants who had developed cancer but

were not diagnosed at the time they were enrolled on study. In addition, a dietary intervention may not have prophylactic effects if a patient is far along the carcinogenesis process. Such subjects may not have a diagnosis of cancer and appear to be eligible for inclusion in the trial but may unknowingly be too far advanced along the carcinogenesis process for the intervention to have any efficacy. Such subjects would be observed to have a diagnosis of cancer within the first few months after their enrollment on study. They may have a similar incidence of cancer as the control subjects during their first few months on study. The impact of such a delayed effect on the evaluation of the intervention is shown in Table 4. Assuming that the study has been designed to continue for five years at the end of which there would be an 80% statistical power associated with a reduction from 3% per year in the control group to a cancer incidence of 1.5% per year in the intervention group. The anticipated reduction in cancer incidence in the active intervention group implicitly assumes that the intervention would be equally effective on all study participants. Table 4 illustrates that the statistical power would be reduced to an observed value of 0.71 if all participants have the same 3% per year cancer incidence during their first year of follow-up on study. Similarly, if the period of delayed effect of the active intervention were to persist during the initial two years, then the statistical power would be reduced to 0.57. This results in slightly better than a 50-50 chance of correctly identifying an active itervention that requires two years of administration before cancer incidence rates are reduced.

SUMMARY

There are similarities but many differences between the design of dietary cancer prophylactic and therapy trials. All clinical trials are based upon the same principles but have different degrees of similarity and difference with regard to methods and logistics of their conduct. Dietary intervention trials have similar methods but require special consideration for the impact of intervention compliance and the duration of time before the intervention shows an effect. Such issues can have substantial impact upon sample size and the ability to draw accurate conclusions from the trial. These and other factors result in substantially higher costs for the clinical evaluation of a dietary intervention. An important consideration is the identification and careful evaluation of less expensive study designs that adequately evaluate the efficacy and resulting acceptability of a dietary intervention by the American population.

TABLE 1

DESIGN OF INTERVENTION TRIALS

Principles

    Efficient Study Design
    Integrity of Study

Ethics

Methods and Logistics

    Selection of Interventions and Subjects
    Assignment of Interventions
    Follow-up
    Compliance
    Sample Size
    Trial Duration
    Evaluation of Endpoint
    Stopping Rule
    Analysis
    Interpretation

Costs

TABLE 2

COMPLIANCE EVALUATION USING RIBOFLAVIN

SPECIMENS REQUESTED

SUBJECTS	1st	2nd	3rd	4th
RETURNING SPECIMENS	24	25	25	25
COMPLIANCE	100%	100%	100%	92%

TABLE 3

IMPACT OF NON-COMPLIANCE ON STATISTICAL POWER

COMPLIANCE	ANNUAL INCIDENCE		STATISTICAL POWER	
	Anticipated	Observed	Anticipated	Observed
100%	1.5%	1.5	.80	.80
50%	1.5%	2.3%	.80	.29
0%	1.5%	3.0%	.80	0

TABLE 4

IMPACT OF DELAYED EFFECT OF
INTERVENTION ON STATISTICAL POWER

STUDY DURATION (YEARS)	PERIOD OF DELAYED EFFECT (YEARS)	STATISTICAL POWER	
		ANTICIPATED	OBSERVED
5	1	.80	.71
5	2	.80	.57

REFERENCES

Haynes, R.B., et al: Patient Compliance to Prescribed Anti-
hypertensive Medication Regimens: A Report to the
National Heart, Lung and Blood Institute, U.S. Dept.
of Health and Human Services, NIH, Publication No.
81-2101, October, 1980.

Magnus, K. and Miller, A.B.: Controlled Prophylactic Trials
in Cancer. JNCI, Vol. 64, No. 4, 693-699, 1980.

Peto, R., Pike, M.C., Armitage, P., Breslow, N.E., Cox,
D.R., Howard, S.V., Mantel, N., McPherson, K., Peto, J.
and Smith, P.G.: Design and Analysis of Randomized
Clinical Trials Requiring Prolonged Observation of Each
Patient, I. Introduction and Design. Brit. J. of Cancer,
34:585-612, 1976.

Staquet, M.: Critical Evaluation of Clinical Trials in
Oncology. Current Concepts in Oncology, 17-22, Winter,
1984.

METHODOLOGIC ISSUES IN CLINICAL TRIALS

Charles H. Hennekens,MD and Sherry Mayrent,PhD

The Channing Laboratory, Departments of Medicine, and Preventive Medicine and Clinical Epidemiology, Harvard Medical School and Brigham
and Women's Hospital, 55 Pond Avenue, Brookline
MA   02146

ABSTRACT

Careful planning of clinical trials is essential to
achieve valid results. If the trial is randomized and well
designed with respect to timing, choice of study population,
completeness of follow-up, high levels of compliance, magnitude of the likely risk reduction, and the accumulation
of sufficient endpoints, it can provide reliable evidence
on the effects of a particular intervention. The Physicians' Health Study, a randomized trial among 21,989 U.S.
male physicians, aged 40 to 84 years, is evaluating beta-
carotene supplementation in the prevention of cancer and
aspirin consumption in the reduction of cardiovascular
mortality, using a 2x2 factorial design. The choice of
physicians as the study population and the implementation
of a pre-randomization run-in period have resulted in 90.2%
compliance with the assigned treatment regimen after two
years, as well as 99.6% morbidity and 100% mortality follow-up. The goal of these methodologic considerations is
to design clinical trials which can clearly prove or refute
the hypotheses being tested.

The eventual success or failure of any clinical trial
is often directly related to the care with which it is designed, since inadequate attention to methodologic issues
can lead to uninformative results. If a trial is well designed and of adequate sample size, random allocation of

283

the exposure achieves control of both known and unknown
confounding variables. If, in addition, follow-up and compliance rates are high, the randomized trial can offer the
most reliable evidence about true effects of an intervention, thus making it the most powerful tool of the epidemi-
ologist (1).

The Physicians' Health Study (PHS), a randomized trial
of beta-carotene in the prevention of cancer and aspirin in
the reduction of cardiovascular mortality among U.S. male
physicians, aged 40-84, was implemented after several years
of planning and pilot studies to resolve methodologic con-
cerns which may have general applicability to other trials.
This report outlines these issues and describes how they
were dealt with in this large-scale trial.

CHOICE OF HYPOTHESIS AND TIMING

Once the possibility of evaluating a particular agent
has been raised, the investigators must consider whether
mounting a trial is appropriate, on the basis of a number
of considerations, including ethics and feasibility. With
respect to ethics, because the researchers themselves determine whether participants do or do not receive a particular intervention, there must be sufficient doubt about the
efficacy of that intervention to permit withholding it from
half of the individuals enrolled and, at the same time,
sufficient belief in its potential to justify exposing the
other half. From a practical point of view, it is optimal
that an intervention not yet have become standard practice,
due to the consequent difficulties in selecting the study
population.

When the PHS was conceived, the aspirin/cardiovascular
disease hypothesis was quite mature, having been derived
from laboratory studies, observational epidemiology, and
a number of randomized trials of secondary prevention (2).
The need for a trial of aspirin among those with no previous history of myocardial infarction was clear, and it
was important to conduct it soon, before a large number of
healthy people began taking aspirin prophylactically on the
basis of the secondary prevention studies. The situation
was very different for beta-carotene, since the possibility
that it might reduce cancer risk was only one of a number
of untested hypotheses concerning chemoprevention of cancer
by micronutrients (3-6). Nevertheless, the use of nutri-

tional supplements was already widespread (7-8) and seemed
likely to continue to increase even in the absence of sound
evidence about possible health benefits. It therefore seemed
important, despite the relative lack of supporting data, to
begin a trial of beta-carotene as soon as possible, since
any delay might have made it less feasible to conduct in
the future.

DESIGN EFFICIENCY

Once it is determined that a trial is both scientifi-
cally justified and timely, another major consideration is
the choice of the optimal design features. In the case of
the PHS, since there was no reason to believe the aspirin
and beta-carotene would interact with each other materially,
it seemed both possible and desirable to study them together without compromising the effect of either. We therefore
decided to implement a 2x2 factorial design (9), in which
participants are assigned at random to treatment A or B to
address one scientific question and within each treatment
group are further randomized to treatment alpha or beta to
address a second issue. The principal advantage of this
factorial design is the ability to answer two unrelated
questions in a single trial for only a marginal increase in
cost. Moreover, the use of this design also allowed us to
couple the relatively immature beta-carotene hypothesis with
the more mature aspirin question, thus resolving the timing
difficulty discussed earlier.

In the PHS, where a reasonable dose and frequency of
the two agents tested seemed to be a single pill every other
day (10), an additional practical advantage of the 2x2 design
was our ability to give participants calendar packs (supplied by Bristol Myers) containing one pill daily, a white
tablet (containing 325 mg Bufferin or its placebo, supplied
by Bristol Myers) on odd-numbered days, alternating with a
red capsule (containing 50 mg Lurotin or its placebo, supplied by BASF) on even numbered days. This regimen enhances
compliance, since it is much easier to get into the routine
of taking a daily pill than to remember to take one ever
other day.

OBTAINING COMPLETE FOLLOW-UP AND CHOICE OF STUDY POPULATION

A second issue to be considered in designing a trial is
ensuring the ability to obtain complete follow-up information

from all participants. Complete follow-up is essential to
the validity of the study results, since high losses to
follow-up render results uninterpretable. In this regard,
our choice of physicians as the study population was important, since they are far less mobile and much easier to
trace than members of the general population. Furthermore,
our pilot studies indicated that over 93% of participating
doctors would return their study questionnaires, that telephone contacts would be effective in obtaining complete
follow-up information from most of the small proportion of
non-respondents, and that death searches could be conducted
to determine vital status for the remainder.

Our choice of physicians as the study population of-
fered several additional advantages. First, because of their
medical knowledge, they are in the best position to give
true informed consent to participation, and to recognize
possible side effects promptly, thus minimizing discomfort
and illness resulting from study treatments. Moreover,
physicians report their medical history and health status
with a greater degree of accuracy than any other population
group, thus ensuring the collection of high quality data.

MAINTAINING HIGH LEVELS OF COMPLIANCE

Another advantage of the enrollment of physicians into
our trial relates to a third area of study design, achieving
high levels of compliance. This is extremely important,
since the power to detect a hypothesized difference between
treatment groups is proportional to the square of the difference in compliance between the groups (10). The optimal
population for a primary prevention trial would be a group
of highly motivated individuals who would clearly understand
and appreciate both the goals of the study and the importance of taking their commitment to it seriously. In this
regard, physicians again seemed an excellent choice (11).

In 1982, we mailed letters of invitation and questionnaires to 261,248 potentially eligible, male U.S. physicians aged 40 to 84, identified from a tape provided by
the American Medical Association. A total of 123,135 doctors returned that questionnaire, with 59,283 indicating
that they were willing to participate in the trial. Of
these, 33,211 were initially eligible and were enrolled in
the trial.

A second major strategy adopted to enhance compliance in the PHS was the use of a run-in period for all subjects prior to actual randomization, during which these 33,211 initially willing and eligible physicians all took their daily pills from calendar packs containing active aspirin and beta-carotene placebo. After approximately 18 weeks, participants were sent questionnaires, and those who reported side effects, the development of an exclusion criterion, a desire to discontinue participation, or inadequate compliance were excluded from the trial. The remaining 21,989 physicians were then randomized to a treatment group. Our pilot studies had shown that when participants were immediately randomized and then followed for two years, virtually all the losses in compliance occurred during the first several months, primarily because of difficulties in remembering to take a daily pill or the development of side effects due to aspirin. On the basis of this experience, it appeared that implementing a run-in period would substantially increase the power of the study by yielding a group of committed compliers for long-term follow-up, even though the actual number of physicians in the study would be lower than if participants were randomized immediately upon enrollment (10).

SIZE OF THE LIKELY RISK REDUCTION

A fourth question in trial design is how to ensure that the study will have adequate power to detect a difference between treatment groups of the order of magnitude likely for the agents being tested. One way to do this is to plan a sufficiently long period of treatment and follow-up. A second strategy, adopted in the PHS, was the collection of pre-randomization blood specimens from participants, to be analyzed for baseline levels of retinol, retinol-binding protein and carotene. The rationale for collecting these samples relates to the possibility that a small overall benefit of carotene, on the order of 10%, might actually result from a much larger reduction in cancer risk (e.g., 50%) confined exclusively to those physicians with initially low serum levels of these parameters. Thus, the availability of these samples increases the sensitivity of the trial to identify which particular subgroup of doctors, if any, stands to benefit the most from dietary supplementation with beta-carotene.

ACCUMULATION OF SUFFICIENT ENDPOINTS

Since the power of a trial is proportional not to the number of individuals enrolled but rather to the number of endpoints they experience, the size of a study population is less important than their likelihood of providing an adequate number of outcomes of interest. This is affected by the length of the follow-up period, the impact of the "healthy volunteer" effect, and the baseline risks of developing an endpoint in the larger population from which study subjects are drawn (12). Planning for a follow-up period of sufficient duration and choosing to study a population at high risk of the disease on the basis of age, sex, or the presence of other risk factors, are therefore crucial to designing a study which will provide truly informative results.

THE EXPERIENCE OF THE PHS

The effectiveness of these strategies can be illustrated by the experience of the PHS to date. As of January 4, 1985, the two-year self-reported compliance among randomized subjects was 90.2% (participants taking both types of study pill regularly), with an additional 4.2% taking at least one type of study pill. In addition, two-year morbidity follow-up is 99.6%, while mortality follow-up is 100%. These figures indicate that as regards compliance and follow-up, the decisions made during the design phase have proven effective.

In conclusion, because of the very large sample size, the choice of physicians as the study population, the run-in period to eliminate poor compliers before randomization, the availability of pre-randomization blood specimens, and the high compliance and follow-up rates, we believe that the PHS will provide definitive answers to the two research questions we have posed, and sound evidence on which future public health policy can be based. That ability is the ultimate goal of all the methodologic considerations outlined. Well-designed, large-scale randomized trials, especially those with simplified protocols which can be conducted at low cost per subject enrolled, can and should play an increasing role in determining whether beta-carotene and other micronutrients can alter cancer risk.

REFERENCES

1. Hennekens CH, Buring JE, Epidemiology in Medicine. Boston: Little, Brown & Co., 1985, in press.

2. Aspirin after myocardial infarction. Lancet 1980; 1:1172-3.

3. Peto R, Doll R, Buckley JO, Sporn MD. Can dietary beta-carotene materially reduce human cancer rates? Nature 1981; 290:201-8.

4. Hennekens CH, Lipnick RJ, Mayrent SL, Willett W. Vitamin A and risk of cancer. J Nutr Ed 1982; 14:135-6.

5. Hennekens CH, Stampfer M, Willett W. Micronutrients and cancer chemoprevention. Cancer Prevention and Detection 1984; 7:147-58.

6. Ames BN. Dietary carcinogens and anticarcinogens. Science 1983; 221:1256-64.

7. Herbert V. The vitamin craze. Arch Intern Med 1980; 140:173-6.

8. Willett W, Sampson L, Bain C, Rosner B, Hennekens CH, Witschie J, Speizer FE. Vitamin supplement use among registered nurses. Am J Clin Nutr 1981; 34:1121-5.

9. Stampfer M, Buring J, Willett W, Rosner B, Eberlein K, Hennekens CH. The 2x2 factorial design: its application to a randomized trial of aspirin and carotene in US physicians. Statistics in Medicine 1985; in press.

10. Buring JE, Hennekens CH. Sample size and compliance in randomized trials. In Sestili MA, Dell JG, eds. Chemoprevention Clinical Trials. Problems and Solutions, 1984. NIH Publ No 85-2715, 1985: 7-11.

11. Hennekens CH, Eberlein KE, for the Physicians' Health Study Research Group. A randomized trial of aspirin and beta-carotene among U.S. physicians. Prev Med 1985; in press.

12. Hennekens CH. Issues in the design and conduct of clinical trials. JNCI 1984; 73:1473-6.

Prevention Trials

DIET AND CANCER PREVENTION

UPDATE ON NATIONAL CANCER INSTITUTE INITIATIVE

Peter Greenwald MD, DrPH

Division of Cancer Prevention and Control

National Cancer Institute, Bethesda, MD 20205

The reduction of cancer mortality to one-half of current levels by the year 2000 has recently been established as a goal by the National Cancer Institute. At least 200,000 lives could be saved each year if this goal is achieved. Diet and lifestyle changes are expected to play a major role in reducing the occurrence of cancer and preventing cancer mortality.

The relationship between diet and cancer incidence has not yet been precisely defined, but epidemiologic and other data increasingly indicate that diet may be a factor in roughly 35 percent of cancers. A variety of studies show that inadequate dietary fiber, excessive fat intake, excessive caloric intake and obesity, and perhaps inadequate consumption of certain micronutrients are associated with higher rates of certain cancers. Evidence to fully characterize the magnitude of these associations and the biological mechanisms involved is still lacking at this time, but dietary components have been associated with cancers of the gastrointestinal tract and some sex hormone-specific sites (breast, prostate, ovaries, and endometrium).

We now believe that a substantial number of lives could be saved each year through changes in national eating habits that include higher levels of dietary fiber and reduced intake of fat. The strategy for reducing the

293

cancer rate by half by the year 2000 will include expanded
programs for educating the public and the professional
community to reverse current dietary trends regarding
dietary fat and fiber. Definitive clinical trials are
also being designed, but results from these will not be
available for a number of years, and it would be a
mistake not to act now on the basis of accumulated
evidence.

Four types of epidemiological studies show a role of
dietary components in cancer: (1) international
correlational studies comparing dietary intakes to cancer
rates, (2) migrant studies comparing cancer rates in
populations that have moved from areas with low cancer
rates to areas with high cancer rates, (3) comparison
of certain low-risk populations in the U.S. (Seventh Day
Adventists, Mormons) to the general populations, and
(4) case-control and cohort studies comparing dietary
patterns in cancer patients to others in the study
population.

High intake of fat is associated with cancers of the
breast, colon, rectum, and prostate, and possibly the
pancreas, uterus, and ovaries. High intake of dietary
fiber, on the other hand, is associated with lower risk
for colon and rectal cancers. Since dietary fat and fiber
levels tend to vary inversely in human diets, it often
is not possible to estimate precisely the relative
contribution of fat or the protection of fiber in the risk
for colon and rectal cancers. Studies suggest that both
contribute, and the protective effects from reducing fat
consumption and increasing fiber intake may be interactive.

CRITERIA FOR EVIDENCE

It is often impossible in human cancer research to
apply rigid laboratory techniques to establish a cause-
and-effect relationship, and exposing humans to potentially
cancer-producing agents to prove causality is clearly
unethical. Therefore, five criteria have been developed
initially to establish epidemiologic evidence of causality
with a very high degree of scientific probablity. These
criteria may be used (1) to determine whether existing
epidemiologic and laboratory data warrant conducting human

trials for cancer prevention, and (2) to determine if the evidence is strong enough to warrant recommending interventions and developing prevention policies. The five criteria are:

1. Consistency of the Association

Diverse methods of approach in the study of an association provide similar conclusions, and the association is repeatedly observed by multiple investigators, in different locations and situations, at different times, using different methods of study.

2. Strength of the Association

The importance of a given factor in the production of disease can be evaluated by determining the ratio of cancer rates for people with the risk factor to those without.

3. Specificity of the Association

Most diseases are influenced by many factors, and a one-to-one correspondence would not be expected; however, the precision with which one component of an associated pair can be utilized to predict the occurrence of the other can be determined.

4. Temporal Relationship of the Association

Exposure to the suspect etiologic factor must precede the disease. Temporality is more difficult to establish for diseases with long latency periods, such as cancer; however, histologic evidence demonstrating premalignant changes among individuals exposed to the agent, but not among unexposed controls, can indicate time sequence.

5. Coherence of the Association

Other possible explanations for the association must
be systematically considered and either excluded or taken
into account. Coherence is clearly established when the
actual mechanism of disease production is defined;
coherence of a lesser magnitude exists when there is
enough evidence to support a plausible mechanism for each
step in the chain of events by which a given etiologic
agent produces disease.

EVIDENCE OF FAT AND FIBER

A number of studies show a relationship between
dietary fat and human cancer. Seventh Day Adventists who
frequently ate fried foods were found to have roughly
twice the risk of breast cancer as Seventh Day Adventists
who less frequently ate these foods (Phillips 1975). A
survey of Hawaiians from five different ethnic groups
showed a strong correlation between breast cancer incidence
and age-adjusted mean daily intake of several different
types of fats (Kolonel 1981). Similar results were found
in a 1981 NCI study. Reliability of dietary surveys is
suggested by the use of several different methods. Thus,
there are similar results from independent investigators
using somewhat different methodologic approaches to the
question of dietary fat in breast cancer.

International comparisons show that countries with
the highest fat consumption also tend to have high breast
cancer mortality unless other dietary factors ameliorate
the problem. A comparison of countries with half the fat
intake of countries with the highest fat intake shows
that the breast cancer mortality for the former is a bit
below half that of the latter. Thus, one might postulate
that reducing calories from fat by half might reduce the
breast cancer mortality rate by at least half.

Solid alternative hypotheses that exclude associating
fat with breast cancer risk are lacking, however, a search
for interacting factors or alternative hypotheses
certainly still is of major importance.

Animal studies have shown that rats on diets high in
corn oil developed many more DMBA-induced mammary tumors

than did rats on diets low in corn oil. The difference was marked at several levels of carcinogen. The study also showed that the primary effect was that of inhibiting promotion, so the major benefit of low dietary fat occurred after injection of the DMBA carcinogen. Many other types of metabolic studies, including those relating to bile steroids and hormones, support the possibility that high fat diets increase cancer risks (Carrol and Khor 1975).

The protective effect of fiber-containing foods has been repeatedly observed by many investigators in different locations and situations at different times using different methods of study. Taken together, these studies make a convincing case for the protective effects of fiber-containing foods.

Research has shown that fiber appears to offer some protection against tumor development in rats given a digestive tract carcinogen (Barboldt and Abraham, 1978). Rats given the carcinogen were fed different amounts of cellulose. Those rats given the least amount of cellulose developed the highest numbers of intestinal tumors, and the observed incidence of tumors decreased as dietary cellulose increased. In other studies, increased dietary fiber was associated with a decrease in co-mutagens in human feces (Reddy et al., 1980), and in vitro studies have shown fiber binds to known, potent food-origin mutagens thereby suggesting a possible mechanism for protection (Barnes et al., 1983).

Human metabolic studies have been performed to consider such mechanisms as the effect of fiber on bile acids and sterols, intestinal transit time, fecal weight or dilution, and the effects on bacteria and mutagens. These studies consistently support the protective effect of fiber and give potential explanations for this effect. A high-fiber diet has been correlated with greater weight of stools (Eastwood et al., 1973), more frequent defecation and more rapid intestinal transit time (Cummings et al., 1976; Eastwood et al., 1982) Furthermore, in 14 of 20 epidemiological studies, including international and within-country correlations as well as case-control and cohort studies, an inverse relationship was seen between high intake of fiber-containing foods and incidence of colorectal cancer. Though the studies

were not standardized, this pattern of research results
is unlikely to have occurred by chance or resulted from
any type of bias.

CLINICAL TRIALS

Clinical trials are a vital component of the NCI
research program, and the rationale for them includes
theoretical and practical considerations. They constitute
the ultimate approach for testing attractive theories to
reveal any flaws, and at the practical level they must
address issues of specificity, clinical relevance of
animal models, questions about participant acceptance, and
the risk/benefit ratio.

Whereas epidemiologic studies often lack specificity
and may have confounding effects, clinical trials may
resolve questions of specificity since intake of a single
nutrient or agent can be manipulated while all other
aspects of the diet are left unchanged. Specificity can
also be addressed in animal studies, but numerous animal
models must first be developed and studied to determine
which ones are most relevant to human disease.

Behavioral research to determine participant
acceptance of specific intervention strategies is an
important component of clinical trials. Much of the
current knowledge about behavior is based on treatment of
persons with illnesses. Participants in cancer prevention
trials would be basically free of illnesses, though they
may represent groups at increased risk for developing
cancer and thus be motivated to accept the intervention.
Developing strategies for long-term adherence to the
intervention diet are important, and NCI will be supporting
research to develop and test strategies for modifying
eating behavior that are efficacious, cost-effective, and
lasting. Clinical trials will also provide the basis for
determining the risk/benefit ratio for each intervention.

An initial human trial aims to study the effects of a
20% fat diet as the intervention compared to the typical
American diet in which approximately 40 percent of calories
are derived from fat. The trial will be of women at high
risk for developing breast cancer; selection criteria used

should result in a population with an annual incidence
of breast cancer of close to one percent. The human
trial will test whether reducing the dietary fat will slow
or halt the promotion phase of carcinogenesis and reduce
the incidence of breast cancer in the study population.
This trial will evaluate the specificity of the
epidemiologic studies and will test whether the impact of
a low-fat diet intervention in humans duplicates animal
model results. This trial will also provide insights
into strategies for influencing eating behaviour and
will document the safety of the study diet.

While we must wait for the results of clinical research
for the most definitive answers, efforts to change diets
now seem prudent in light of our existing knowledge.
Though it is not possible at this time to quantify the
precise contribution of diet to overall cancer risk or to
estimate with absolute confidence the reduction in cancer
mortality to be expected from dietary modifications,
international and migrating population data suggest that
significant reductions in cancer incidence or mortality
are possible.

The following dietary guidelines for Americans have
been recommended by the Departments of Health and Human
Services and Agriculture. They are in keeping with good
dietary habits for general health and may reduce overall
cancer mortality as well. Health professionals should
counsel all their patients to do the following:

o Eat a variety of foods.
o Maintain ideal weight.
o Eat foods with adequate starch and fiber.
o Avoid too much fat, saturated fat, and cholesterol.
o Avoid too much sugar.
o Avoid too much sodium.
o If you drink alcohol, do so in moderation.

In addition to dietary recommendations, the National
Cancer Institute's Cancer Prevention Awareness Program,
an information campaign designed to increase public
awareness about cancer prevention, was launched this past
year. A national survey conducted recently by NCI
indicated that 46 percent of Americans believe "there is
not much a person can do to prevent cancer," and 49 percent

failed to identify cancer as a disease affected by life-
style choices. Through the Cancer Prevention Awareness
Program, the National Cancer Institute will work with
physicians, health professionals, private companies, and
local organizations to make cancer prevention information
widely available to the general public and especially to
populations most at risk.

REFERENCES

Barbolt TA, Abraham R. The effect of bran on
dimethylhydrazine-induced colon carcinogenesis in the
rat. Proc Soc Exp Biol Med 157:656-659, 1978

Barnes WS, Maiello J, Weisbuerger JH. In vitro
binding of the food mutagen 2-amino-3-methylimidazo-(4,5-f)
quinoline to dietary fibers. JNCI 70:757-760, 1983

Carroll KK, and Khor HT. Dietary fat in relation to
tumorigenesis. Progr Biochem Pharmacol 1975:308-353

Eastwood MD, Baird JD, Brydon WG, Smith JH, Helliwell
S, Pritchard JL. Dietary fiber and colon function in a
population aged 18-80 years. In Dietary Fiber in Health
Disease pp 23-33, Vahouny and Kritchensky ed, Plenum,
New York, 1982

Eastwood MA, Kirkpatric JR, Mitchell WD, Bone A,
Hamilton T. Effects of dietary supplements of wheat bran
and cellulose on feces and bowel function. Br Med J,
4:392-394, 1973

Kolonel LN, Hankin JH, Lee J, Chu SY, Nomura AMY,
Ward-Hinds, MW. Nutrient intakes in relation to cancer
incidence in Hawaii. Br J Cancer 44:332, 1981

Phillips RL. Role of life-style and dietary habits
in risk of cancer among Seventh-Day Adventists. Cancer
Res 35:3513-3522, 1975

Reddy BS, Chand S, Wynder E. Fecal factors which
modify the formation of fecal co-mutagens in high- and
low-risk population for colon cancer. Canc Letters 10:123-
132, 1980

THE CHEMOPREVENTION PROGRAM OF THE

NATIONAL CANCER INSTITUTE

William D. DeWys, M.D.
Winfred F. Malone, Ph.D.
Mary Ann Sestili, Ph.D.
Gary J. Kelloff, M.D.
Charles W. Boone, M.D., Ph.D.

National Cancer Institute

Bethesda, Maryland

In 1982 the National Cancer Institute initiated a new
program involving chemoprevention clinical trials. For many
years the institute had supported laboratory research and
epidemiologic research involving identification of carcinogenic factors and identification of agents which would inter-
rupt or reverse the carcinogenic process. By 1982 this
laboratory and epidemiologic research had reached a stage of
maturity which provided the scientific basis for the development of intervention clinical trials.

Early in the development of the chemoprevention program
an implementation plan was developed to provide a framework
for the development of the chemoprevention research area.
The first step in this planning process involved identification of the objectives of the chemoprevention plan which are
shown in outline form in Table 1. One objective involved
reviewing research which had been done in animal models of
carcinogenesis in order to identify and characterize agents
which had been found to have cancer preventing activity.
Another objective involved reviewing epidemiologic research
results to identify agents such as dietary components which
might have protective effects against carcinogenesis. Agents
identified from either laboratory research or epidemiologic
research might require additional studies of efficacy in
animal models followed by preclinical pharmacologic and

toxicologic testing prior to introduction into clinical
trials. Initial human studies would involve evaluation
of toxicity and tolerable doses as well as pharmacologic
evaluation. Based on the results of these initial human
studies, phase III clinical trials would be developed.
The final objective of the chemoprevention plan was to
apply the results from the clinical trials to the general
population.

TABLE 1 - OBJECTIVES OF CHEMOPREVENTION PLAN

1. Identifying and characterizing agents with proven
   activity in preventing carcinogenesis in animals.
2. Identifying agents based on epidemiologic studies.
3. Pharmacologic and toxicologic testing of such agents
   to select the most promising agents.
4. Phase III Clinical Trials of potential chemoprevention agents.
5. Application of research results to the general population.

The principles underlying the development of the
plan are shown in Table 2. An increasing body of epidemiologic information supported the importance of diet and
nutrition and specific dietary components as risk factors
factors for cancer development and prevention. A second
principle was that further development of this research
area would involve multi-disciplinary collaboration
between scientists with backgrounds in epidemiology,
laboratory research, and clinical trials. An important
principle in the development of the plan was to maintain
a balance between investigator initiative and the development of research according to a preconceived strategy.
It was recognized that research vigor and enthusiasm is
engendered when the investigator follows his research
interests and initiative in the development and implementation of a research plan. However, balancing this is the
need to allocate resources to meet specific strategic
objectives.

TABLE 2 - PRINCIPLES UNDERLYING DEVELOPMENT OF PLAN

1. Relative role of diet and nutrition in cancer etiology
2. Multidisciplinary approach to cancer prevention
3. Balance between investigator initiative versus research
   according to a preconceived strategy.

The research plan which was developed is shown in skeleton in Figure 1. Laboratory research relevant to cancer prevention can be broadly divided into basic research and applied research. The chemoprevention program does not actively support basis research but rather monitors the results from basic research in order to identify promising leads to be further developed in applied research in the laboratory. Leads from epidemiologic research may also be carried into the experimental laboratory enriching interaction between laboratory research and epidemiologic research. When results from laboratory research or from epidemiolgic research support the possibility of cancer prevention, these leads are considered for further study in clinical trials. If the results of clinical trials are positive, the emphasis then shifts to wide application of these results to the relevant segments of the general population.

Epidemiologic research relevant to chemoprevention may be viewed as passing through two stages. An initial stage is largely descriptive and identifies dietary factors and chemopreventive factors for further study. Related to this stage the National Cancer Institute is supporting the development of an International Food Composition Data System to facilitate epidemiologic research within individual countries and comparative research involving more than one country. Hypotheses emerging from initial epidemiologic studies must then be subjected to further testing and refinement in prospective epidemiologic research. The National Cancer Institute is currently supporting several activities involving prospective followup of population cohorts in which hypotheses are being further tested. We are also supporting analysis of serum factors which may provide leads for future prevention studies.

FIGURE 1

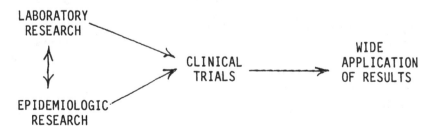

The laboratory research plan is divided into three stages. The initial stage involves a review of available research information both published and archived in order to select and evaluate potential agents. We are currently developing an information management system which has identified approximately 450 candidate chemopreventive compounds. About half of these have been found to have some affect in preventing cancer in animal models and the other half show evidence of inhibition of transformation or inhibition of mutagenesis in vitro. Based on an initial survey of these candidate compounds we have selected 100 of the most promising agents on which comprehensive monographs are being developed to further assess the priorities for evaluating these compounds. Stage II of the laboratory flow involves performance of initial studies of efficacy as well as initial pharmacologic and toxicity testing. This stage involves both in vitro and in vivo testing. In vitro screening systems can be divided into two broad categories. One category involves chemical carcinogenesis including initiators and promoters (Table 3) and the endpoint of these screening systems is inhibition of transformation or inhibition of synthesis of new proteins having structural, secretory or enzymatic functions. In several of these systems colonies can be documented to be tumorigenic by transplantation into appropriate hosts.

TABLE 3 - IN VITRO CHEMOPREVENTION SCREENING SYSTEMS

Cell System	Initiator	Promoter	Endpoint: Inhibition of
C3H/10T1/2	DMBA, 3-MC UV light	TPA, phenobarb, Saccharin, none	Transformed foci
BALB-3T3	3-MC	TPA, cigarette tar, none	Transformed foci
Mouse epidermal cells (JB-6)	none, or DMBA	TPA, cigarette smoke condensates	Growth of colonies in soft agar
Mouse epidermal cells (SENCAR)	none	TPA	Synthesis of new proteins
Human foreskin cells	MNNG, Aflatoxin B	TPA, estradiol anthralin	Growth colonies in soft agar
Tracheal organ culture	DMBA	TPA	Colonies transformed cells

The second broad category involves oncogene and growth factor aspects of carcinogenesis. The endpoints involve inhibition of transformation, inhibition of growth, or differentiation of cells (Table 4). In vivo chemoprevention screening systems are displayed in Table 5, and indicate that a spectrum of carcinogens, a spectrum of target sites, and a spectrum of types of cancer are involved in the initial in vivo screening for chemoprevention activity.

TABLE 4 - IN VITRO CHEMOPREVENTION SCREENING SYSTEMS

Cell System	Onc gene/ growth factor	Endpoint: Inhibition of
BALB-3T3 carrying ts Mutant	ras, abl, sis	Transformed Foci, other
HL-60 Human pro-myelocytic leukemia	myc, abl, ras	Differentiation into myeloid cells
T24 Human bladder cancer	ras	Growth of colonies in soft agar, other
A-431 Human skin cancer	erbB	Growth of colonies in soft agar, other
NRK	TGF	growth of colonies in soft agar
NIH-3T3	TGF	growth of colonies in soft agar

TABLE 5 - IN VIVO CHEMOPREVENTION SCREENING SYSTEMS

Species	Carcinogen	Target organ	Endpoint: Inhibition of
Mouse	DMBA/TPA	Skin	Papillomas
Mouse	3-MCA	Lung	Squamous cell carcinomas & adenocarcinomas
Mouse	OH-BBN	Bladder	Transitional cell carcinomas
Mouse	Balb 3T3 cells on plastic plate	Connective tissue	Fibrosarcoma
Rat	DMBA or NMU	Mammary gland	Adenocarcinomas
Rat	AOM	Colon	Adenocarcinomas

The third stage of the laboratory flow involves expanded studies of efficacy particularly looking at comparisons between potentially active agents and investigation of combinations of agents. Stage III also involves formal preclinical toxicology of chemopreventive agents. Studies which are currently in progress in this stage of our activities are shown in Table 6. The agents being studied represent a number of different chemical classes. Some studies involve a comparison between several different agents, while others are evaluating agents in combinations. Agents which will be undergoing formal preclinical toxicology evaluation include sodium selinite and selenomethionine in an effort to further decide between these two agents in terms of development of future clinical trials.

TABLE 6 - ANIMAL MODELS FOR EFFICACY STUDIES

Chemopreventive Agent(s)	Inducing Agent	Target Organ
B-Carotene	OH-BBN	Bladder
B-Carotene	NMU	Lung
Piroxicam	AOM	Colon
4-Hydroxyphenyl Retinamide	NMU	Mammary
4-HPR + Tamoxifen	NMU	Mammary
Sodium Selenite + 4-HPR	OH-BBN	Bladder
Sodium Selenite, Selenomethionine	3-MCA	Lung
4 HPR + Selenium	Asbestos + 3-MCA	Lung
4 HPR (measure intermediate endpoints)	OH-BBN	Bladder
4 HPR, α tocopherol, ascorbic acid, selenium (factorial design)	NMU AOM	Breast Colon

Agents which have passed through the laboratory research studies and meet certain decision criteria are then candidates for initial clinical studies. Initial human studies focus on development of information about toxicity and acceptance of the agent in phase I pharmacologic studies. These studies are currently being conducted in both the intramural and extramural components of our program. Agents having an acceptable pattern of toxicity become candidates for phase III clinical trials.

The reasons for the conduct of clinical trials in cancer prevention are summarized in Table 7. Epidemiologic studies often lack specificity in terms of correlating an outcome with a specific dietary factor. Diets which are high in one protective factor may be high in others, and it is difficult to evaluate the relative contributions of specific factors. Although animal models are currently being used to select agents for clinical trials, we have reservations about the predictive value of animal models for human application. This issue will be further evaluated in the future by comparison of clinical trial results with animal model results. A third reason for conducting clinical trials is to evaluate the participant acceptance of the intervention. And finally, the clinical trials will will evaluate the risk benefit relationships and the relationship between cost and benefit.

TABLE 7- REASONS FOR CLINICAL TRIALS IN CANCER PREVENTION

1. Evaluate the specificity of epidemiologic observations.
2. Determine the clinical relevance of animal models and other laboratory research.
3. Evaluate participant acceptance of the intervention.
4. Evaluate the risk/benefit ratio and the cost/benefit ratio.

The objectives and endpoints of cancer prevention clinical trials currently in progress are summarized in Table 8. Several studies are focusing on preneoplastic lesions with the intent of either reversing precursor lesions or preventing their progression to malignancy. Other studies are focusing on the prevention of precursor lesions as well as the prevention of overt malignancy. Although the studies will have the greatest statisitical power related to change in incidence, many of the studies will also be able to reach conclusions regarding reduction in mortality due to malignancy and to evaluate an impact on total mortality.

TABLE 8 - OBJECTIVES OF A CANCER PREVENTION CLINICAL TRIAL

1. Prevent precursor lesions
2. Reverse precursor lesions
3. Prevent progression of precursor to malignancy
4. Reduce incidence of malignancy
5. Reduce mortality due to malignancy
6. Reduce total mortality

Chemoprevention intervention studies which are currently in progress or about to be activated are displayed in Table 9. A spectrum of risk groups have been identified for these studies. A range of inhibatory agents are included in these studies including naturally occuring micronutrients as well as synthetic analogs. Many of the investigators involved in these studies will be making presentations later in this program and therefore I will not elaborate in any more detail on these studies.

Many of the clinical trials are evaluating serum levels of micronutrients for their correlation with subsequent development of cancer, and/or as a monitor of the compliance with the chemopreventive intervention. To assist in the development of the highest quality in these assays, the National Cancer Institute is supporting an inter-laboratory proficiency testing program designed to: 1) evaluate the current level of analytical accuracy; 2) identify analytical problems that affect accuracy; 3) make recommendations on methodology; and 4) establish criteria for acceptable range of accuracy. This activity will involve distribution of standard solutions and unknown samples, and will also involve periodic workshops aimed at enhancing laboratory proficiency.

Future directions within the chemoprevention clinical trial area will involve emphasis on development of studies which are either oriented toward specific sites, specific agents, or specific risk groups. As an example it is noteworthy that there is only one chemoprevention study in breast cancer, and there is a need for additional studies with this tumor site. As new agents are identified through the laboratory research activities and readied for clinical trials, there will be a need for the development of studies which are oriented to the further development of a specific agent. As epidemiologic studies identify additional high risk groups it may be of interest to develop studies focusing on specific risk groups.

We are entering an exciting new era in cancer research. We have the possibility of identifying interventions which may significantly reduce the incidence of cancer. If such agents are identified, we will then have the opportunity for wide application of these research results to the general population.

TABLE 9 - CHEMOPREVENTION INTERVENTION STUDIES

Target Site/ Organ	Target/Risk Group	Inhibitory Agents	Investigator/Inst.
Bladder	Superficial bladder cancer	4-Hydroxyphenyl retinamide (4-HPR)	E. Milroy U. of London, England
Breast	Breast cancer	4-Hydroxyphenyl retinamide (4-HPR)	U. Veronesi NCI, Milan, Italy
Cervix	Cervical dysplasia	Retinyl acetate	E. Surwit U. of Arizona
Cervix	Cervical dysplasia	Retinyl acetate	S. Romney Albert Einstein
Cervix	Cervical dysplasia	Folic acid	J. Chu Fred Hutchinson CRC
Colon	Familial polyposis	Vitamins C, E, & Wheat bran	J. DeCosse Memorial Hospital
Colon	Adenomatous polyps	Beta carotene	P. Bowen U. of Illnois, Chicago
Colon	Adenomatous polyps	Beta carotene Vitamins C, E	E. R. Greenberg Dartmouth Med. School
Colon	Normal volunteers	Vitamin C, E	T. Colacchio Dartmouth Med. School
Esophagus	Dysplasia patients	Multiple vit. & minerals	P. Taylor, W. Blot Nat'l Cancer Institute
Esophagus	General population from high risk area	Multiple vit. & minerals	P. Taylor, W. Blot Nat'l Cancer Institute
Lung	Chronic smokers	Vitamin B12 folic acid	C. Krumdieck U. of Alabama, Birmingham

TABLE 9 – (Continued)

Site	Population	Agent	Investigator / Institution
Lung	Asbestosis	Beta carotene Retinol	G. Omenn Fred Hutchinson CRC
Lung	Cigarette smokers	Beta carotene Retinol	G. Goodman Fred Hutchinson CRC
Lung	Middle age smoking males	Beta carotene Vitamin E	D. Albanes/J. Huttunen NCI/National Public Health Institute, Finland
Lung	Smoking males	Beta carotene	L. Kuller U. of Pittsburgh
Lung	Asbestos exposed	Beta carotene Retinol	J. McLarty U. of Texas at Tyler
Skin	Basal Cell Carcinoma (Albino)	Beta carotene	J. Luande Tanzania, Africa
Skin	Basal cell carcinoma	Beta carotene Vitamins C & E	B. Safai Memorial Hospital
Skin	Basal cell carcinoma	Beta carotene	E. R. Greenberg Dartmouth Med. School
Skin	Basal cell carcinoma	13-cis retinoic acid	J. Tangrea NCI
Skin	Actinic keratoses	retinol	T. Moon U. of Arizona
Skin	Basal cell carcinoma	retinol, 13-cis retinoic acid	F. Meyskens U. of Arizona
All sites	Physicians	Beta carotene aspirin	C. Hennekens Peter Bent Brigham
All sites	Dentists	Retinyl palmitate Sodium selenite Vitamins B_6 and E	C. Hennekens Peter Bent Brigham

NUTRITION INTERVENTION STUDIES OF THE

ESOPHAGEAL CANCER IN LINXIAN, CHINA

Jun-Yao Li

Department of Epidemiology, Cancer Insti-

tute, Chinese Academy of Medical Sciences

The highest worldwide incidence and mortality for cancer of the esophagus occurs in China.(1,2) Linxian, in Henan Province, is the epicenter of this maligancy and may indeed be the world's highest risk area, where the cumulative death rates (0-74yr) are 32.5% for males and 20.4% for females. Reasons for such exceptional risk of esophageal cancer are not yet known, but a series of investigations carried out in Linxian suggests that the population may be enhanced susceptibility to specific carcinogens because of deficiencies of multiple nutrients, especially vitamins and minerals. (3,4,5) To test an hypothesis that multiple vitamin/mineral deficiencies may contribute to Linxian's high rates and that supplementation may reduce the cancer risk, the Cancer Institute, Chinese Academy of Medical Sciences in collaboration with the National Cancer Institute, NIH, in U.S.A. are carring out two intervention trials in Linxian using multiple vitamin-mineral supplements. One trial will be conducted in patients diagnosed with esophageal dysplasia and the other in the general population.

In this paper, I will briefly introduce the research protocol for the on going nutrition inter-

vention trials of the esophageal cancer in China
and present the results of a fesibility study conducted in 1983.

A. Specific aims

The specific aims of two intervention trials are
to examine the effects of daily vitamin-mineral
supplements on age-specific incidence and death
rates of esophageal cancer among patients diagnosed
with esophageal dysplasia and the general population who have not previously had cancer. In addition, these two studies will also evaluate the effects of those supplements on regression/progres-
sion of dysplasia, age-specific incidence and death
rates of total cancer and total causes of death.
We propose to do these by conducting 2 5-year randomized, double-blind, placebo-controlled trials
among 3200 participants with esophageal dysplasia
and about 30000 adults (aged 40-69) of general
population. Intervention trials will be conducted
in 3 communes in north part of Linxian. Linxian,
a rural county with population 800,000, was selected because it has the highest rate of esophageal cancer in the world and because there is
suspicion that the population's chronic deficiencies
of multiple nutrients may be etiologically involved

B. Significance

Although China is a developing country, cancer
has gradually become one of the main causes of death
since 1970s.(6,7) According to the data from a national mortality survey during 1973-1975, cancer
was the second leading cause of death among males,
and the third among females.(8) In some areas, the
mortality of cancer now ranks first among deaths
from all causes. In 1973-1975, of 900 million Chinese surveyed, approximately 700,000 died of cancer
each year, one in every 40 seconds, including
160,000 deaths of stomach cancer, 156,000 of e-

sophageal cancer and 100,000 of liver cancer, the
three most common causes of cancer deaths in the
nation. Cancer has different effects in different
age-groups, taking a heavy toll of lives among the
people in the prime of life. While increases in
cancer survival rates and decreases in mortality
have been achieved for some types of cancer, the
burden of the disease remains high, and the impact
of cancer on the nation's health care system and
economy is likewide significant. Serious attention
must be paid, therefore, to cancer prevention and
control, and to all aspects of cancer research.
Coordinated and innovative approaches must include
research to develop and test effective cancer prevention and control strategies.

Among the common cancers in China, esophageal
cancer is the second leading cause of cancer death,
accounting for 27% of all cancer deaths in males
and 20% in females. Although elevated mortality is
seen in several parts of the country, the most prominent cluster forms in north central China, particularly in the Taihang mountain area on the border
of Henan, Hebei, and Shansi provinces. Within this
area in Henan Province is Linxian, a county where
the annual incidence rates of esophageal cancer
were $140.9/10^5$ in males and $107.3/10^5$ in females
during 1980-1983. Although there are only limited
historical data, it appears as if esophageal cancer
has long been a problem in these areas and that
there has been little change in the death rates
from 1959 to 1983.

Abnormalities thought to represent esophageal
cancer precursor lesions are common in Linxian.
Past cytologic and endoscopic surveys in Linxian
indicate that only about 20% of the adult population
have "normal" esophageal epithelia. The remaining
80% have some degree of esophagitis, including approximately 25% with esophageal dysplasia.(9)

Numerous epidemiologic and laboratory intestig-
ations have been conducted in areas at high and
low risk of esophageal cancer. Evidence from correlational study indicated that areas of the world
elevated esophageal cancer rates have corn or wheat
as the dietary staple, with low intake of riboflavin, ascorbic acid, niacin, zinc, and other
nutrients.(10) A number of analytic epidemiologic

studies also show that patients with epithelial
cancers, including those of the esophagus, often
had diets characterized by reduced intakes of certain foods, especially fruits and fresh vegetables.
(11,12) These results are consistent with the Linxian's data, which indicate that there were a series of clues to etiology in Linxian high risk
area of esophageal cancer, but have not yet con-
clusively pinpointed a specific carcinogen responsible for the elevated esophageal cancer rates.

Rather extensive laboratory studies suggest that
the low nutrient intake may be involved in the high
risk of cancer and the incidence of certain cancers
can be reduced by increased intake of certain micronutrients, such as retinol (13), beta-carotene(14),
riboflavin (15), vitamin C (16), vitamin E (17),
magnesium (18), molybdenum (19), selenium (20), and
zinc (21). The combined epidemiologic/laboratory
evidence does not seem specific enough, however,
to single out one or two nutrients as solely explained for the clustering of esophageal cancer
in Linxian. Thus, a broader hypothesis has been
raised that multiple vitamin/mineral deficiencies
may contribute to Linxian's high rates and that
supplementation may reduce the cancer risk.

Although further observational studies of these
agents are warranted, the only way to determine
with any reliability whether micronutrients themselves or which ones have any protective effect
would be a large, randomized intervention trial.
Consequently, a clinical trial in Linxian now seems
both relevant and timely. If micronutrients do appear to be anti-tumor agents in humans, it would
become a prescribable cancer prophylactic for people, particularly for high risk group. From a public
health point of view, such knowledge that a readily
available, safe, multiple vitamin-mineral supplement
could reduce cancer risk would have an enormous
public health impact, particularly as people may
be more willing to accept prescription of an anticancer substance than proscription of carcinogens.

C. pilot study

To assess the feasibility of such trials in Linxian, pilot studies were undertaken in 1973. The
specific questions the pilot studies were designed
to answer included:
(1) Can sufficient numbers of persons from the
general population be recruited?
(2) Can sufficient numbers of dysplasia patients
be identified and recruited?
(3) How compliant will participants be?
(4) Can the administrative logistics of patient
recruitment, information collection, pill delivery,
and follow-up be managed?
(5) What is the current nutritional status of
the population?
(6) Will supplementation with U.S. Recommended
Daily Allowance (RDA) levels of vitamins improve
low or deficient states?

Two pilot trials were conducted, the first involving the general population and the second involving persons diagnosed with severe esophageal
dysplasia.

For the general population pilot, twenty-one
production teams(villages) were randomly selected
from two communes(Yaocun and Rencun) in northern
Linxian. A central census roster listed 937 names
of persons aged 40-69. Sixty-two (7%) proved to be
ineligible for the following reasons:
- Suffering from esophageal cancer 7
- Suffering from other cancers 2
- Suffering from other debilitating diseases..5
- Had already died 18
- Temporarily assigned work outside the county16
- Other (incorrect age, erroneous or duplicate
  listing, etc.) 14
852 of the 875 eligible subjects (97%) agreed to
enroll in the general population pilot trial. For
the dysplasia pilot trial, 91 persons from Yaocun
and Rencun communes most recently discovered by
balloon-swallow cytology examination to have severe
dysplasia were recruited. All 91 agreed to participate. All participants in the pilot studies were
given One-A-Day (Miles Laboratory) multiple vitamin
tablets for six months.

Barefoot doctors visited the subjects monthly
during the trial to distribute pill packs. The obtained results show the losses to follow-up during

the course of the trial. Losses were generally due
to death, cancer or other debilitating diseases
occurring among participants, or to movement away
from the study area. At the end of the 6-month
trial, losses were about 3%, refused rates were
2.5%, taking at least some pills were 95%. In addition to counting unused pills, compliance was
also assessed using a urine test. Randomly selected
participants were adminstered loading-dose tests
for urinary riboflavin prior to pill-taking and at
either 3,5,9,11 and 16 weeks after the start of
supplementation. The results show that average
levels of riboflavin were marketly higher after
than before supplementation.

Nutritional assessments involving 24 hour recall
of diet intake (only at the outset of the study)
and laboratory assays of blood and urine were conducted prior to the start of and 4 months after
supplementation. The assessments were carried out
on 100 randomly selected individuals taking daily
pills, 48 patients with dysplasia, and (as a control) on 51 similarly aged individuals from commune
production teams not participating in the pilot
study. Nutritional assessment results using 24 hour-
recall measure indicated that in April 1983, the
intake of protein, phosphorus, thiamin and iron
apparently was adequate in the Linxian population,
whereas the mean intake of calories, calcium, riboflavin, niacin, Vitamin C and Vitamin A was inadequate. The intake of Vitamin A, riboflavin, and
calcium was particularly poor, with more than 90%
of subjects studied comsuming less than two-thirds
of either Chinese or U.S. recommended intakes. The
results of blood and urine assays also showed that
at the outset of the trial, the mean plasma ascorbic acid level was 0.26-0.29mg/dl. Approximately
half of all subjects were classified as deficient.
The mean 4-hour riboflavin excretion post loading
dose was about 740mg, 40-50% of the study population was deficient.(22) The mean plasma retinol
level was 24-27mg/dl, 20-35% of the individuals
were lower than 20mg/dl which are considered either
low or deficient. The mean plasma beta-carotene
level was 8-12mg/dl, about half of the people surveyed had values 10mg/dl and almost 90% of the individuals had values 20mg/dl. (β-carotene levels

were also low with mean values from 1.2 to 2.0mg/
dl), the mean plasmaα-tocopherol levels ranged
from 700 to 737mg/dl, about half of the individuals
either low or deficient. As expected subjects taking a daily pill showed improved nutritional status
during the study.(5, 23)

The pilot study thus suggests that a vitamin intervention trial will be well accepted in Linxian.
Indeed compliance, as judged by pill counts, was
exceptionally high. Of course, the disappearance
of a pill from the pill pack does not guarantee
that the pill was actually taken by the participant,
but our initial laboratory analyses provide biochemical confirmation from both urine tests (reflecting recent pill taking) and blood tests (reflecting longer-term pill taking) that compliance
was high. Therefore, the present study also firmly
establishes the deficiencies of several vitamins
in Linxian and demonstrates that the nutritional
status can be improved by daily supplementation
with vitamin tablets. The pilot study also led to
the establishment of an organizational system which
can be readily expanded to accommodate a larger
trial. In summary, progress to date indicates that
a population-based nutritional intervention study
of esophageal cancer in Linxian is feasible. Pilot
study results have clearly shown that: patients
can be identified and recruited; compliance is excellent; administrative logistics can be handle;
nutritional deficiencies are common; and low dose
vitamin supplementation improves nutritional status.

D. Experimental design

(1) Study population. Truncated death rates
(40-69 yrs) of esophageal cancer for total Linxian
is 470/10^5, for 3 Linxian's Northern Communes(Yaocun, Rencun, and Donggang are the Linxian's highest
risk areas of esophageal cancer where the intervention study is to take place) 760/10^5. It clearly
demonstrats that the rates in Linxian, especially
in Northern Communes are much higher than those for
total China(56/10^5) and for U.S.(while-5/10^5, Black-
19/10^5).(24):.Although rates of esophageal cancer

are extremely high in the general population of
Linxian, there is a subgroup for whom the rates
are extraordinary. This is a group of persons with
severe dysplasia of the esophagus. A mass screening
survey in 1974 identified, via cytologic means,
over 2000 persons with severe esophageal dysplasia.
Preliminary data on follow-up through 1982 indicate
that their subsequent risk of esophageal cancer
($1775/10^5$) may be 3 to 4 times greater than those
without severe dysplasia($510/10^5$).

In consideration of the possibility of the intervention may be too late and the practical difficulty
of assembling large number of dysplasia patients,
two intervention trials will be advanced. One trial
is involved a fixed sample of persons with recently
diagnosed prevalent dysplasia and other trial would
be persons selected from the remainder of the Linxian population. The latter trial has advantage of
covering the entire high risk population.

Participants in dysplasia trial are recruited
from among residents of Yaocun, Rencun, and Donggang communes identified as having severe esophageal dysplasia in the December 1973 balloon swallow cytology screening. There are 3489 persons with
severe esophageal dysplasia among 13049 residents
screened. So far, we have already completed the
pre-study evaluation which includes having a physical examination and filling out a short questionnaire asking about demographic information, diet,
and esophageal cancer risk factors, and obtained
an informed consent from every eligible dysplasia
subjects.

Participants in general population trial will be
recruited from census lists of eligible residents
aged 40-69 from three communes(excluding those already taking part in the dysplasia component). Census figures indicate that the current population
of the 3 target communes for males and females age
40-69 is 33,643. The pre-study evaluation for these
subjects is expected to take 3 months and will be
started from March, 1985.

For both trials, randomization will be conducted
in Beijing and the key will be kept at NCI so as
to keep the study double-blind for all involved
persons in Linxian and Beijing.

(2) Intervention plan. The dysplasia trial

will use a simple two-group design with one-half
the patients assigned to receive multivtamin-multi-
mineral pills to be taken daily. The other one-
half participants will receive placebos identical
in appearance to the active pills. For the general
population trial, a factorial design will be used.
The form of design to be used is a one-half replicate of a 2^4 factorial design.

The 4 proposed factors include:

A. - Vitamin A, beta-canotene, Zinc
B. - riboflavin, niacin
C. - Vitamin C, molybdenum
D. - selenium, Vitamin E

A full 4-factor factorial design would include
2^4-16 different treatment groups (show below):

Placebo	A	B	AB
C	AC	BC	ABC .
D	AD	BD	ABD
CD	ACD	BCD	ABCD

One-half repetition includes only 8 treatment
groups (the 8 underlined above).

For both trials participants will receive various
combination of vitamins and minerals in doses between one and three-times the U.S. Recommended Daily Allowances (RDA).

(3) Toxicity. No toxicity is expected in administration of vitamins and minerals given at 1-
3 times RDA levels. The proposed levels of micronutrients are shown in table 1.

Though unexpected, allergic reactions to fillers
or coatings of vitamin pills could occur. Barefoot
doctors will be intructed in the signs and symptoms of potential adversd reactions to the pills.
If an allergic reaction or other potential drug
effect is suspected, the pills will be stopped.
Patients may be re-challenged in one month if the
reaction was mild and reversible.

(4) Compliance. Compliance will be assessed
in two ways: pill counts for all participants, and
biochemical tests for a sample of them. The procedure of compliance assessment is the same as that
in pilot study. Approximately 400 randomly selected
study subjects per year will be checked for compliance in each of the 5 years. Groups of 100 will

be assessed at quarterly intervals. Each group of
100 will be composed of 20 dysplasia and 80 general population subjects.

(5) Measures of efficacy(end points). The
primary endpoints in both the dysplasia and general
population trials are esophageal cancer mortality
and incidence. Although intermediate endpoints can
be considered, to fully evaluate the role of vitamins and minerals upon cancer risk the actual occurrence of cancer must be monitored. In addition
to esophageal cancer, total cancer mortality and
incidence, total mortality, and the onset rates of
some common medical conditions will be ascertained,
including the infective and other diseases. The
time period of ascertainment will be at least 5-
year, if the nutritional supplementation truly affects the late stages of the carcinogenesis process,
a downward trend in incidence might be detectable
within the 5-year period.

Some intermediate endpoints will be assessed for
those enrolled in the dysplasia trial and a sample
of those enrolled in the general population trial.
Therefore, several ancillary assessment will also
be made. These include: a, reviewing cytologic regression and/or progression at 18, 36 and 60 months
in all patients in the dysplasia trial and a sample
of the participants in the population trial. b,
endoscoping a sample of 400 dysplasia patients before starting pill and again after 18 or 24 months
of pill-taking to assess: (1) Endoscopically observed esophagitis; (2) Histologically diagnosed
esophagitis; (3) Ability of the tritiated thymidine
incorporation in various cells layers; (4) The pre-
valence of positive esophageal fungal cultures; (5)
The micronucleus test as applied to exfoliated
esophageal cells; (6) Observe the concordance between endoscopic and histologic scoring of esophagitis; and (7) Observe the concordance between the
histologic results from either the balloon cytologic
examination at baseline or the endoscopic examination at baseline or 24 months. (8) Ear information
detection using auricular needling to detect the
cases with severe dysplasia and cancer of esophagus
before starting pill and again after 18, 36, 54
months. c, obtaining 24-hour urine collections on
a sample of individuals after the start of pill

Table 1
Proposed dosages for the nutrition intervention trials in Linxian

Nutrient	Dysplasia trial		General pop.trial	
	Dose	%RDA	Dose	%RDA
Vitamin A(as acetate)	10000IU	200	5000IU	100
Beta-carotene	25mg	-	25mg	-
Riboflavin	4.8mg	300	3.2mg	200
Niacin(as niacinamide)	40mg	200	40mg	200
Vitamin C(as ascorbic acid)	180mg	300	120mg	200
Vit.E(as dl-α-tocopheryl- acetate)	20mg	200	20mg	200
Selenium(as sodium selenite)	50mcg	-	50mcg	-
Zinc(as Zinc sulfate)	45mg	300	22.5mg	150
Molybdeum(as sodium molybdate)	30mcg	-	30mcg	-

taking 24 months to evaluate the effect of vitamin
C on nitrosamine formation. d, obtaining toe nail
clippings on a sample of individuals before and
after pill-taking for future analysis of trace element. e, obtaining an initial blood sample from
each participant and separating into plasma and
cells stored in freezer(-80°C) for the future analyses.
  During the coure of the study barefoot doctors
will identify all deaths to study subjects. We have
experience in monitoring mortality and cancer incidence in Linxian. We will use the Linxian Cancer
Registry System (established in 1959) for standardized ascertainment of cancer cases, plus we will
have immediate notification from the barefoot doctors of all deaths occurring among trial participants. Information from medical records will be
abstracted to include date and cause of each death.
Incident cancer cases will also be identified. Date
of diagnosis and type of cancer will be determined.
Annually, in collaboration with NCI, the CI will
calculate age and sex specific rates of mortality
from all causes and rates of mortality and incidence

from esophageal and all other cancers among study
participants, stratified by treatment group (with
the code identifying placebo and treatment groups
broken only if there are highly significant differences).

A biochemical/nutritional surveillance program
will be included in both trials to provide information on background of nutrients for trial participants before the interventions, to assess compliance, and to allow us to measure seasonal and
secular variation during the interventions.

During the trials 400 study subjects per year
will be selected at random to have blood and urine
collected and have a dietary history and anthropome-
tric measurements taken. Blood will be analyzed for
the various vitamins and minerals being administered
during the trials and urine will be analyzed for
nitrosamines. This surveillance will include participants from both trials and will be performed
throughout the year (100 persons every 3 months;
20 from dysplasia trial, 80 from general population
trial).

The laboratory analysés for this surveillance
program will be performed in China with a 10% sample
being sent to the U.S. for simultaneous analysis
as a part of an ongoing quality control program.

(6) Statistical considerations. **A**, Sample
size. The total population aged 40-69 in the 3
communes in which the study will be conducted numbers 33,643, based on the national census conducted
in China in 1982. As mentioned above, in December
1983, a mass screening of esophageal cytology by
balloon swallow was conducted among 13049 adults
age 40-69 in these communes. 3489 patients were
identified as having severe dysplasia (Grade I-
2685, Grade II-804). It is proposed to enroll all
eligible persons in the general population and in
the dysplasia trials. From our pilot study, we estimate that 90% will be eligible and willing to
participate in the trials. Thus, there will be about
28000 participants in the general population trial.
We have already completed the pre-study evaluation
procedure of subjects with dysplasia of esophagus.
There are about 3000 eligible dysplasia subjects
for dysplasia trial. **B**, Power. The following
assumption were made in the power calculations:

(1) The annual crude esophageal cancer mortality rate in persons aged 40-69 in the genreal population trial is 650×10^{-5} (or 0.65% per year). (2) The annual mortality from esophageal cancer in patients with severe dysplasia age 40-69 is 1.78% (3) Excluding events in the first 6 months, the cumulative incidence for the following 4.5 years will be 2.9% for the general population and 8.0% for those with dysplasia. (4) The effect of dropouts and competing risk is ignored; and (5) Alpha error(one-sided) is set at 0.05.

For the dysplasia trial, with P=0.08 and 1500 persons in each treatment arm, the detectable differences and power are shown below:

P_1	Decrease due to intervention	Power
0.064	20%	52%
0.060	25%	69%
0.056	30%	84%
0.052	35%	93%
0.048	40%	98%

For the general population trial, with P_0=0.029 and 14,000 per treatment arm and assuming a 2 group trial for simplicity of calculation: detectable differences and power are:

P_1	Decrease due to intervention	Power
0.0247	15%	72%
0.0232	20%	92%
0.0218	25%	99%

These estimates are based on the formula.(25)

Thus, the dysplasia trial will be able to detect with high power a 35% reduction in esophageal cancer rates associated with the intervention, and the general population trial, a 20% reduction. The power

of the general population trial (which will use a
fractional factorial design) to detect difference
associated with individual factions will vary under
various possible alternative outcome, but will be
high to evaluate differences of 20%-30% due to each
factor under a number of plausible outcomes. C,
Data analysis. The methods of analysis to be applied to the data collected during these trials
include simple contingency table analysis and Cox's
method of regression analysis for survival data.
The use of regression methods will allow for incorporation of variables stratified on at randomization and adjustment for risk factors which are
found by the initial interview to be nonrandomly
distributed between treatment groups.
   Analysis of the dysplasia trial data will allow
us to make a statement about the effect of the combined multivitamin-multimineral preparation only,
while in the general population trial we will be
able to separate out the effects of the several
factors.
   (7) Quality control procedures. A high level
of quality control will be maintained throughout
the course of the trials. Quality control procedures include the follow:
   a. monitoring the performance of all field staff
   b. verifying that all coding of data is accurate;
   c. ensuring that all blood, urine, nail specimens
are collected, processed, and stored completely,
validly and accurately.
   d. ensuring that proper quality control procedures
are carried out for all laboratory work;
   e. sending 10% of blood and urine samples to a
U.S. lab. for duplicate analysis.
   f. recovering used pill packs with unconsumed
pills left in the package. A random sample of these
will be returned to the U.S. for chemical analysis,
as a way of verifying the appropriate formulation
and assuring that subjects are receiving the correct pills.

   E. Conclusion

The important relationship of diet and nutrition

in the development of cancer has become well known
through various research effects. Some kinds of
nutrients have also been implicated to have cancer
preventive potential, but their significance in
cause and prevention remain to be confirmed. Many
studies of cancer use experimental animals or cells
and experimentally contrived conditions to observe
the effects of manipulating one or two diet and
nutrition agents. Although such studies represent
a good starting point for new hypotheses, it is
clear that, ultimately, these ideas must be examined in human living situation. This project offers
an outstanding opportunity to evaluate the prophylactic roles of multiple nutrients or which ones
in the carcinogenesis of human esophageal cancer,
because: (1) the study population has very high
risk of esophageal cancer. (2) Patients with severe
dysplasia of esophagus can be identified and recruited; (3) the dietary pattern of residents is
simple and predictable. The people consume whatever
they produce so that food effects on cancer are not
confounded by the effect of a broad distribution
of food. (4) The population is relatively stable,
the rural families usually do not move, (5) nutritional deficiencies are common and low dose vitamin supplementation improve nutritional status.
(6) Compliance of participants is excellent. (7)
The local health organizations are experienced in
epidemiological studies, maintaining a high quality
cancer registry system. We are confident that this
collaborative project will not only be mutually
rewarding to both of China and U.S. but, obtained
results should lead to a better understanding of
human cancer cause and prevention.

References

1. Li Jun-Yao: Epidemiology of Esophageal Cancer in China. Natl Cancer Inst Monogr 62:113-120, 1982.

2. Yang CS: Research on esophageal cancer in China: a review. Cancer Res 40: 2633-2644, 1980.

3. Zheng SF: Copper, iron, magnesium, and zinc contents in hair of peasants in high and low incidence areas of esophageal cancer. Chin J Oncol 4: 174-177, 1982.

4. Yang CS,etal:Diet and Vitamin nutrition of the high esophageal cancer risk population in Linxian, China. Nutr.Cancer 4: 154-164, 1982.

5. Yang CS,etal:Nutritional Status of the high esophageal cancer risk population in Linxian, China: effects of vitamin supplementation and seasonal variations. Presented at the 4th Symposium on Epidemiology and Cancer Registries in the Pacific Basin, Kona, Hawaii. January 15-20, 1984.

6. Li JY,etal: Atlas of Cancer mortality in the People's Republic of China-An aid for cancer control and research. Int. J. Epid. 10: 127-133, 1981.

7. Li JY, etal:Atlas of cancer mortality in the People's Republic of China. The China Map Press, Peking, 1981.

8. Li JY   Investigation of geographic patterns for cancer mortality in China. Natl. Cancer Inst MonogrNo. 62:17-42, 1981

9. Munoz N. Crespi M. Grassi A. Wang GQ, Shen Q, Li ZC: Precursor lesions of esophageal cancer risk population in Linxian China Lancet 1: 876-879, 1982.

10. Van Rensburg ST: Epidemiology and dietary evidence for a specific nutritional predisposition to esophageal cancer. J Natl Cancer Inst. 67:243-251, 1981

11. International Agency for Research on Cancer: Final report: Etiology of esophageal cancer in Caspian littoral of Iran.

Lyon.IARC, 1981.
12. Mettlin C, Graham S, Priore R, Marshall J, Swanson M:Diet and cancer of the esophagus. Nutr.Cancer 2: 143-147, 1980.
13. Sporn MB, Newton DL:Chemoprevention of cancer with retinoids. Fed Proc 38: 2528-2534, 1979.
14. Peto R, Doll R, Buckley JD, Sporn MB: Can dietary beta-carotene materially reduce human cancer rates. Nature 290: 201-208, 1981.
15. Foy H, Mbaya V: Riboflavin. Prog Fd Nutr Sci 2: 357-394, 1977.
16. Shamberger RJ: Vitamins and Cancer: Current controversies. Cancer Bull 34:150-154, 1982.
17. Shaklar G: Oral mucosal carcinogenesis in hamsters: inhibition by vitamin E. J Natl Cancer Inst 68:791-797, 1982.
18. Blondell JM: The anticarcinogenic effect of Magnesium. Med Nypoth 6: 863-871, 1980.
19. Luo XM, Wei MJ, Yang SP: Inhibitory effects of Molybdenum on esophageal and forestomach careinogenesis in rats. J Natl Cancer Inst. 71:75-80, 1983.
20. Medina D: Selenium and murine mammary tumorigenesis. Cancer Bull 34:162-164,1982.
21. Fong LY, Sivak A, Newberne PM: Zinc deficiency and methlybenzylnitrosamine-induced esophageal cancer in rats. J Natl Cancer Inst 61:145-150, 1978.
22. Ershow AG, etal: Compliance and nutritional status response during a feasibility study for an intervention trial in China. (in press)
23. Li JY, etal: A pilot vitamin intervention trial in Linxian.Presented at Hawaii conference, 1984.(see ref.5)
24. Blot WJ, Li JY: Some considerations in the design of a nutrition intervention trial in Linxian, China. Presented at Hawaii conference, 1984(see ref.5)
25. Rothman KJ, Boice JD: Epidemiologic analysis with the programmable calculator, NIH Publication No. 79-1649, 1979.

CHEMOPREVENTION STUDIES IN FAMILIAL POLYPOSIS

FREEDMAN, L.S., Ph.D., GROSHEN, S., Ph.D.

MILLER, H.H., M.S., and DeCOSSE, J.J., M.D.

MEMORIAL SLOAN-KETTERING CANCER CENTER

NEW YORK, NY 10021

INTRODUCTION

Familial polyposis is a classic prototype of hereditary human precancer. Patients with polyposis coli were chosen for our studies of chemoprevention because the precursors and histology of sporadic large bowel cancer are mirrored and truncated in time by polyposis. One of several clearly defined precancerous lesions of genetic origin, polyposis, is characterized by the development of numerous adenomas of the large bowel at a young age, with a risk approaching 100% of eventually developing single or multiple adenocarcinomas (1). Familial polyposis is transmitted as an autosomal-dominant disorder with a high degree of penetrance (2), and occurs at an expected frequency of 1 in 6850 to 1 in 23,790 live births (2,3). The study of environmental factors in the more dynamic setting provided by polyposis may identify modes of chemoprevention relevant to sporadic large bowel cancer, as well as provide this information in less time. Thus, it is hypothesized that the important genetic mutational event requires subsequent promotional events for the induction of adenomas and cancer and that these promotional events can be blocked by chemopreventive agents.

There exists evidence that antioxidants and fiber may have effective antitumor activity against colon cancer in animals and man. The theoretical basis for our present chemopreventive trial involving ascorbic acid, alpha-

tocopherol, and fiber dietary supplements has evolved from
numerous studies in this area.

Several studies have demonstrated that ascorbic acid
and alpha-tocopherol inhibit experimentally-induced colon
tumors (4,5,6,7). Both of these antioxidants have also
been shown to inhibit other experimental tumors (8-15).
Ascorbic acid reduced the formation of N-nitroso compounds
from nitrite precursors (16-18), and alpha-tocopherol
inhibited nitrosamine formation from nitrite in a model
system (19). Ascorbic acid has both inhibited 3-methyl-
cholanthrene-induced morphological transformation and
reversed the transformed phenotype in mouse embryonic cell
cultures (20), and it has suppressed the in vitro growth
of human leukemic cells (21). Bruce and Dion (22) observed
that when volunteers were given daily dietary supplements
of ascorbic acid (4g) or alpha-tocopherol (400mg) or both,
there was a sharp decrease in fecal mutagenic activity;
the greatest effect followed administration of both
agents.

Studies in humans have suggested that wheat fiber has
the best association with a reduction in carcinogenesis.
In the case control studies of Modan et al (26) and the
population studies of Jensen and MacLennan (27) fiber
protected against large bowel cancer. We have reviewed 18
studies of insoluble fiber in 17 publications. All used
the rat as the experimental model and dimethylhydrazine
(DMH) or azoxymethane (AOM) as the carcinogen.
Carcinogenesis was inhibited by wheat bran in 7 of 9
studies, by nonspecified insoluble fiber in 1 of 2, by
cellulose in 5 of 6, and by hemicellulose in 1 study.
Hence, protection against large bowel carcinogenesis was
observed in 14 of 18 experiments. We have inferred from
this review that the insoluble components of fiber provide
some protection against experimental large bowel
carcinogenesis. In contrast, soluble fibers such as
pectin had no value in 3 of 4 experiments (23,24,25).

In an initial study by our group, ascorbic acid 4g
day was administered to a small group of patients with
familial polyposis. A reduction in rectal polyps was
observed (28). In a subsequent randomized double blind
trial of ascorbic acid 4g/day among 47 polyposis patients,
a suggestion of a reduction in polyp area was observed in

the ascorbic acid group (29). The present trial is based on this experience and is designed to assess the effects of ascorbic acid in combination with alpha tocoperhol and high fiber dietary supplements.

METHODS

The current chemoprevention phase II-III cancer control study which began in November 1982 is a three arm randomized, double blind, controlled clinical trial. The goal of this study is to assess the effect of combined administration of ascorbic acid and alpha-tocopherol alone or with wheat fiber in the diet in patients with familial polyposis who had previously undergone colectomy and ileorectal anastomosis. The three treatment arms are (i) ascorbic acid, 4g/day, plus alpha-tocopherol, 400 mg/day with a high fiber, 22.5g/day supplement; (ii) ascorbic acid, alpha-tocopherol and a low fiber, 2.2g/day supplement (iii) placebo: inert placebo pills and low fiber.

Eligible patients were randomized to one of the three treatment arms. At the end of a three-month stabilization period of placebo drug only, during which time patients were discouraged from taking any supplementary ascorbic acid or alpha-tocopherol, the treatment allocations were begun. This second visit represented the baseline for the study. Patients are seen at three month intervals. At these visits, we (i) assess polyp number, area, and location (ii) evaluate vitamin and fiber compliance by interview and laboratory tests (iii) collect information about dietary intake (iv) evaluate by hematologic tests the safety and toxicity of treatment. On an annual basis, a biopsy of rectal mucosa is obtained to determine the proportion of rectal epithelial labeling by tritiated-thymidine.

Safety, toxicity and compliance issues are an important focus of our trial. At each visit possible side effects are reviewed with each patient. The hematologic evaluation screen for safety and toxicity includes tests for bleeding time, prothrombin time, white blood cell count, hemoglobin, hematocrit, platelets, red blood cell morphology, and serum calcium. In addition, serum ascorbic acid and alpha-tocopherol levels are periodically assessed.

In order to be able to fully evaluate the effects of the dietary treatment allocations, dietary intake information has been collected and entered into the study data base. At each visit, a 3 day complete diet inventory is collected. This nutritional data base will allow us to evaluate total dietary fiber intake and to assess whether administered fiber might alter other components of the dietary such as fat, thus introducing confounding variables.

With the aim of developing a more complete profile of our polyposis patients other studies have included: (i) psychosocial studies related to participation and compliance (ii) development of a polyposis registry and genetic analysis of the pedigrees of polyposis families (iii) upper gastrointestinal endoscopy (iv) measurement of intestinal transit times.

RESULTS

Accrual: Since the trial began, 72 eligible patients have consented to participate. The first group of patients entered in November 1982 and total accrual occurred over five trial sessions. The study was closed to patient entry in November 1983 with 62 patients. The characteristics of the evaluable patient sample is presented in Table I. Of the 72 patients who began the protocol, 14 have withdrawn. Four dropped out between the first and second visit and thus did not begin treatment; 4 more dropped out between their second and third visits. The remaining 6 withdrawals include 1 patient who was diagnosed as having carcinoma of the duodenum or pancreas and 1 who developed a psychiatric illness.

As of the last study session in November 1984, 58 patients remained on protocol. However, the interim analysis, started in August 1984, was based on a study sample of 60 patients, of whom 26 had been on treatment allocation for 18 months, 34 for 15 months, 45 for 12 months, 50 for 9 months, and 60 for 6 months.

Table 1

Comparison of Three Study Arms at Visit 2 (Baseline)

	Placebo	Low Fiber	High Fiber
Number of Patients	22	18	20
Sex (M/F)	10/12	7/11	6/14
Median Interval from Colectomy (Years)	3.1	3.4	5.3
Number with Prior Polypectomy	8	2	7
Prior Vitamin C Usage	27.3%	31.3%	15.0%
Prior Vitamin E Usage	9.1%	18.8%	0.0%
Median Age at Start Protocol (Years)	32.0	29.9	32.4
Median Dietary Fiber (G/da)	8.5	8.0	8.2
Median Labelling Index (%)	6.6%	5.4%	6.5%
Median Number of Polyps	4.1	7.8	3.0
Median Total Area Polyps (mm^2)	23.7	31.5	18.2

Compliance and Safety: Few studies have examined the effects of the long term administration of ascorbic acid, alpha-tocopherol, and high fiber supplements in humans. Throughout the trial there has been no symptom or side effect which could be attributed either to the vitamins or to the low or high fiber supplement. Patient-reported symptoms such as headache, dizziness, and diarrhea occurred equally often in all treatment groups. All hematologic tests remained within normal limits. We have observed a decline in serum calcium during the course of the trial. The decrease was thought to be more prominent in the "high fiber" study group but subsequent analysis showed the decrease to be distributed evenly among all three groups. The calcium levels remain in the normal range. Further analysis of the relationship of this finding to total diet intake and specifically fiber consumption is underway.

Fiber and vitamin compliance has been monitored throughout the trial (Table II). With respect to patient-reported as well as clinically-evaluated compliance, there was no evidence of significant differences among the groups. During the past year, patient reported compliance with vitamins or placebo has been 80% or better in over 80% of the patients and satisfactory (60-79% compliance) in an additional 10%. Compliance with fiber supplements has been more difficult, averaging in excess of 80% of compliance in approximately 55% of the patients and averaging between 60-79% in an additional 15% of the patients.

Main Response Variables: The main response variables of the trial are total polyp number and area and the ratio of total polyps area and/or number to baseline values. Final analyses will be performed after all patients have been on treatment for a minimum of 36 months. As indicated previously, at the time of our interim analysis in August 1984, patient time on trial varied from 6-18 months. Analysis of these preliminary data on polyp status indicated no statistically significant differences among the 3 treatment arms. In spite of the limited followup, exploratory plots and various descriptive tables and figures suggest there may emerge inherent treatment effects, even though statistical analyses have not yet confirmed them. The full evaluation of the biological

Table II
Overall Compliance for the November 1984 Trial
and the 5 Previous Trials

	AUG '83	NOV '83	FEB '84	MAY '84	AUG '84	NOV '84
FIBER:						
GOOD	48%	56%	61%	53%	51%	51%
SAT	24%	13%	12%	17%	17%	13%
POOR	27%	31%	28%	31%	32%	36%
N	33	45	51	59	59	53
VITAMINS:						
GOOD	92%	83%	91%	79%	80%	79%
SAT	7%	8%	5%	12%	10%	11%
POOR	2%	10%	3%	9%	10%	9%
N	42	52	61	58	59	53

GOOD=80-100% COMPLIANCE, SAT=60-70% COMPLIANCE,

POOR=0-59% COMPLIANCE, N=THE NUMBER OF PATIENTS ON WHICH

COMPLIANCE WAS BASED

effects of the treatment allocations await complete
followup of these polyposis patients.

Labeling Index: The tritiated-thymidine labeling
index provides a measure of rectal epithelial DNA
synthetic activity. Thirty-three patients have undergone
both pre and post treatment biopsies. A comparison of
change in annual labeling index among treatment arms shows
no significant difference, but there is a suggestion of a
treatment effect in the "high fiber" group.

Intestinal Transit Time: Intestinal transit time was
assessed following administration of a carmine marker to
patients before and several months after initiation of
dietary fiber supplementation. There has been no
significant difference between findings for low and for
high fiber groups. Previous data of changes in transit
time related to fiber probably reflects the effect of
fiber of the intact large bowel. The negative findings
may be a result of the fact that the large bowel is
virtually absent in our patient sample because of prior
colectomy and ileorectal anastomosis.

DISCUSSION

The present trial will provide information not only
on the effects over time of the vitamin and fiber
supplements on rectal polyps, but also on the natural
history of the syndrome in our sample of patients. There
exists little information on the time required for dietary
interventions to express a preventive effect on rectal
adenomas in humans. Completion of followup in our study
patients will afford us the opportunity to fully evaluate
the biological findings of this chemoprevention trial.

Our experience has indicated that a randomized,
double-blind controlled clinical trial can be established
and maintained in patients with familial polyposis. We
have demonstrated that these patients can maintain
acceptable levels of vitamin and fiber compliance during
the trial and that there has been no adverse safety or
toxicity findings related to long-term administration of
ascorbic acid and alpha-tocopherol.

Many questions remain. Can variations of measurement be reduced? A persistent problem has been the difficulty of accurately counting and measuring polyps in the rectal mucosa. If polyp counts are under ten, the assessment is reasonably trustworthy. However, when counts are high, there may be substantial degree of error. This range of error in measurement is, of course, common to all three treatment groups. In an effort to reduce it, we have obtained and begun to use a Welch Allyn video sigmoidoscope, which provides us with lasting visual records. The use of videoendoscopic procedures should enable us to make more accurate counts and comparisons between successive visits of a given patient.

Can the results of these studies be applied to the much larger population of patients with sporadic large bowel cancer? Clearly, this is our ultimate objective. The hypothesis is that patients with familial polyposis have a truncated form of large bowel carcinogenesis wherein the genetic mutation has provided a biological amplification system but environmental or promotional events are still necessary. The following findings argue for environmental or promotional events that may possibly be subject to therapeutic interventions: the 10 year average interval between onset of polyps and onset of cancer; the frequent spontaneous regression of rectal polyps; and the regular occurrence among these patients of cancer in the left side of the colon rather than throughout the large bowel. Moreover, the observation of a waxing and waning of polyps even in the control group, yields another hint that environmental influences are at work and may perhaps be modified. It is possible, of course, that the genetic mutation is powerful enough to overwhelm any efforts at blocking the action of environmental carcinogens. Nevertheless, it remains our hypotheses that these environmental events can indeed be blocked, and that what we can learn from the study of familial polyposis will prove applicable over a far longer time frame to the larger population of patients at risk for sporadic adenomas and sporadic large bowel cancer.

Acknowledgement: This research has been supported in part by USPHS Grant CA 31711.

REFERENCES

1. Bussey HJR. Familial Polyposis Coli. Baltimore, Hopkins University Press, 1975.

2. Reed TE and Neel JV. A genetic study of multiple polyposis of the colon (within appendix deriving a method of estimating relative fitness). Am J Human Genet 7:236-263, 1955.

3. Veale AMO. Intestinal Polyposis. Cambridge, Cambridge University Press, 1965.

4. Logue T and Frommer D. The influence of oral vitamin C supplements on experimental colorectal tumor induction. Aust N E J Med 10:588, 1980.

5. Reddy BS and Hirota N. Effect of dietary ascorbic acid on 1,2-dimethylhydrazine-induced colon cancer in rats. Fed Proc 38:714, 1979.

6. Jones FE, Komorowski RA, Condon RE. Chemoprevention of 1,2-dimethylhydrazine-induced large bowel neoplasms. Surgical Forum 32:435, 1981.

7. Cook MG and McNamara P. Effect of dietary vitamin E on dimethylhydrazine-induced colonic tumors. Cancer Res 40:1329, 1980.

8. Haber SL and Wissler RW. Effect of vitamin E on carcinogenicity of methylcholanthrene. Proc Soc Exp Biol Med 111:774, 1962.

9. Harman D. Dimethylbenzanthracene induced cancer, inhibiting effect of dietary vitamin E. Clin Res 17:125, 1969.

10. Jaffe W. The influence of wheat germ oil on the production of tumors in rats by methylcholanthrene. Exp Med Surg 4:278, 1946.

11. Yamafuji K, Kakamur Y, Omura H. Antitumor potency of ascorbic, dehydro-ascorbic or 2,3-diketogulonic acid and their action on deoxyribonucleic acid. A Krebsforsch 76:1, 1971.

12. Shamberger RJ. Increase of peroxidation in carcinogenesis. J Natl Cancer Inst 48:1491, 1972.

13. Shamberger RJ and Rudolph G. Protection against cocarcinogenesis by anti-oxidants. Experientia 22:116, 1966.

14. Schlegal JU, Pipkin GE, Mishimura R et al. The role of ascorbic acid in the prevention of bladder tumor formation. J Urol 103:155, 1970.

15. Rustia M. Inhibitory effect of sodium ascorbate on ethyl urea and sodium nitrite carcinogenesis and negative findings in progeny after intestinal innoculation of precursors into pregnant hamsters. J Natl Cancer Inst 44:1389, 1975.

16. Kamm JJ, Dashman T, Conney AM, Butns JJ. The effect of ascorbate on amine nitrate hepatoxicity. In: N-Nitroso Compounds in the Environment, IARC, Lyon, France 1974, pp 200-204.

17. Marquardt M, Rufino F and Weisburger JH. Mutagenic activity of nitrite-treated foods: Human stomach cancer may be related to dietary factors. Science 196:1000, 1977.

18. Mirvish SS, Wallcate L, Eagen M et al. Ascorbate-nitrite reaction: Possible means of blocking the formation of carcinogenic N-nitroso compounds. Science 177:65-68, 1972.

19. Mergens WJ, Kamm JJ, Newmark HL. Alpha-tocopherol: Uses in preventing nitrosamine formation. In: Walker EA, Castegnaro M, Gricinte L, Lyle RE Eds. Environmental Aspects of N-Nitroso Compounds. (IARC Scientific Publications) No. 19, Lyon, France, 1978.

20. Benedict WF, Wheatley WL, and Jones PA. Inhibition of chemicaly induced morphological transformation and reversion of the transformed phenotype by ascorbic acid in C3H/10T 1/2 cells. Cancer Res 20:2796, 1980.

21. Park CH, Amare M, Savin MA and Hoogstraten B. Growth

suppression of human leukemic cells in vitro by L-ascorbic acid. Cancer Res 40:1062, 1980.

22. Bruce WR, Dion PW. Studies relating to a fecal mutagen. Am J Clin Nutr 33:2511, 1980.

23. Bauer HG, Asp N-G, Oste R, Dahlqvist A, Fredlund PE. Effect of dietary fiber on the induction of colorectal tumors and fecal B-glucuronidase activity in the rat. Cancer Res 39:3752, 1979.

24. Bauer HG, Asp N-G, Dahlqvist A, Fredlund PE, Nyman M, Oste R. Effect of two kind of pectin and guar gum on 1,2-dimethylhydrazine initiation of colon tumors and on fecal B-glucuronidase activity in the rat. Cancer Res 41:2518, 1981.

25. Freeman HJ, Spiller GA, Kim YS. A double-blind study on the effects of differing purified cellulose and pectin fibre diets on 1,2-dimethylhydrazine - induced rat colonic neoplasia. Cancer Res 40:2661, 1980.

26. Modan B. Barell BA, Lubin F et al. Low-fiber intake as an etiologic factor in cancer of the colon. J Natl Cancer Inst 55:15-18, 1975.

27. Jensen OM and MacLennan R. Dietary factors and colorectal cancer in Scandinavia. Israel J Med Sci 15:329-334, 1979.

28. DeCosse JJ, Adams MB, Kuzma JF, LoGerfo P, Condon RE. Effect of ascorbic acid on rectal polyps of patients with familial polyposis. Surgery 78:608, 1975.

29. Bussey JR, DeCosse JJ, Deschner EE, Eyers AA, Lesser ML, Morson BC, Ritchie SM, Thomson PS, Wadsworth JV. A randomized trial of ascorbic acid in polyposis coli. Cancer 50:1434, 1982.

Chemoprevention of Lung Cancer with Retinol/Beta-Carotene

G.E. Goodman, G.S. Omenn, P. Feigl, M.D., G.D. Kleinman,
B. Lund, D.D. Thomas, M.M. Henderson, R. Prentice

Swedish Hospital Tumor Institute, Fred Hutchinson
Cancer Research Center, University of Washington
Seattle, WA

Introduction

Lung cancer is a major health problem in the USA. It is estimated that in 1982, greater than 110,000 deaths were directly attributable to lung cancer.[1] In addition to being the most common cause of cancer death in man (and in 1985, women also), lung cancer is unique in that the primary causative agent has been identified. Epidemiologic studies have clearly shown that cigarette smoking is a major etiologic factor in the development of pulmonary neoplasia.[2,3,4] Although the public is well aware of this relationship, there has been little success in primary prevention. In general, anti-smoking campaigns are met with apathy and tobacco abuse continues. Because the primary prevention of lung cancer has not yet been possible, alternative methods of prevention are needed for those who are unable or unwilling to give up smoking. The availability of a "chemoprevention drug" for this population would be of significant public health interest.

Epidemiologic studies of cancer patients and matched controls as well as retrospective analysis of dietary ;histories and serum samples from cardiovascular/hypertension trials have suggested an increased incidence of cancer in subjects having low serum retinol and beta-carotene concentration.[5,6,7,8,9] Although more recent studies have not always confirmed this inverse correlation between serum

concentrations of retinol/beta-carotene and the incidence
of cancer[10], there does appear to be a correlation between
dietary intake of fresh fruits and vegetables (beta-caro-
tene-rich food) and the incidence of cancer.

In addition to these epidemiologic trials, animal work
suggests a relationship between cancer and the family of
synthetic and naturally-occurring Vitamin A compounds col-
lectively referred to as the retinoids. These compounds
have been shown to cause tumor regression, inhibit the
growth of established tumors, and prevent the occurrence of
many naturally-occurring and carcinogen-induced animal
tumors.[12,13] A number of these studies have been presented at this meeting and will not be detailed here.

There are few human studies evaluating the chemopreventive effects of the retinoids and beta-carotene. Two
studies of particular importance to our planned trials will
be discussed. Gouvia et al studied the effect of the synthetic retinoid, etretinate on the incidence of bronchial
metaplasia in chronic cigarette smokers.[14] They enrolled
70 chronic smokers on a trial of 25 mg of the etretinate
daily for six months. Previous to treatment all patients
had bronchoscopy with biopsies taken from 10 specified
points in the bronchial mucosa. The degree of metaplasia
was graded by a strict grading criteria. Six months after
treatment, all patients were re-bronchoscoped and had repeat biopsies. Eleven patients were analyzed in their
recent report. Ten of 11 patients showed a significant
decrease in the degree of metaplasia with a P value of <
0.01. Reportedly, all patients continued to smoke while
on treatment. This trial suggests that the retinoids may
be effective in reversing previously established metaplasia
induced by cigarette smoking.

Stitch et al have performed a somewhat similar study
in the Philippines with subjects who were chronic betel-nut
quid chewers.[15] These subjects have a high incidence of
oral cancers. The end point the investigator used was the
percent of micronuclei observed in Pap stains of a scraping
of the oral mucosa. Micronuclei represent chromosomal fragments and may indicate nuclear damage induced by a potential carcinogen. Patients were treated orally with retinol
50,000 units twice a week and beta-carotene 150,000 units
twice a week. Patients had mucosal samples for micronuclei

determination pretreatment and at 1, 2 and 3 months after the start of treatment. On the right side of the cheek, the results were $5.2 \pm 1.8\%$, $2.7 + 1.2\%$, $2.0 \pm 1.1\%$ and $0.8 \pm 0.6\%$ respectively, a gradient fall in the percent micronuclei with continued treatment. The authors felt that this study gave evidence that beta-carotene and retinol in combination can decrease the incidence of chromosome damage caused by beetle-nut quid chewing.

Intervention Trials

With the available animal and epidemiologic studies, we feel it is reasonable to consider the initiation of a trial of beta-carotene and retinol in subjects at high risk for developing epithelial malignancies. In Seattle, Washington, under the auspices of an NCI-funded Cancer Prevention Research Unit, we have initiated two trials to evaluate the affect of beta-carotene and retinol in the prevention of lung cancer. Two high-risk populations will be studied: 1) Heavy cigarette smokers; and 2) Patients with asbestosis.

Smokers Pilot

To determine the sample size requirement to test an intervention on the incidence of lung cancer, we have made the following assumptions: 1) The incidence of lung cancer in subjects age 50-67 with a history of more than 20 pack-years will be approximately 100 per 100,000 man years;[3] 2) We wish to detect the difference between treatment and nontreatment of 33%; 3) Subjects will be followed for 8 years; 4) The power of this trial will be 80%. With these assumptions, it will be necessary to enroll 15,000 subjects randomized between treatment and nontreatment.

Prior to the initiation of this large scale trial, we are conducting a pilot study to determine the feasibility of such a trial. The specific objectives of this pilot trial are as follows: 1) To evaluate the methods of enrollment of subjects into this study; 2) To evaluate incidence of and methods of monitoring beta-carotene and retinol side effects; 3) To evaluate differences in side effects of long term therapy with retinol, beta carotene or a combination of both; 4) To evaluate subject adherence in a) taking the agents, b) completing the follow-up questionnaires, c) reporting to the clinic for follow-up examinations. 5) To initiate retinol/ beta-carotene treatment in a group of subjects who will be closely followed for side effects. This group will serve as a vanguard group for the proposed phase III intervention trial. 6) Evaluate the accuracy of a dietary history in predicting, retinol and beta carotene serum concentrations.

The eligibility criteria for this trial are seen in Figure 1, below:

Figure 1: Smokers Pilot Eligibility Criteria

1) Age 50-67
2) Smoking history of 20 pack-years or greater
3) Current smokers or those who have quit less than six years previously
4) No history of cirrhosis or hepatitis within the past 12 months
5) Supplemental retinol intake of 5000 units or less
6) No beta-carotene supplementation
7) No diagnosis of cancer within the past five years (other than skin cancer)
8) SGOT and alkaline phosphatase must be within the 99th percentile

Population

The population for this trial will be drawn from subscribers of King County/Blue Shield, a local Puget Sound health insurance group. Blue Shield has agreed to send out introductory letters to all subscribers between the ages of 50 and 67. This letter will introduce the basic concept of this study and ask questions as pertains to eligibility. Subjects interested in this trial will respond directly to the study offices. From the questionnaires returned, we will re-contact those who are both eligible and interested in participating in this trial.

King County/Blue Shield has currently around 40,000 subscribers aged 50 to 67. In a pilot mailing to 1000 subscribers in May of 1983, we received 687 return questionnaires. This included both questionnaires from subscriber and spouse. In total, of the 1000 letters sent, approximately 13% were eligible and willing to participate in this trial. With this population, we feel that we will have an adequate sample size for the pilot trial.

Treatment Plan

Four treatment groups will be evaluated:

1. Retinol placebo and beta-carotene placebo
2. Retinol 25,000 IU/day + beta-carotene placebo;
3. Retinol placebo + beta-carotene 30 mg/day;
4. Retinol 25,000 IU/day + beta-carotene 30 mg/day.

230 subjects will be randomized to each of the four groups. All subjects will be followed for two years of treatment.

Enrollment

After contacting subjects with the preliminary mailing, those interested and eligible will be contacted by phone and given an appointment to the prevention clinic. At the time of the clinic visit, study nurse-practitioners will aid the subjects in filling out the questionnaire. A side-effects questionnaire will also be completed in this pre-treatment period. Since many of the side effects of the retinoids and beta-carotene are subjective, it will be imperative to have a pre-study evaluation. A limited physical exam will also be done. Subjects will be given a side-effects information sheet for beta-carotene and retinol which will be explained.

If subjects agree to participate, informed consent will be obtained and pre-study blood samples will be drawn. These will consist of four aliquots of serum, (three for long-term storage and one for immediate analysis of beta-carotene, retinol, the retinyl esters and screening chemistry profile) and two plasma samples (both for long-term storage). Patients will then receive a two-months' supply of retinol and beta-carotene placebo capsules for the 2 month run-in period. They will then be given an appointment for a two-month follow-up visit.

At the two-month follow-up, the side-effect interview and physical exam will be repeated (after 2 months of placebo.) Levels of compliance will be determined by pill count and history taking. If compliance is greater than 75%, the patient will be randomized onto the trial. Subject will be stratified by the following criteria: 1) Age 50-60 or age >60; 2) 20-40 pack years or >40 pack years. Subjects will then be randomized to one of the four treatment arms and given a five-month's supply of drug.

Follow-up visits will be at 4-month intervals and consist of a repeat of the side-effect interview and physical physical examination. Blood samples will be drawn at four-to eight-month intervals for retinoid and beta-carotene content and screening laboratories as well as long-term storage. Between clinic visits at four-month intervals, subjects will be contacted by phone to determine compliance and side effects. The standardized side-effects questionnaire will be administered by phone.

This pilot trial will continue for a total treatment duration of two years. At the end of this two year period, the four arms will be compared in terms of compliance and occurrence of side effects. During this pilot, we will also determine methods to improve adherence and participation by the subjects. The methods for evaluating side effects and the incidence of side effects in this population will be determined. The treatment best tolerated and with the highest adherance will then be proposed for the phase III intervention trial.

Asbestosis Trial

In parallel with the smokers pilot, we are conducting a phase III intervention trial in subjects with asbestosis-related lung disease. Because this group as a whole is more aware of their increased risk for developing pulmonary neoplasms and their potential adherence and participation will hopefully be excellent, we feel we are justified in initiating an intervention trial. Eligibility for the asbestosis trial are seen in Figure 2, below:

Figure 2: Asbestosis Eligibility Criteria

1) Age 45-74
2) Greater than or equal 15 years since first exposure
3) Chest X-ray positive for pleural changes and/or interstitial fibrosis OR Chest X-ray neagative and at least five years in a high risk trade

The subjects for this trial are being recruited from: 1) pulmonary physicians within the Seattle area; and 2) the membership of unions with a historically high exposure to asbestos, i.e., ship scalers, pipefitters, shipyard workers, boilermakers, etc. Once subjects are identified by their source, they are contacted by a direct mailing. If a return letter indicates eligibility and interest, they are contacted and a clinic appointment is given.

The intervention in this group is retinol 25,000 units per day and beta-carotene 15 mg. per day. Subjects will be randomized between the combination or placebo. Stratification includes: 1) Current smoker or never smoked; and 2) less than 25 years since exposure to asbestos or greater than 25 years since exposure to asbestos.

The followup of the subjects in this trial is identical to that in the aforementioned smokers pilot. The forms and side effects evaluations for both trials are identical. We anticipate enrollment of 2000-2500 subjects with a followup of 8-10 years.

Discussion

Both these trials are ambitious undertakings. To determine if these interventions alter the incidence of lung cancer both populations will require a followup of from 8 to 10 years. In the asbestosis trial although the incidence of lung cancer is significantly higher than smokers a total randomized population of at least 2000 will be necessary to statistically detect a 33% difference in the incidence of cancer. Adequate recruitment of this highly selected population will be a major goal of this trial.

While recruitment of the population in the smokers pilot trial will not present a problem, recruitment of 15,000 subjects required for the intervention trial will present a major undertaking, especially if this trial remains localized to the Puget Sound area. We are hopeful this trial can be expanded to other areas of the country to recruit the required population.

Other major questions to be answered in these trials relate to adherence: While patients diagnosed with asbestosis are at high risk for developing cancer, their motivation and adherance in taking a daily capsule is unknown. Smokers are a completely different group. These subjects are "well" and do not regard themselves as ill. It is difficult to know if this population will take a capsule daily for a period of 8 to 10 years. Hopefully we will gain some insights into these questions during the pilot trial.

The specific choice of agents in these trials is somewhat empiric. Although animal studies suggest that retinoids will reverse pre-neoplastic lesions, there are few human studies. In addition, most of the synthetic retinoids currently available have a low therapeutic index. Retinol itself is toxic in high doses, and it is unknown if low-dose supplementation will be effective. While animal studies have shown the retinoids to be effective in nutritionally-depleted animals, it is unknown if low-dose supplementation will have any efficacy in a nutritionally normal population. There is some rationale for a somewhat moderate dose of retinol, however. Such a dose would correct subjects who may be marginally deficient in retinol intake and increase the serum concentration of the retinyl esters which have been shown to be chemopreventive in animal studies.

The use of beta-carotene is somewhat more empiric. While epidemiologic studies suggest its value few animal studies are available. The dose-response relation of beta-carotene is unknown. Some preliminary human studies by Stitch have suggested that beta-carotene acts mainly through its conversion to retinol. However, in vitamin A loaded subjects beta carotene appears to have an independent action on its own. This may relate to intracellular conversion to retinol. Hence there is rationale for combining beta-carotene and retinol in clinical trials.

As additional chemoprevention compounds become introduced and evaluated in the laboratory they will undoubtedly require clinical evaluation. We are hopeful that these pilot trials, in addition to evaluating retinol and beta-carotene, will provide useful information for the successful conduct of future trials.

References

1. Silverberg, E. Cancer Statistics. CA 30:2338, 1980.

2. Hammond, E.C. and Horn, D. Smoking and death rates: Report on 44 months of follow-up of 187,783 men. I: Total Mortality. JAMA 166:1159-1172, 1958.

3. Hammond, E.C. and Horn, D. Smoking and death rates: Report on 44 months of follow-up of 187,783 men. I: Total Mortality. JAMA 166:1159-1172, 1958.

4. Doll, R. and Hill, A.B. Lung cancer and other causes of death in relation to smoking. 2nd report on mortality of Brish doctors. BMJ 2:1071-1081, 1956.

5. Bjelke, E. Dietary vitamin A and human lung cancer. Int. J. Cancer 33:119-121, 1979.

6. Basu, T.K., Donaldson, D., Jenner, M., Williams, D.L. and Sakula, A. Plasma vitamin A in patients with bronchial carcinoma. Br. J. Cancer 33:119-121, 1979.

7. Kark, J. D., Smith,A.H., Switzer, B.R. and Hames, C.G. Serum vitamin A (retinol) and cancer incidence in Evan County, Georegia. JNCI 66:7-16, 1981.

8. Shekelle, R.B., Liu, S., Raynor, W.J.Jr., Lepper, M., Maliza, C., Rosseof, A.H., Oglesby,1 P., Shryock, A.M. and Stamler, J. Dietary vitamin A and risk of cancer in the Western Electric study. Lancet Nov.28:1185-1190, 1981.

9. Wald, N., Idle, M. and Boreham, J. Low serum-vitamin A and subsequent risk of cancer: Preliminary Results of a prospective study. Lancet Oct.18:813-815, 1980.

10. Willett, W.C., Polk, B.F., et al. Relation of serum vitamins A and E and carotenoids to the risk of cancer. NEJM Feb.16: 430-434, 1984.

11. Trown, P.W., Buck, M.J. and Hansen, R. Inhibition of growth and regression of a transplantable rat chondrosarcoma by three retinoids. Cancer Treat Rep 60:1647-1652, 1976.

12. Sporn, M.B. and Newton, D.L.   Chemoprevention of can
     cer with retinoids.   Fed. Proceed. 38:2528-2534, 1979.

13. Editorial: Vitamin A, retinol, carotene and cancer
     prevention.   Brit. Med. Journal 281:957-959, 1980.

14. Gouveia, J., Hercend, T et al.   Degree of bronchial
     metaplasia in heavy smokers and its regression after
     treatment with a retinoid.   Lancet Mar.27:710-712,
     1982.

15. Stitch, H., Rosin, M. and Vallejera, M.   Reduction
     with vitamin A and beta-carotene administration of
     proportion of micro-nucleated buccal mucosal cells in
     Asian betel nut and tobacco chewers.   Lancet 1:1204-
     1206, 1984.

HIGHLIGHTS OF METHODOLOGICAL APPROACHES: A CASE-CONTROL STUDY OF DIET AND BREAST CANCER

Moseson M., Shore R.E., Lazaro C.M.

New York University Medical Center

New York, N.Y. 10016 U.S.A.

Methodologic problems encountered in an epidemiologic study of diet and breast cancer will be discussed. This ongoing case-control study is investigating the hypotheses that breast cancer risk is increased by ingestion of fats, and is decreased by ingestion of retinol, beta-carotene, ascorbic acid, alpha tocopherol, zinc, selenium, dietary fiber, cruciferous vegetables, and foods containing protease inhibitors. The subjects will consist of about 500 breast cancer cases screened at a breast diagnostic center in New York City between 1981 and 1986 and 750 randomly-selected controls without breast cancer screened at the same center, and frequency matched with the cases on year of screening. Information is being obtained through a highly structured telephone interview which takes about an hour and a half.

The interview is administered by trained interviewers who are unaware of the case or control status of the respondent at the start of an interview. Information about dietary intake is elicited for the "reference year" --the interval one to two years preceding the detection year of the cases and the matched screening year of the controls. This recent time period was decided upon, rather than the more distant past, because there are indications that certain dietary factors may have late-stage promoting (or anti-promoting) effects on carcinogenesis (1,2). Questions are asked about the average frequency of ingestion and portion size of about 135 food

items during the reference year. Information on frequency
of ingestion of vitamin supplements is also obtained, as
well as information about known risk factors for breast
cancer, demographic factors and physical activity. Nutrient indices will be computed using a large nutrient data
base.

Extensive developmental work was necessary before
interviewing could commence. The methodologic issues
which needed to be addressed in the preliminary phase of
the study and which will be discussed in this paper
include the following:
- How to estimate food portion sizes in a telephone interview, a situation in which three-dimensional food models
were out of the question.
- How to develop a comprehensive measuring instrument
short enough to encourage compliance.
- How to ask the questions in unambiguous terms that could
be easily answered by the population in this study, and
that would result in more valid responses.

ESTIMATION OF PORTION SIZE

Questionnaires which ask only about frequency but not
portion size have been widely used in epidemiologic
studies (3-7), although a recent paper showed that food
frequency alone was an inadequate estimate of nutrient
intake (8). Studies which obtained information about
amounts of foods consumed, as well as frequency of
ingestion have generally used three-dimensional life-sized
food models of a single size for each food item (9,10).
One recent study used reduced-in-size photographs of three
portion sizes for each item (11). We decided to develop a
set of food photographs which would be mailed in advance
to the participants to help them estimate their portion
sizes. Different versions of food photos were compared in
pilot experiments to assess their ease of use and accuracy
when compared with actual food samples. First, a single
photo for each food item, which required the subject to
estimate multiples and fractions, was compared with
several photos of different sizes for each item, for which
only a simple visual choice between sizes was required.
Second, reduced photos of foods on dishes were compared
with life-sized photos without dishes. (Life-sized photos
on dishes, though desirable, would require an impractical-

ly large size of paper.) A single food photo was found to be the least accurate way to estimate portion size. Multiple reduced photos of foods on dishes were intermediate, while multiple life-sized photos were the most accurate.

Next, decisions were made regarding which foods to photograph. Some food items having a generalizable shape and texture were selected because their photographs could be used for more than one item; mixed vegetables and pineapple chunks (Figure 1) are examples. Also included were items of unique shape which are very variable in size, and therefore require their own photos, such as broccoli stalks and wedges of cake. Photos of fresh fruit were not included; a medium size was assumed.

Three photo sizes were used for most items. Four sizes were used where the range of possible portion size was greater. Determination of medium portion sizes was based mainly on USDA estimates (12). Large and small portion sizes were defined so as to be sufficiently different from the medium sizes to permit easy discrimination between them. Very large portion sizes were included for snack items such as cookies and potato chips in order to encourage respondents to report their true intake without embarassment. Chicken portions were estimated by using photos of six parts of an average-sized roasting chicken (Figure 2) to allow reporting of various combinations eaten at a single meal. Butter portions were photographed on knives to simplify estimation of size.

The final version consisted of 27 black and white sets of life-sized photographs. The photos were printed in an 8 1/2 by 11 inch booklet and arranged in the order in which they were first referred to in the interview.

REDUCING THE LENGTH OF THE QUESTIONNAIRE

The length of a telephone interview is of particular concern because a participant can easily terminate an interview before its completion by hanging up the telephone. Because of the many dietary hypotheses being investigated in this study, developing an interview of feasible length while retaining its comprehensiveness presented a problem.

Generating an abbreviated list of food items for

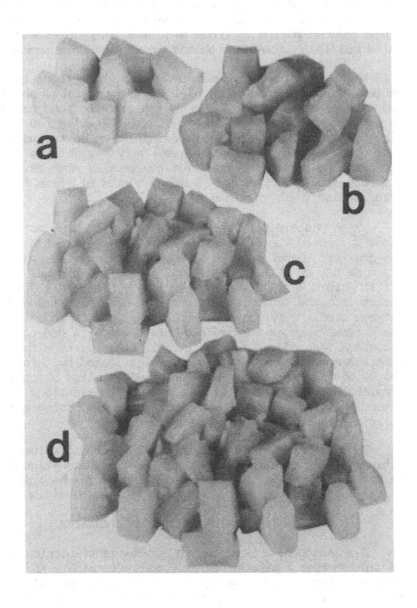

FIGURE 1. Photo Booklet - Illustration of Multiple
           Portion Sizes. (Reduced in size)

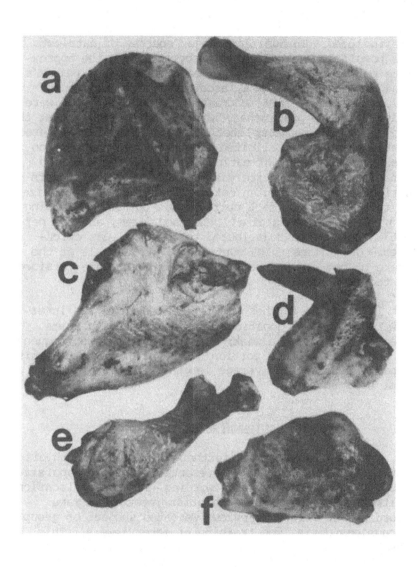

FIGURE 2. Photo Booklet - Illustration of Chicken Parts.
(Reduced in size)

inclusion in the questionnaire was the first step in
development of the questionnaire. Foods found to be
related to breast cancer in other epidemiologic studies
were included. In addition, major sources of nutrients in
this population were identified by obtaining the approximate per cent contribution by each item to the person's
total intake of vitamin A, ascorbic acid, alpha tocopherol, total fats, fiber and zinc. To do this, data were
analyzed from a preliminary study of women screened at the
same center who had completed a lengthy self-administered
questionnaire which elicited frequency, but not portion
size. The frequency of eating of each of the 180 food
items in the quesionnaire was multiplied by the amounts of
nutrients contained in an estimated average portion size.
The total intake of each nutrient was obtained by adding
the nutrient contents of all the food items, and the per
cent which an item contributed to the total was calculated. Only items which contributed at least 1% of the
intake of one or more nutrients of interest were retained
for the present study.

In order to further reduce the length of the interview, portion size questions were restricted to items
eaten at least once a week; for items eaten less frequently, estimated average portion sizes were were used. This
probably reduced the average length of the interview by at
least half an hour.

QUESTIONNAIRE REFINEMENT

The questionnaire was further developed through pilot
testing on about 75 women representative of the population
to be studied. Revisions in wording, format and location
of items were made after each pilot interview. Tape
recordings of pilot interviews were the subject of group
discussions during the training of interviewers. This
phase of interviewer training was closely linked with
pilot testing the interview, since the interviewers' expe-
riences with questions were the main source of information
on needed revisions. A number of open-ended questions
were included in the pilot interviews in order to determine whether food items commonly eaten in this population
had been omitted from the original list. These open-ended
questions were deleted from the final version and replaced
by some of the previously omitted items, in order to

standardize the interview. A manual was developed which consists of detailed interviewing and coding instructions as well as standardized probes. This manual is used for training interviewers and also serves as a record of coding decisions made as the study progresses.

SOME APPROACHES AIMED AT IMPROVING VALIDITY

A number of approaches have been developed with the aim of aiding recall and improving the validity of the data.

Setting the Time Frame

The problem of obtaining valid retrospective data is inherent in all dietary studies because of the difficulty of recalling past diets. Recall is made more difficult because dietary patterns have been changing in recent years as a result of media publicity concerning diet and health. Several studies have reported that estimates of retrospective dietary intake are influenced to some extent by current dietary habits (13-15). In an attempt to reduce this problem, the subject in our study is asked whether her diet during the reference year differed from her current diet, and our lack of interest in her current diet is emphasized. In order to underscore the reference year, a strong effort is made in the interview to set the time frame for that year in the mind of the subject in terms of where she was living at that time, who was living in her household, who did the cooking, whether she was working outside her home, and so on. The woman is reminded repeatedly throughout the interview of the reference year of interest. The subjects often repeat the year in the course of their responses, correcting themselves when they stray into the wrong year.

Information is also obtained about the stability of a subject's diet with regard to some major food groups. If a drastic dietary change occurred during the reference year, an earlier year is chosen which is representative of several years prior. This change in reference year is coded and will be considered at the time the data are analyzed.

Wording and Format of Questions

The wording of questions influences the validity of dietary information obtained. Interpretation of a question may differ, depending on the population studied and its dietary patterns. We experimented with different wordings and formats of questions to make certain they were actually eliciting the desired information. Those found to be the least ambiguous and easiest to answer were incorporated into the questionnaire.

Our usual question format was to ask how often a subject ate a food and what the portion size was. Subjects whose diets were quite variable found it difficult to report how often they ate bread products when asked in this manner. We found the best format for eliciting information about bread products to be the number of slices, rolls or bagels eaten in a day or in a week.

With regard to combination dishes, there exists an almost unlimited variety of Italian, Chinese, and Hispanic dishes having varying components. Many subjects could not give their frequency of intake of such combination dishes because there was much alternating of different dishes. The approach which proved easiest was to ask about the frequency of intake of the general category of an ethnic food (e.g., Italian dishes), followed by estimation of the per cent of the time the ethnic food contained such components as meats, fish and seafoods, cheeses, or vegetables. This generic approach had the advantage of greatly reducing the number of questions which needed to be asked. In addition to generic questions about combination dishes, specific combination dishes found to be commonly eaten by the pilot population were included on the list as separate food items.

Questions were also asked about the per cent of the time a food item was eaten in a specific form, such as per cent of the time fruits or vegetables were eaten with peels, per cent of the time bread was wholewheat or toasted, per cent of the time meats, fishes, or eggs were eaten fried, and so on. The use of per cents was possible in this generally well-educated study population, but might not succeed in a less educated study population.

Dietary Context of Food Items

In order to aid recall, food items have been placed in a dietary context where possible. For example, to elicit information about the ingestion of mayonnaise, there are two separate questions--mayonnaise as a spread on breads and mayonnaise added to foods. For butter a third question is asked about its use in cooking. To elicit the information about spreads in their dietary context, the questions about spreads follow the questions about breads and are asked in terms of the number of slices of bread on which the spread was used.

Separation of Food Items from Groupings

Grouping similar food items in a question often did not save interview time because respondents had to separate out and itemize the individual foods mentally in order to estimate the frequency and portion size of their intake. For example, turkey and chicken are not grouped together in this interview, despite their similar nutrient content, because they require different photographs to estimate portion sizes and because they are eaten in different dietary contexts (e.g., in our population, turkey is usually eaten in sandwiches for lunch, whereas chicken is generally eaten for dinner). Moreover, respondents sometimes tend to fixate on a particular item in a grouping, while ignoring the rest of the items, resulting in reporting errors.

Sequence of Food Items

The sequence of items in an interview can influence responses. Some subjects tended to include several subtypes of foods in the first question asked, if it was perceived as a more general category. For example, when the question about butter was placed before margarine in our interview, some respondents included margarine in their answer for butter. Then, when the question on margarine was asked, the original answer had to be revised, adding time to the interview and leading to inaccuracies. It was therefore found best to ask about margarine before butter.

Similarly, when beef was placed before other meats, some respondents tended to include chicken and all meats in their response for beef, because for some people in this population, the term beef refers to meat in general. Therefore, chicken, veal, liver and other meats appear before beef in the questionnaire.

Summary Questions to Check on Consistency of Responses

We have found it useful to insert consistency checks into the interview. These take the form of summary questions following certain categories of foods such as cereals, delicatessen meats, beef, cakes and pastries, and vegetables. For example, we ask how often a subject ate cooked vegetables of any type and how many were eaten at a meal. When the summary response is discrepant with the tally of the frequencies of individual items, the discrepancy is pointed out by the interviewer and possible sources of the apparent under- or overreporting are suggested to the respondent through the use of standard questions. The respondent is then encouraged to revise either the summary response or the frequencies of individual items in order to make the responses correspond more closely. ·

As another consistency check, a tally is computed of main dishes containing meat, fish or cheese. If this tally is discrepant with the expected seven lunches and seven dinners a week, standard probes are used to ascertain whether some meals were skipped, whether more than one protein dish was eaten at some meals, whether protein foods were sometimes eaten as snacks between meals, and so on. If under- or overreporting has actually occurred, the respondent is encouraged to revise the frequencies of individual items. When discrepancies are found after the interview has ended, the woman is called back to resolve them.

The validity and reliability of dietary methodologies need to to be assessed in order to be able to evaluate the findings of a completed study. In addition to assessment of validity and reliability of data that have already been gathered, methods are needed to improve the quality of data while they are being gathered. In this paper we have described several approaches aimed at this goal. We hope that other researchers will report on the problems they have encountered and the different approaches that have been useful, so that methodologic advances will be achieved in this difficult area.

ACKNOWLEDGEMENTS

The assistance and suggestions of Dr. Sharon Kolasinski, Denise Heimowitz, Anita Redrick, Marguerite Holmes, Sylvia Cotton, Karen Koenig, Dana Friedman, Ann Shore, and LaVerne Yee are gratefully acknowledged.

This work was supported in part by PHS Grants CA-32194 and CA-34280 from the National Cancer Institute to the Institute of Environmental Medicine, New York University Medical Center, and by PHS Center Program Grants ES-00260 and CA-13343 to the Institute.

REFERENCES

1. Davidson, M.B., and Carroll, K.K. Inhibitory effect of a fat-free diet on mammary carcinogenesis in rats. Nutr. Cancer, 3: 207-215, 1982.
2. Moon, R.C., McCormick, D.L., and Mehta, R.G. Inhibition of carcinogenesis by retinoids. Cancer Res. (Suppl.), 43: 2469s-2475s, 1983.
3. Graham, S., Dayal, H., and Swanson, M., Mittelman, A., and Wilkinson, G. Diet in the epidemiology of cancer of the colon and rectum. J. Natl. Cancer Inst., 61: 709-714, 1978.
4. Mettlin, C., Graham, S., and Swanson, M. Vitamin A and lung cancer. J. Natl. Cancer Inst., 62: 1435-1438, 1979.
5. Modan, B., Barell, V., Lubin, F., Modan, M., Greenberg, R., and Graham, S. Low-fiber intake as an etiologic factor in cancer of the colon. J. Natl. Cancer Inst., 55: 15-18, 1975.
6. Haenszel, W., Kurihara, M., Segi, M., and Lee, R.K.C. Stomach cancer among Japanese in Hawaii. J. Natl. Cancer Inst., 49: 969-988, 1972.
7. Bjelke, E. Dietary vitamin A and human lung cancer. Int. J. Cancer, 15: 561-565, 1975.
8. Chu, S.Y., Kolonel, L.N., Hankin, J.H., and Lee, J. A

comparison of frequency and quantitative dietary
methods for epidemiologic studies of diet and disease.
Am. J. Epidemiol., 119: 323-334, 1984.

9. Sorenson, A.W. Methodology and strategies for nutri-
tional epidemiology studies using a diet and colon
cancer model. In: J. Cairns, J.L. Lyon, and M.
Skolnick (eds.), Banbury Report 4: Cancer Incidence in
Defined Populations, pp. 51-67, Cold Spring Harbor
Laboratory, 1980.

10. National Center for Health Statistics. Dietary Intake
Source Data (HANES) United States, 1971-1974. (DHEW
Publ. No PHS 79-1221). Washington, D.C.: U.S. Govt.
Printing Office, 1979.

11. Hankin, J.H., Kolonel, L.N., and Hinds, M.W. Dietary
history methods for epidemiologic studies: application
in a case-control study of vitamin A and lung cancer.
J. Natl. Cancer Inst. 73: 1417-1422, 1984.

12. Page, L., and Raper, N. The USDA Pocket Guide:
Calories and Weight. Science and Education Administra-
tion. (Agriculture Information Bulletin Number 364)
Washington, D.C.: U.S. Govt. Printing Office, 1981.

13. Byers, T.E., Rosenthal, R.I., Marshall, J.R., Rzepka,
T.F., Cummings, K.M., and Graham, S. Dietary history
from the distant past: a methodological study. Nutr.
Cancer, 5: 69-77, 1983.

14. Rohan, T.E., and Potter, J.D. Retrospective assessment
of dietary intake. Am. J. Epidemiol., 120: 876-887,
1984.

15. Garland, B., Ibrahim, M., and Grimson, R. Assessment
of past diet in cancer epidemiology. (abstract)
Fifteenth Annual Meeting of the Society for Epidemiologic Research, p. 37, 1982.

TREATMENT

ASCORBIC ACID AND CANCER

Dr. Alfred Hanck

Unit of Social and Preventative Medicine

University of Basel, Basel Switzerland

ABSTRACT

Ascorbic acid has been used in the treatment of cancer since the vitamin became available. The effect of ascorbic acid on cancer has been studied in vitro, in animals and in patients. Conversely, the influence of cancer on ascorbic acid status has also been investigated as has the influence of cancer and cancer treatment on ascorbic acid status. In early studies treatment was with milligram amounts, only later doses in the gram range were used. Significant inhibition of a variety of carcinogens, environmental pollutants and endogenously-formed carcinogens was demonstrated.

Stimulation of immune defence due to the immuno enhancing effect of high doses of ascorbic acid was reported, but the significance of this effect in cancer is still disputed. On the basis of retrospective studies, it was reported that high doses of ascorbic acid prolonged survival in patients with terminal cancer. These findings have not been confirmed in prospective clinical studies, in untreatable terminal cancer patients, one of which was in patients with adenocarcinoma of the large bowel - one of the most resistant cancers. In one prospective double-blind study, ascorbic acid appeared to reduce pain and improve quality of life, as was reported in earlier studies.

A dose-related analgesic effect and anti-inflammatory activity after high doses of ascorbic acid have been confirmed in animals. In some cancer patients significant well-being and pain relief was achieved. Ascorbic acid also improved tolerance of conventional cancer therapy e.g. irradiation and chemotherapy. It has also been reported to potentiate the in vitro cytotoxicity of several chemotherapeutic agents. This indicates that further studies are needed, especially when considering the extremely good tolerance of high doses of ascorbic acid, i.v. administration being even better tolerated than oral.

ASCORBIC ACID AND CANCER

The history of a therapeutic use of ascorbic acid in cancer treatment dates back to the times when ascorbic acid was synthesized for the first time by Reichstein in 1933 (37). A year later when Jorissen and Belinfante observed a considerable degradation of lactic acid by ascorbic acid, the question was raised about possible effects of ascorbic acid in cancer (23).

First investigations of malignant tumours showed that the tumours contained ascorbic acid and that the vitamin reserves in the tissues of guinea pigs on a scorbutic diet were exhausted more rapidly if the animals were supporting rapidly growing tumours (48). As early as 1939, vitamin C balance studies were carried out in patients with tumours including those of Hodgkin's disease. These patients were actually deficient in the vitamin, and required up to 5 g of ascorbic acid for saturation of the tissue. The daily utilization of vitamin C, after balancing the deficit was up to 400 mg., depending on the severity of the disease (46). These findings were repeatedly confirmed (27), the deficit being even greater when x-ray therapy had been applied. Studying the influence of vitamin C on the growth of Brown-Pearce rabbit carcinoma of the testicle, subcutaneous injections of 50 mg/kg of ascorbic acid for 5 days were found to inhibit growth of the tumour (20). In 1940 doses of up to 4 g of ascorbic acid per day were administered to cancer patients for several days, and showed a remarkably beneficial effect on the general condition of cancer patients and an improvement in their ability to tolerate exposure to x-rays (17).

The known hypovitaminosis of tumour patients was explained by the increased consumption of vitamin C of the tumour cells resulting from an increased vital function. Effective x-ray therapy resulted in liberation of vitamin C from the tumour cells and an increased excretion in the urine. On that basis administration of ascorbic acid was thought to be contraindicated in tumour patients (42).

In experiments in mice with transplantable tumours (melanosarcoma S 39, Watts sarcoma and sarcoma 180), both a stimulatory effect on tumour growth as well as an inhibitory effect were reported (5). But in mice with spontaneous mammary tumours, repeated injections of 1-5% solutions of ascorbic acid retarded tumour growth slightly and prolonged survival time.

Insufficient oxidation was found to be the most characteristic metabolic disturbance in carcinomatous metastases. Treatment with quinones and ascorbic acid improved the condition (24).

In patients with cancer, lower levels of ascorbic acid in plasma were found than in healthy individuals, 0.48 mg/100 ml compared to 0.8 mg/100 ml respectively, scorbutic levels being thought to be lower than 0.2 or 0.1 mg/100 ml (2). This was confirmed later also in white cells, which have proven to provide the best index of tissue levels of ascorbic acid (1).

The majority of patients with malignant disease at different sites showed leukocyte levels less than the lower limits of the normal range (18-50 µg/10^8 W.B.C.) and more than 50% showed very low levels (<12.5 µg/10^8 W.B.C.). Signs of subclinical scurvy, such as decreases in capillary fragility were frequent (26). Recently a clear case of clinical scurvy was reported even though a blood level of 0.4 mg/100 ml plasma was found (18).

On the basis of decrease of plasma ascorbic acid to 0.3-0.01 mg/100 ml after x-ray therapy, up to 8 g ascorbic acid per day were recommended during x-ray therapy of patients suffering from cancer of the uterus (53). Patients with carcinoma of the oesophagus were found deficient in nearly all vitamins but especially in ascorbic acid. To replenish ascorbic acid levels in these patients before

surgery one gram per day for 5 consecutive days was
recommended (41).

Inhibition of respiration and glycolysis of Ehrlich
ascites tumour cells was achieved by ascorbic acid and
copper ions (40), and a marked decrease of catalase
activity was found as a common characteristic in tumorous
livers (32).

In the 70's the main emphasis shifted to prevention of
cancer by ascorbic acid. Schlegel reported that bladder
cancer induced by 3-hydroxyanthranilic acid, a natural
metabolite of tryptophan was prevented by oral administration of ascorbic acid (39).

Efficacy of ascorbic acid in preventing tumour induction
by the most common carcinogens has been confirmed by several
other investigators as well. A mechanism for the antitumour
effects could be through the inhibition of the formation of
carcinogenic N-nitrosocompounds (28).

The formation of endogenously occurring nitrosamines
was also efficiently blocked by ascorbic acid, thus preventing cancer formation (12, 19, 22, 38, 49).

In these experiments mostly carried out in rats, cancer
induction was only inhibited when ascorbic acid could act
on precursors. To inhibit cancer induction by ascorbic acid
was no longer possible when nitrosamines were already
formed. Also, carcinogenic effects of other environmental
chemicals like benzo (a) pyrene were shown to be inhibited
by ascorbic acid when given in high doses (25). These
findings were of great significance as these carcinogens are
present in a great variety of food and luxury items like
beer, wine, cigarette smoke, etc., and in environmental
pollutants (51).

At the same time a steady trend in increased cancer
mortality was reported (7,30), which in the future, hopefully may reverse (11) (figure 1, figure 2). In the U.S.A.,
40 to 60% of malignancies may be associated with diet.
Increased awareness of the significance of nutrition could
contribute to lower cancer incidence (21).

However, we may be faced here with a choice between

two evils. If we increase intake of polyunsaturated fat
we promote a decrease of cholesterol in serum thus protecting against arteriosclerosis. At the same time fecal
neutral and acid sterols may be increased, which in turn
may augment tumourigenesis in the intestine (4).

Polyposis coli, especially familial polyposis, endangers
the patient to develop cancer of the colon. In a prospective
randomized trial in 49 patients lasting two years, oral
ascorbic acid treatment with 3 g daily resulted in a significant reduction in rectal polyp area, 74% compared to 31% in
controls, and a tendency to decreased polyp counts at 9 and
12 months (74% and 83%) (6). Positive results achieved by
3 g ascorbic daily given to patients with active rectal
adenomatous polyp formation had been reported earlier (15).
In 1977, a reduction in number and size of residual rectal
polyps had been reported in 8 patients with familial polyposis maintained on ascorbic acid, 3 g/day for 22-30 months
(16).

Broad interest in the role of ascorbic acid in the
cancer process, despite the long standing history of research in that field, was only created when Cameron and
Campbell (8) and later Cameron and Pauling (9) reported on
a significant increase in survival time in terminal cancer
patients treated only with 10 g ascorbic acid daily. The
mean survival time in 100 ascorbic acid treated patients
was in the average 4.2 times greater than in the controls.

These findings were vehemently criticized with regard
to the historical controls used. To address the criticisms
this retrospective study was re-evaluated with matched
controls. Again, the patients taking ascorbic acid after
being judged to be untreatable, showed a significant increase
in mean survival time, about 300 days greater than that of
the controls (10) (figure 3, figure 4).

Similar results were reported from Murata and co-workers
(31) (figure 5). At two different clinics, 130 terminal
cancer patients received either low (less than 4 g ascorbic
acid per day or high (more than 5 g ascorbic acid per day,
average 25 g per day) doses of ascorbic acid. An increase
in survival time was reported for the high ascorbate
patients. The average factor of life prolongation by high
versus low ascorbic acid intake was 2.4 in one and 5.6 in

the other clinic. The least benefit was seen in cancer of
lung and bronchus (4.4) and the greatest in cancer of the
uterus (14.6).

These beneficial findings could not, however, be
confirmed in two prospective randomized placebo controlled
trials. In the first trial 150 terminal cancer patients
with advanced cancer from a variety of primary sites
received either 10 g ascorbic acid per day or placebo
(figure 6). A criticism of this study was that most of
the patients had previously received radiation therapy or
chemotherapy to which they no longer responded. Consequently
their immune system was most probably destroyed. Fifty
percent of the patients were already dead about 1.5 months
after start of the trial (14).

In the second trial carried out by the same investigators 100 patients with advanced colorectal cancer were
randomly assigned to treatment with either 10 g ascorbic
acid per day or placebo. All were beyond any reasonable
hope of potentially curative surgery or radiation therapy.
Contrary to the first trial at study entry, the patients
were judged to be still in good general condition (figure 7).

Ascorbic acid 10 g daily proved not to be superior to
placebo in adenocarcinoma of the large bowel, one of the
most resistant cancers known (29).

In an open, non randomized study in women with early
breast cancer, 21 patients received 3 g ascorbic acid during
10 months, and 22 served as untreated controls. No influence
of the treatment on five year survival was seen (34) (table 1).

In several studies, the study of Creagan et al. included,
ascorbic acid appeared to provide minor symptomatic improvement, a beneficial influence on quality of life and a
reduction of pain (43).

High doses of ascorbic acid may be of significance in
tumour treatment on 3 different levels. Certain cellular
immune responses are potentiated, selective cell death may
be achieved and pain may be mitigated. Ascorbic acid
increases lymphocyte blastogenesis and increases recall
antigen reactivities. Lymphocyte responses were normalized
in peripheral blood lymphocytes from patients with

subnormal responses (52). Patients with Chediak-Higashi
syndrome, with deficient natural killer cell function,
showed normalized killing while taking 6-8 g ascorbic
acid daily (33). Lymphocyte reactivity was reported to
correlate well with the prognosis of cancer-bearing
patients (13,44).

Selective cell death may be achieved by high doses of
ascorbic acid through interaction with hydrogen peroxide
detoxification. Tumour cells may accumulate much higher
condentration of ascorbic acid than normal cells (50).
Ascorbic acid in high concentration inhibits catalase, thus
becoming toxic to peroxidase deficient cells (figure 8).
At the same time ascorbic acid may induce hydrogen
peroxide formation. In normal cells there is no danger for
toxicity from such a mechanism. The cells don't take up
such high amounts of ascorbic acid and are well equipped
with catalase and peroxidases. In some tumours low
peroxidase activity was shown. Under these circumstances
selective killing of tumour cells may be achieved. Pain
may be mitigated by high doses of ascorbic acid. This could
be demonstrated in rats.

Anti-inflammatory and analgesic activities were assessed
with the rat paw carrageenan induced edema test. The
determinations were carried out always 4 hours after
induction of edema. To test prophylactic activity drugs
were administered 0.5 hours before initiation of inflammation. In all trials the test drugs were administered only
once, with the exception of one trial, the results of
which were compared with a known analgesic or anti-inflammatory agent, and with placebo. To determine dose levels
at which the vitamins were effective, an ascending dose
schedule was used.

The anti-inflammatory and analgetic effect of oral
vitamin C is shown in table 3. There is a dose-dependent
significant reduction of pain and inflammation after
administration of vitamin C. The prophylactic efficacy of
vitamin C is shown in tables 4 and 5. To achieve an
analgesic effect, higher doses of vitamin C are necessary
than for its anti-inflammatory effect.

Table 6 shows the anti-inflammatory effect of vitamin
C after 15 to 60 minutes of irritation after a daily oral
intake for 8 consecutive days. There was a significant

anti-inflammatory effect of vitamin C. The dose-effect
relation of vitamin C as an anti-inflammatory agent is
shown in figure 9 and that of its analgesic action in
figure 10.

This effect was demonstrable also in patients with pain
caused by bone metastases in breast cancer and in osteosarcoma. The tolerance of high doses of ascorbic acid
especially when administered i.v. proved to be extremely
good. In contrast to oral intake intravenous infusion
provided up to 100 times normal plasma levels. Under
these conditions two apparent elimination half-life times
are noticed; there is a rapid elimination with a $t_{1/2}$ =
0.47h and a slower phase with $t_{1/2}$ = 2.8h, plasma levels
after 24h still being in the range of 2 mg pro 100 ml
(figure 11).

Preliminary data show that oral intake of 15 g ascorbic
acid induces a rise of the plasma concentration from about
3 mg/l to 30-50 mg/l. In the 24h urine samples levels of
ascorbic acid were raised from undetectable to about 1-2 g.
Under these high intakes of ascorbic acid the blood levels
could be maintained in the above mentioned range for
several months.

No significant change was noticed during that time
with respect to blood pressure, pulse rate, temperature,
altertness, sleep pattern, appetite or fatigue. The
status of vitamin A, vitamin E, β-carotene, vitamin B_1,
vitamin B_2, vitamin B_6, was not significantly influenced,
nor was the concentration of sodium, potassium, iron and
zinc in plasma. In no case was a rise of interferon α-A
beyond the threshold of detection seen.

Uric acid in plasma decreased, and a tendency for
bilirubin and cholesterol to decrease was also noted.
LDH, alk. phosphatase, SGOT, SGPT, γ-GT, creatinine, urea,
serum albumin, triglycerides and fasting blood sugar were
essentially unaltered, as was ESR, Hb and differential
blood picture. No protein or glucose was detected in the
urine. Diarrhea was a transitory side effect and one
patient interrupted intake of ascorbic acid for that
reason. No other side effects were noticed. These findings
demonstrate an extremely good tolerance of 15 g ascorbic
acid daily given orally for several months.

A last aspect is the combination of ascorbic acid with other agents. Very interesting clinical results were reported recently. By treatment with a combination of gamma-linolenic acid with ascorbic acid, the mean duration of survival in 11 patients with histologically verified primary liver cancer rose to 90 days compared to mean his - torical survival time of only 42 days. One patient was still surviving after 314 days of treatment. This patient also showed tumour nodule regression of 34 mm after treatment(45) (table 7). Earlier on a potentiation of the growth inhibitory effects of certain agents on neuro-blastoma cells in culture by ascorbic acid was reported (36). Potentiation of the effect of 5-fluorouracil, x-irradiation and bleomycin was seen.

Also reported was a reduction of the cytotoxic effect of methotrexate. Recently a growth inhibiting effect of hydroxocobalamin and ascorbic acid on solid tumours in mice was reported (35) (table 8). For treatment of malignant melanoma a combined regimen of ascorbic acid and copper was recommended (3). In man the resolution of desmoid tumors by treatment with indomethacin and ascorbic acid was also reported (47).

In summary, for the time being in the field of ascorbic acid and cancer the data available demonstrate that the use of ascorbic acid for inhibition of the formation of several important environmental carcinogens seems to be reasonable. This is supported by in vitro and in vivo studies, and by studies in man. There are several sound reasons, primarily derived from in vitro and animal studies, that high doses of ascorbic acid may inhibit growth of certain malignant cells preferentially, although therapeutic use of ascorbic acid in terminal cancer patients judged to be no longer conventionally treatable has in prospective trials up till now not fullfilled expectations.

One explanation for the unsuccessful trials may be that 10 g ascorbic acid per day given orally, most probably are insufficient to generate in man cytotoxicity for tumour cells. However further work at these concentrations is justifiable in view of the extremely good tolerance of ascorbic acid.

The deficit of ascorbic acid formed in cancer patients, due to the stress of the disease and partially due to specific treatment calls for high extra ascorbic acid intake. High doses of ascorbic acid cause a significant immuno-stimulation, the relevance of which is not yet fully understood in the cancer process.

Within the scope of the subjective beneficial impressions about the action of high doses of ascorbic acid certain analgetic and anti-inflammatory actions of ascorbic acid should be discussed. The combination of ascorbic acid with conventional therapy to reduce side-effects and possibly to increase efficacy, seems to be warranted. When used, the combined treatment has to be considered carefully and the needs of the individual patient carefully evaluated.

REFERENCES

1. Bartley, WH, Krebs, A, O'Brin, JRP. Medical Research Counsil Special Report. No. 280, London: H.M.S.O. 1953.
2. Bodansky, O, Wroblewski, F, Markardt, B. Concentrations of ascorbic acid in plasma and white cells of patients with cancer and non-cancerous chronic disease. Cancer Res, 11: 238, 1951.
3. Bram, S, Froussard, P, Guichard, M, Jasmin, C, Augery, Y, Sinoussi-Barre, F, Wray, W. Vitamin C preferential toxicity for malignant melanoma cells. Nature 284: 629-631, 1980.
4. Broitman, S. Polyunsaturated Fat, Cholesterol and Large Bowel Tumorigenesis. Cancer 40, (Suppl. 5): 2455-2463, 1977.
5. Brunschwig, A. Vitamin C and Tumour Growth. Cancer Res. 5: 550-553, 1943.
6. Bussey, JJR, DeCosse, JJ, Deschner, EE et al. A Randomized Trial of Ascorbic Acid in Polyposis Coli. Cancer 50: 1434-1439, 1982.
7. Cairns, J. Sci Am, 233: 64, 1975.
8. Cameron, E, Campbell, A. The orthomolecular treatment of cancer. II. Clinical Trial of High-Dose Ascorbic Acid Supplements in Advanced Human Cancer. Chem Biol Interactions 9: 285-315, 1974.
9. Cameron E. Pauling, L. Supplemental Ascorbate in the Supportive Treatment of Cancer: Prolongation of Survival Times in Terminal Human Cancer. Proc Nat Acad Sci 73: 3685-3689, 1976.
10. Cameron, E, Pauling, L. Supplemental Ascorbate in the Supportive Treatment of Cancer: Reevaluation of prolongation of Survival Times in Terminal Human Cancer. Proc Natl Acad Sci 75: 4538-4542, 1978.
11. Celentano, DD. Trends and patterns in cancer mortality in Baltimore. In: Advances in Cancer Control: Epidemiology and Research, 235-244, Alan R. Liss, Inc., 150 Fifth Avenue, New York, NY 10011, 1984.
12. Chan, WC, Fong, YY. Ascorbic Acid Prevents Liver Tumour Production by Aminopyrine and Nitrite in the Rat. Intern J. Cancer 20: 268-270, 1977.
13. Chretien, PB, Crowder, WL, Gertner, HR, Sample, WF, Catalona, WJ. Surg Gynec Obstet. 136: 380-384, 1973.
14. Creagan, ET et al. Failure of High-Dose Vitamin C (Ascorbic Acid) Therapy to Benefit Patients with Advanced Cancer. New Engl J Med. 301: 687-690, 1979.

15. DeCosse, JJ, Adams, MB, Kuzma, JF et al. Surgery (USA) 7815: 608, 1975.
16. DeCosse, JJ, Condon, RE, Adams, MB. Cancer 40: 2549, 1977.
17. Deucher, WG. The vitamin C economy in tumor patients. Strahlentherapie 67: 143-151, 1940.
18. Ellis, CN, Vanderveen, EE, Rasmussen, JE. Scurvy: A Case Caused by Peculiar Dietary Habits. Arch Dermatol 120: 1212-1214, 1984.
19. Fong, YY, Chan, WC. Effect of ascorbate on amine nitrite carcinogenicity. I.A.R.C. Sci Publ. 14: 461-464, 1976.
20. Gentetsu Ryo. The influence of vitamin C on the growth of Brown-Pearce rabbit carcinoma of the testicle. J Chesen Med Assoc 29: 1184-1192, 1939.
21. Gori, G. Krebs-Prophylaxe. Ernahrungsrisiko ausschalten. Selecta 19: 347, 1977.
22. Ivankovic, S, Zeller, WJ, Schmahl, D, Preussmann, R. Verhinderung der pranatal carcinogenen Wirkung von Aethylharnstoff und Nitrit durch Ascorbinsaure. Naturwissenschaften 60: 525-527, 1973.
23. Jorissen, WP, Belinfante, AH. The induced oxidation of lactic acid by ascorbic acid and the cancer problem. Science 79: 13, 1934.
24. Jorissen, WP. Induced oxidation in carcinoma cases. Chem Weekblad 51: 705-506, 1955.
25. Kallistratos, G, Fasske, E. Inhibition of benzo(a) pyrene carcinogenesis in rats with vitamin C. Folia Biochim Biol Graeca 16: 15-30, 1979.
26. Krasner, N, Dymock, EW. Ascorbic Acid Deficiency in Malignant Diseases: A Clinical and Biochemical Study. Br J Cancer 30: 142-145, 1974.
27. Minor, AH, Ramirez, MA. The utilisation of vitamin C by cancer patients. Cancer Res 2: 509-513, 1943.
28. Mirvish, SS, Wallcave, L, Eagen, M, Shubik, P. Ascorbate-Nitrite Reaction: Possible Means of Blocking the Formation of Carcinogenic N-Nitroso Compounds. Science 177: 65-68, 1972.
29. Moertel, ChG. Fleming, TR, Creagan, ET et al. High-Dose Vitamin C versus Placebo in the Treatment of Patients with Advanced Cancer who have had no Prior Chemotherapy. New Engl J Med 312: 137-141, 1985.
30. Munro, H. Nutrition USA - 1977. Food Technol 31: 24-27, 1977.

31. Murata, A, Morishige, F, Yamaguchi, H. Prolongation of Survival Times of Terminal Cancer Patients by Administration of Large Doses of Ascorbate. In: A. Hanck (Edit.): Vitamin C. New Clinical Applications in Immunology, Lipid Metabolism and Cancer. Hans Huber Publishers, Bern, Stuttgart, Vienna: 103-113, 1982.

32. Ono, T. Biochemistry of cancer in the host. Ed. Miyakawa, Masasumi, Asakura Publ Co, Tokyo, 164-167, 1966.

33. Panush, RS, Delafuente, JC, Katz, P, Johnson, J. In: Hanck, A, Ritzel, G (Edit.) "Vitamin C. New Clinical Applications in Immunology, Lipid Metabolism and Cancer" p. 35, ff: Hans Huber, Bern, 1982.

34. Poulter, JM, White, WF, Dickerson, JWT. Ascorbic Acid Supplementation and Five Year Survival Rates in Women with Early Breast Cancer. Acta Vit Enzymol 6: 175-182, 1984.

35. Poydock, E. Growth-inhibiting Effect of Hydroxocobalamin and L-Ascorbic Acid on two Solid Tumors in Mice. IRCS Med Sci 12: 813, 1984.

36. Prasad, KN, Sinha, PK, Ramanujam, M, and Sakamoto, A. Sodium ascorbate potentiates the growth inhibitory effect of certain agents on neuroblastoma cells in culture. Proc Natl Acad Sci 76: 829-832, 1979.

37. Reichstein, T, Grussner, A, Oppenauer, R. Helv Chim Acta 16: 1023, 1933.

38. Rustia, M. Inhibitory Effect of Sodium Ascorbate on Ethylurea and Sodium Nitrite Carcinogenesis and Negative Findings in Progeny After Intestinal Inoculation of Precursors Into Pregnant Hamsters. J Natl Cancer Inst 55: 1389-1394, 1975.

39. Schlegel, JU, Pipkin, GE, Riyuichi, N, Shultz, GN. Role of ascorbic acid in the prevention of bladder tumor formation. J Urol 103: 155-159, 1970.

40. Schon, R, Menke, KH, Negelein, E. The influence of heavy metal ions on the Ehrlich ascites tumor cells of mice and the effect of cysteine. Z Physiol Chem 323: 155-163, 1961.

41. Sung, WH. Ascorbic Acid in Carcinoma of the Oesophagus. Annals of Academy of Med (Singapore) 3: 232-234, 1974.

42. Szenes, T. The action of ascorbic acid in Rontgen irradiation of tumors and tumorous proligerations. Strahlentherapie 71: 463-471, 1942.

43. Tschetter, L, Creagan, ET, O'Fallon, JR et al. A
    Community-Based Study of Vitamin C (Ascorbic Acid)
    Therapy in Patients with Advanced Cancer. Proc Am
    Soc Clin Oncol. 2, 19 Meet, p.92, 1983.
44. Twomey, PL, Catalona, WJ, Chretien, PB. Cancer 33:
    435-440, 1974.
45. Van der Merwe, CF. The reversibility of cancer. Sa
    Med J 65: 712, 1984.
46. Vogt, A. The utilization of vitamin C in tumor patients
    and in lymphogranulomatosis. Strahlentherapie 65: 616-
    623, 1939.
47. Waddell, WR, Gerner, RE. Indomethacin and Ascorbate
    Inhibit Desmoid Tumors. J Surg Oncol 15: 85-90, 1980.
48. Watson AF. The chemical reducing capacity and vitamin
    C content of transplantable tumors of the rat and
    guinea pig. Brit J Exp Pain 17: 124-134, 1936.
49. Weisburger, JH, Raineri, R. Dietary Factors and the
    Etiology of Gastric Cancer. Cancer Res 35: 3469-3474,
    1975.
50. Wilson, CWM. Clinical Pharmacological Aspects of
    Ascorbic Acid. Ann New York Acad Sci 258: 355-376, 1975.
51. Wynder, EL. Nutrition and cancer. Fed Proc 35: 1309-
    1315, 1976.
52. Yonemoto, RH. Vitamin C and Immune Responses in Normal
    and Controls and Cancer Patients. In: Hanck, A,
    Ritzel, G (Edit.) "Vitamin C, Recent Advances and
    Aspects in Virus Diseases, Cancer and in Lipid
    Metabolism." p 143 ff: Hans Huber, Bern 1979.
53. Zalchikova, KN, Vladinurovo, VS. Use of ascorbic acid
    for cancer of cervix of uterus. Vestnik Rentgenol
    Radiol 32: 4-5, 1957.

TABLE 1

Five year survival and development of metastatic disease in patients with early breast cancer: effect of administration of 3 g ascorbic acid (AA) per day

Patients		DEAD	Local Recurrence	Skeletal Recurrence	Alive N.S.R.
Controls	No.	7	3	2	12
Percentage		29	12.5	8.5	50
Receiving AA	No.	12	1	1	13
Percentage		44	3.7	3.7	48

* N.S.R. - no sign of recurrence.

According to Poulter et al. 1984

TABLE 2

Anti-inflammatory and analgesic effect of sodium acetylsalicylate
(AcSal) or/and vitamin C (C)
'Therapeutic test': Two hours after paw injection
(Trial R 23/82; N = 10 rats per group)

Parameter: Four hours after local carrageenan injection (0.1 ml; 1 % sol.)	Control Untreated	Sodium Acetylsalicylate; Vitamin C Oral route per kg body weight		
		100 mg AcSal	100 mg C	100 mg AcSal + 100 mg C
Anti-inflammatory effect:				
Mean increase of dot/plan paw diameter (mm)	1.86	1.23***	1.46*	1.02***
SEM+	0.08	0.09	0.05	0.10
Inhibition (per cent)		33.9 %	21.5 %	45.2 %
Analgesic effect:				
Mean improvement of pain tolerance (g)	35.00	14.00***	22.00**	13.00***
SEM+	2.69	2.67	2.49	2.60
Inhibition (per cent)		60.0 %	37.1 %	62.9 %

+ Difference between injected and non-injected paw
* Significant (p < 0.05)   in comparison with untreated controls
** Significant (p < 0.02)
*** Significant (p < 0.01)

TABLE 3

Anti-inflammatory and analgesic effect of vitamin C 'Therapeutic test': Two hours after paw injection (Trial R 25/82; N = 10 rats per group)

Parameter: Four hours after local carrageenan injection (0.1 ml; 1% sol.)	Control Untreated	Vitamin C Oral route per kg body weight		
		50 mg	100 mg	200 mg
Anti-inflammatory effect:				
Mean increase of dor/plan paw diameter (mm)	1.73	1.50*	1.40***	1.12***
SEM+	0.09	0.06	0.05	0.06
Inhibition (per cent)		13.3 %	19.1 %	35.3 %
Analgesic effect:				
Mean improvement of pain tolerance (g)	36.00	26.00ns	15.00***	14.00***
SEM+	3.40	4.00	3.42	3.06
Inhibition (per cent)		27.8 %	58.3 %	61.1 %

+ Difference between injected and non-injected paw
* Significant ($p < 0.05$) in comparison with untreated controls
*** Significant ($p < 0.01$)
ns Not significant

TABLE 4

Anti-inflammatory and analgesic effect of vitamin C
'Prophylactic test': 0.5 hour before paw injection
(Trial R 6 /81; N = 10 rats per group)

Parameter:	Control	Vitamin C Oral route per kg body weight			Phenylbutazone Oral route
Four hours after local carrageenan injection (0.1 ml; 1 % sol.)	Untreated	62.5 mg	125 mg	250 mg	20 mg
Anti-inflammatory effect:					
Mean increase of dor/plan paw diameter (mm)	2.05	1.97^{ns}	1.61^{***}	1.28^{***}	0.88^{***}
SEM+	0.06	0.04	0.07	0.06	0.06
Inhibition (per cent)		3.9 %	21.5 %	37.6 %	57.1 %
Analgesic effect:					
Mean improvement of pain tolerance (g)	38.00	36.00^{ns}	35.00^{ns}	31.00^{ns}	21.00^{***}
SEM+	2.01	1.51	3.00	3.32	2.44
Inhibition (per cent)		5.3 %	7.9 %	18.4 %	44.7 %

+ Difference between injected and non-injected paw
ns Not significant in comparison with untreated controls
*** Significant ($p < 0.01$)

TABLE 5

Anti-inflammatory and analgesic effect of vitamin C
'Prophylactic test': 0.5 hour before paw injection
(Trial R 4 /81; N = 10 rats per group)

Parameter:	Control Untreated	Vitamin C Oral route per kg body-weight			Phenylbutazone Oral route
		250 mg	500 mg	1000 mg	20 mg
Four hours after local carrageenan injection (0.1 ml, 1% sol.)					
Anti-inflammatory effect:					
Mean increase of dor/plan paw diameter (mm)	2.04	1.30***	1.04***	1.04***	0.85***
SEM+	0.05	0.04	0.07	0.07	0.06
Inhibition (per cent)		36.3 %	49.0 %	49.0 %	58.3 %
Analgesic effect:					
Mean improvement of pain tolerance (g)	37.00	30.00ns	17.00***	15.00***	20.00***
SEM+	2.13	1.49	2.13	3.42	2.11
Inhibition (per cent)		18.9 %	54.0 %	59.5 %	46.0 %

+ Difference between injected and non-injected paw
ns Not significant in comparison with untreated controls
*** Significant (p < 0.01)

TABLE 6

Anti-inflammatory effect of vitamin C (C)
Daily oral application during eight consecutive days
'Prophylactic test': 15, 30 and 60 minutes after local paw injection of
hyaluronidase (125 USP units/0.05 ml NaCl-sol.) on day nine

Anti-inflammatory effect + after irritation	Control, untreated	Oral application, daily during eight days		
		250 mg C per kg body weight	500 mg C per kg body weight	Phenylbutazone 2 mg per kg
15 minutes	1.94 0.13	1.72 0.18 11.3 %	1.09 0.16 43.9 %	1.40 0.11 27.7 %
30 minutes	2.10 0.12	1.69 0.14 19.6 %	1.27 0.15 39.3 %	1.26 0.10 40.0 %
60 minutes	1.49 0.06	1.26 0.16 15.4 %	0.94 0.11 36.9 %	0.87 0.10 41.6 %

+ Difference between injected and non-injected paw (mm $\pm$ SEM)

TABLE 7

Survival of patients with primary liver cancer, treated
with ð-linolenic acid * and ascorbic acid **

Patient	Survival (days)
1	19
2	28
3	57
4	57
5	60
6	69
7	77
8	79
9	104
10	130
11	314 ***

*   x = 27 capsules Efamol-G/day

**   x = 6.5 g per day

***   Patient still alive at the date of report.
        Normal mean duration of survival is 42 days.
                    According to van der Merwe 1984.

TABLE 8

Inhibition of tumour growth in mice by a combination of
hydroxocobalamin (HC) and ascorbic acid (AA).
Size (cm^3) after one week treatment (mean $\pm$ SD; n = 25)

Tumour	Test group	Control group
Krebs 2	0.13 [a]	1.63 $\pm$ 0.47
Ehrlich	0.00 [b]	2.19 $\pm$ 0.58

a) Mean of only 2 tumours which developed (0.1 and 1.2 cm^3)
b) No tumour developed; controls all developed tumours
Treatment: 240 mg/kg b.wt.daily (25 mg AA, 200 mg CaAA,
15 mg HC) in 8 ml H_2O.

According to Poydock, E. 1984

FIGURE 1

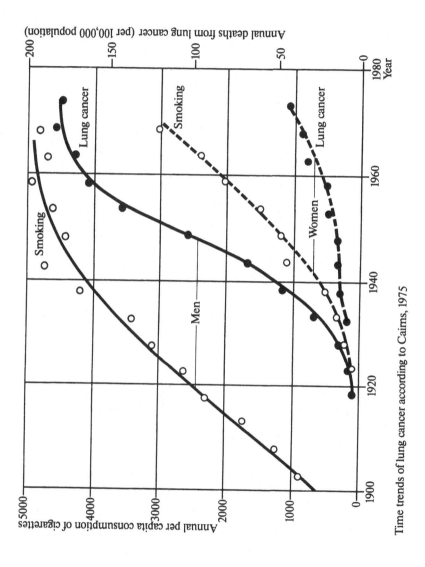

Figure 1

Time trends of lung cancer according to Cairns, 1975

Figure 2

Time trends in cancer mortality
Age-adjusted rates per 100,000 population:
Baltimore City, 1969–1980

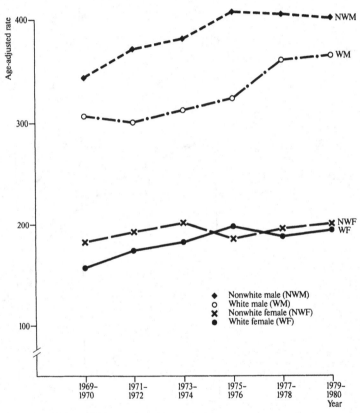

According to Celentano, 1984

Figure 3

Survival times after date of onset of terminal stage (untreatability) of ascorbate-treated cancer patients (kidney, rectum, bladder, ovary) compared with that of matched controls (10 per ascorbate-treated patient).

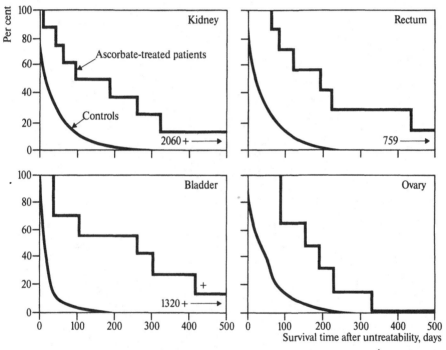

According to Cameron and Pauling, 1978

FIGURE 4

Figure 4

Survival times after date of onset of terminal stage (untreatability) of ascorbate- treated cancer patients (colon, stomach, bronchus, breast) compared with that of matched controls (10 per ascorbate-treated patient).

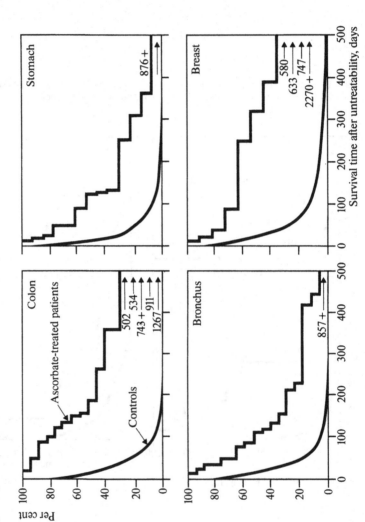

According to Cameron and Pauling, 1978

Figure 5

Survival times after date of onset of terminal stage of ascorbate-treated cancer patients (< 4 g versus > 5 g ascorbic acid daily).

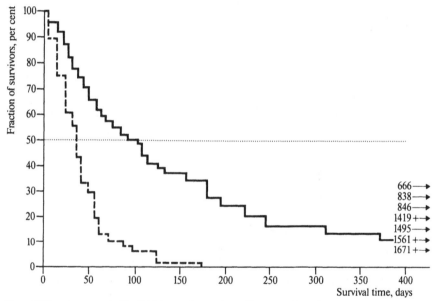

The solid line shows survival in 55 high-ascorbate patients. The dashed line shows survival in 44 low-ascorbate patients. The sign + indicates that some of the patients were still alive.

According to Murata et al., 1982

Figure 6

Survival results in patients with advanced cancer. 10 g ascorbic acid daily versus placebo

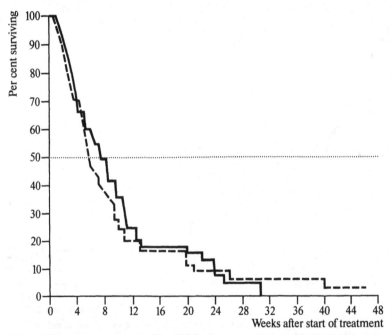

The solid line shows survival in 60 patients given ascorbic acid. The dashed line shows survival in 63 patients given the lactose placebo.

According to Creagan et al., 1979

Figure 7

Survival times after date of onset of terminal stage of ascorbate-treated patients with adenocarcinoma of the large bowel.

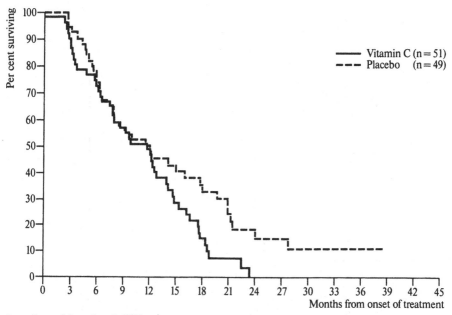

According to Moertel et al., 1985

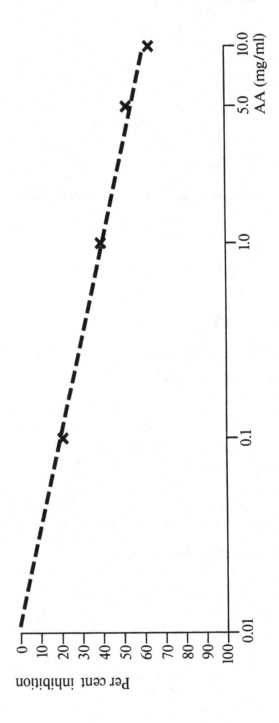

Figure 8

Inhibition of catalase in blood by ascorbic acid (AA)

Figure 9

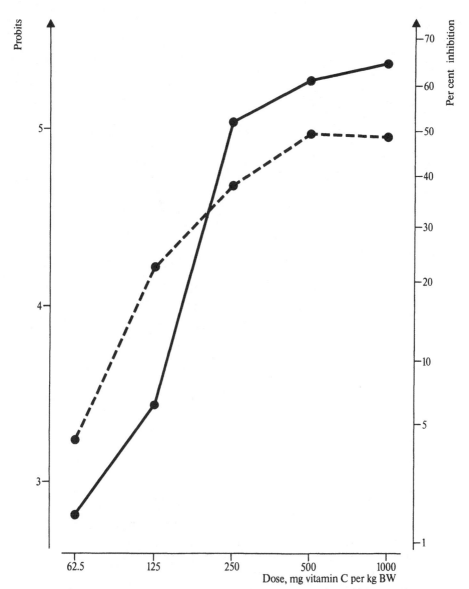

Vitamin C: Anti-inflammatory effects oral route. Inhibition per cent (probits)
Irritation by 0.1 ml carrageen 1% single oral application per kg body-weight (BW)

●━━━● Prophylactic assay: ½ hour before paw injection
●———● Therapeutic assay: 2 hours after paw injection

(n = 10 rats per group)

Figure 10

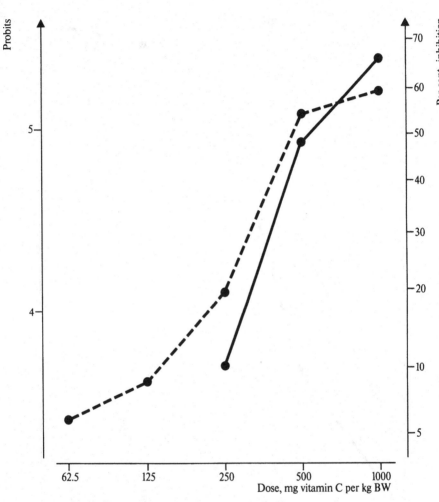

Vitamin C: Analgesic effects oral route. Inhibition per cent (probits)
Irritation by 0.1 ml carrageen 1% single oral application per kg body-weight (BW)

● ─ ─ ─ ● Prophylactic assay: ½ hour before paw injection

● ━━━━ ● Therapeutic assay: 2 hours after paw injection

(n = 10 rats per group)

11

e of ascorbic acid (AA) in plasma after infusion of 25 g AA in 250 ml glucose solution within
in man.

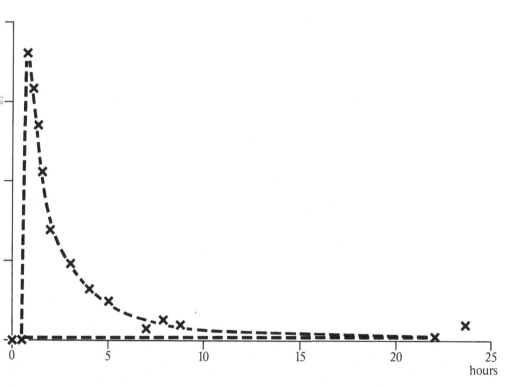

THE ROLE OF VITAMIN C IN TUMOR THERAPY (HUMAN)

Fukumi Morishige, M.D., Dr. Med. Sci., Ph.D.
Takahide Nakamura, M.D., Dr. Med. Sci.
Naoko Nakamura, M.D.
Noritsugu Morishige, M.D.

Fukuoka Nakamura Memorial Hospital

Fukuoka, Japan

INTRODUCTION

About thirty years ago, I started administering large doses of vitamin C to post-operative patients. Its primary aim was to improve the healing of surgical wounds. During that time, I recognized that vitamin C supplemented patients very rarely suffered from post-operative and post-transfused hepatitis. This finding is from observations made on many post-operative patients especially in Kyushu district.

During the 1975 International Congress on Microbiology held in Tokyo, we presented a report of our clinical observations for the period from 1967 to 1973. The observations indicated that, the use of large doses of vitamin C remarkably reduced the occurrence of post-operative hepatitis.

In 1975, we invited Dr. Pauling to Fukuoka and had discussions about orthomolecular nutritional treatment (especially, mega-vitamin C therapy) of various diseases including cancer. Since then, we started a systematic administration of large doses of vitamin C to patients with advanced cancer. My interest was gradually attracted by the basis and clinical problems related to the mechanism of action of vitamin C against cancer.

REVIEW OF OUR STUDIES

1. Use of Vitamin C in the Treatment of Advanced Cancer
    Patients

    I described here the results of the treatment of all
patients with terminal cancer who were first admitted to
the hospital with the diagnosis of cancer during the five-
year period from January 1, 1973 to December 31, 1977 (9).

    We conclude, in agreement with Cameron and Pauling
(2), that supplemental vitamin C in large dosages have
sufficient benefit for patients with advanced cancer. We
have noticed, in agreement with Cameron and Campbell in
1974 (1), that in many patients the administration of
vitamin C seems to improve the state of well being, as
indicated by better appetite, increased mental alertness
and desire to return to ordinary life.

2. Influence of Oral Supplementation of Vitamin C upon
    the Induction of MNNG Gastric Carcinoma in Rats

    To study this prolongation of survival times of human
cancer, we researched (5) about the influence of oral
supplementation of vitamin C upon the induction of MNNG
gastric carcinoma in rats.

    The summary is given here. The influence of megadose
ascorbate intake upon the induction of gastric cancer in
rats. By feeding with the ascorbate-supplemented diet,
though the incidence of gastric cancer was not effectively
inhibited, the infiltrative growth was significantly
repressed. Mega-ascorbate intake was more beneficial in
alleviating the development of gastric cancer when it was
commenced after the middle of a long-term experimental
period (initiation of adenomatous hyperplasia but no
appearance of malignant lesions) rather than from the
beginning of MNNG drinking. The aim of mega-ascorbate
intake was to reinforce the surrounding conncective tissues
to retard the malignant growth.

3. Enhancement of Antitumor Activity of Vitamin C by
    Copper/GGH Complex (6)

In summary, it will be stated that, when in contact with tumor cells, the physiochemically stable copper/GGH complex is easily decomposed due to its high peptide-cleavaging activity (12). In such circumstances, even such an inert copper complex liberates free copper ions in the medium surrounding tumor cells and causes synergistic killing of tumor cells by ascorbate.

4. Changes in Paramagnetic Species of Blood Plasma Following a Mega-Vitamin C Intake (10)

Ascorbic acid is known to be an essential reducing agent in biology. Having a moderately low redox potential, ascorbic acid readily reduces both cupric and ferric ions. The ESR spectrum of blood plasma frozen in liquid nitrogen exhibits three major paramagnetic species (3, 11, 4): organic free radical at about g=2.00, cupric ions bound to ceruloplasmin (CPL) - its perpendicular component at g=2.05 and ferric ion bound to transferrin(TRF) at g=4.2. These ESR signals might be changeable due to a large intake of vitamin C.

Ascorbic acid is readily autoxidized to dehydro-ascorbic acid in an oxygen-containing aqueous solution. It proceeds through a semiquinine intermediate of which the free radical(AFR) of substantial life time is demonstrable on ESR spectrum at room temperature (8, 7). Ascorbic acid, which undergoes free radical formation in vitro under conditions within the physiological range, may be expected to behave similarly in vivo.

This paper deals with elucidation of changes of these ESR-demonstrable paramagnetic species of human blood plasma following a large intake of vitamin C.

The summary of this report is as follows: Measurements of ESR spectra of blood plasmas, frozen in liquid nitrogen, reveal higher cupric and lower ferric ion signals both in vitamin C deficient guinea pigs and in a considerable number of cancer patients. An in vitro addition of an excess amount of vitamin C, which is capable of reducing free cupric and ferric ions, does not decrease these signals of blood plasmas to an appreciable extent. A large dosage of vitamin C in vivo decreases these signals significantly.

An aqueous solution of vitamin C exhibits a stable
free radical during its autoxidation process. Blood
plasmas of the rabbit, rat and monkey show the ESR signal
of ascorbic free radical, whereas plasmas of adult human
beings, chimpanzees and guinea pigs do not. A large dose
of vitamin C given to patients significantly increases this
ESR signal, which may be considered as a finding suggestive
of an abundance of these antioxidant in quenching destructive free radicals in the body.

CURRENT STUDIES OF OUR HOSPITAL ON TUMOR THERAPY USING VITAMIN C

With this background, a randomized clinical trial was
undertaken in our hospital. Usage of vitamin C in tumor
therapy has been as follows:

(1) When the patients possessed low NK activity of
depressed PWM-blastogenesis of lymphocytes, they were
given together or separately, large doses of vitamin C and
900,000 U. of interferon. Chart 1 shows the direct plaque
forming cells induced by PWM in patients of various ages
to whom vitamin C was not adminsitered. It is noticeable
that many cancer patients do not necessarily always show
PFC (plaque forming cells).

In chart 2, you can see the activity of natural
killer cells as a target of K-562 cells in patients of
various ages not taking vitamin C. In our laboratory,
the normal range of NK activity is from sixty percent
upwards. Cancer patients later on often show low NK
activity. Elderly persons do not always show low NK
activity.

Chart 3 represents PWM stimulated PFC assay of cancer
patients before and after administration of anticancer drug
plus i.v. infusion of vitamin C. Some cases show downhill
courses and the others uphill.

In chart 4, you can see the NK activity in cancer
patients who received i.v. vitamin C infusion before and
after anticancer drug administration. Most cases show
downhill courses and a few cases uphill or stationary
levels. When the patients show lower NK activity, they are
given i.v. infusion of 10g or more vitamin C. If the

patients continued to show low NK activity despite vitamin C injection, 900,000 U. of interferon were injected every day. In our experience, the daily dosage of about 1,000,000 U. (1 million units) of interferon injection has shown no side effects on the patients.

In chart 5, one can see the change of both NK activity and PFC induced antibody production. When chemotherapy was carried out, IgG produced a B cell function showed a rapid decrease. On the other hand, NK activity recovered despite chemotherapy. This is suspected to be the influence of interferon.

In the course of receiving chemotherapy, the cancer patients show a lower NK activity. Interferon injection is given to activate NK cells. Chart 6 shows the NK activity did not take decline in spite of the chemotherapy. Even if the patients had lower NK activity, they would speedily recover after daily doses of about one million units of interferon.

(2) When the radical mastectomy of cancer patients is unavailable, the combination therapy of a mega-dose of chemotherapy, frozen autologous bone marrow transplantation and vitamin C plus nucleic acid intake, is carried out (Table 1). As of now, one hundred and ninety patients with advanced solid cancer have been subjected to treatment with mega-doses of ascorbate plus chemotherapy. Of the 190 cases, all were given ascorbate 10g per day or more, 109 received the frozen autologous bone marrow transplantation(FABMT) 160 times. Thirty-four of the 109 patients received a second treatment, and five of the 34 received a third treatment with a mega-dose chemotherapy following FABMT.

Of the 109 patients, 84 (77%) showed subjective and/or objective remissions; however, 59 (54%) died from the original solid cancer, 27 (25%) from the profound acquired immune deficiencies, and the remaining 18 cases are still being followed. Comparative studies between patients who received the mega-dose chemotherapy after FABMT and those who received only the chemotherapy because of no remarkable myelosuppression will be effected in the future.

We saw some important cases in which ascorbate plus

FABMT played a decisive role to rescue the marrow abrasion
from anticancer drug toxicity. After the mega-dose chemotherapy, patients still showed myelosuppression in spite
of vitamin C administration.

Chart 7 shows CFU-C (colony forming units in culture),
which represents the hematopoietic function. It gradually
decreased in cancer patients after chemotherapy. Here,
bone marrow cells were separated by Ficoll-paque density
gradient.

Nowadays, vitamin C plus nucleic acid is given for
such cases. Chart 8 shows the influence of a drug called
Nuclear C_D which is a mixture of vitamin C plus nucleic
acid. Cancer patients who received Nuclear C_D did not
often show any decrease of leucocytes, NK activity and PWM
induced antibody production despite chemotherapy.

In chart 9, one can see that the patients who received
only nucleic acid had larger amounts of uric acid in their
blood. In contrast, the group that received Nuclear C_D
had a normal range. The patients who received Nuclear C_D
for a longer period did not show large amounts of uric acid
in their blood (see Chart 10). It would seem that vitamin
C inhibits the formation of uric acid.

We feel certain that nucleic acid-ascorbate plus FABMT
could accelerate hematopoietic recovery in cancer patients
after the mega-dose chemotherapy plus ascorbate. Although
ascorbate plus FABMT is still in a clinical trial stage
in specialized hospitals, we are inclined to think that it
is an interesting approach to provide hope for the advanced
cancer patients who have failed to respond to conventional
chemo and radiotherapies. If we had no knowledge of
ascorbate plus FABMT, we would not have applied the mega-
dose chemotherapy used in this study to our patients.

In Chart 11, the effect of the intravenous injection
of vitamin C can be seen. This patient was suffering from
metastatic liver tumor. The patients received 20g of
vitamin C injection every day, and despite the anticancer

drug injection, bone marrow did not show myelosuppression.

Chart 12 shows the effect of vitamin C after autologous bone marrow transfusion. After marrow transfusion, leucocytes and platelets increase very rapidly. It is suspected that vitamin C stimulates bone marrow function.

(3) For the enhancement of antitumor activity of vitamin C, we often use copper-glycylglycylhistidine complex. Next, I would like to show one case which we reported in the Journal of Nutrition, Growth and Cancer, 1983.

Patient, M.H., a 34-year old housewife and mother of two young children, began to have an intolerable pain in the upper arm in October, 1980. Analgestic drugs failed to relieve her pain. The pain and paresis of her left arm increased gradually. On November 27, she was admitted to the hospital. From the bone x-ray films and antiograms, osteosarcoma in the left upper arm was suspected. The x-ray film made on December 11 indicated a destructive bone lesion. At this time, ^{67}Ga uptake was very high on this region. She began to take 10g of vitamin C by intravenous drip infusion and orally 20mg of cupric sulfate (5mg as copper) per day.

On December 7, the dose of vitamin C for injection was increased to 20g per day. At the end of December, her bone pain began to decrease gradually. As mentioned, remarkable palliative effects. In early January, however, no remarkable repair of the lesion was noted on x-ray films and isotope bone scan.

On January 16, we began injecting the Cu/GGH solution selectively into the tumor region from the artery under the left clavicle. Twenty ml of Cu/GGH solution was injected by a continuous infusion pump for two days. This injection was continued twice a week, together with an intravenous injection of 20g of vitamin C, up to the end of March.

Examinations of the isotope bone scan and x-ray films (Figure 1) made in early February, indicated that ^{67}Ga uptake decreased significantly and the calcification of tumor lesion was remarkable. She had no more pain at this time. X-ray film (Figure 2) made on April 7, indicated a

complete regression of the tumor lesion. In early April,
the dose of vitamin C for injection was reduced to 10g per
day. Arterial infusion of Cu/GGH was stopped. She began
to take orally 20mg of cupric sulfate per day.

On April 29, she was discharged and has since been
receiving 6g vitamin C and 20mg cupric sulfate per day
orally. At the present time (as of August 10, 1982), she
has no symptoms nor pain in her arm. X-ray shows complete
regression of the tumor lesion.

(4) For the inoperable tumor tissues, lesions are locally
frozen by liquid nitrogen. In order to facilitate the good
recovery of necrotic tissues, large doses of vitamin C are
given. Up to now, 53 cases of advanced malignant tumors
have been treated with cryosurgery plus ascorbate. After
cyrosurgery, a mega-dosage of vitamin C is administered
for the enhancement of immune responses and of connective
tissue formation (Table 2). We made examinations weekly
for the natural killer activity(NK), monthly for the
pokeweed mitogen(PWM) induced antibody production and before
and after cryosurgery for tuberculin(PPD) reaction.
Following cryosurgery plus ascorbate intake, NK, PWM and
PPD respecitvely increased in eight cases (50%), 11 cases
(60%) and 4 cases (40%) (Charts 13, 14 and 15).

Vitamin C is related to the formation of connective
tissue. There is one case who suffered from liver
metastasis with gastric cancer. Chart 16 shows the
patient's protocol in autopsy. This liver autopsy
(Figure 3) revealed that a thick connective tissue formation surrounded the liver tumor which had a mega-dose of
vitamin C for 90 days. In spite of the high dosage of
chemotherapy, connective tissue formation was not
inhibited. We strongly suspect the predominant role of
vitamin C in the formation of the connective tissue.

Acknowledgement. We would like to thank our co-workers:
Shigeaki Morifuji, M.D., Shiro Matsumoto, M.D., Yashuhiko
Sato, M.D., DR.MED.SCI., Yoshiko Sakai, Tomoko Arima and
Jun-ichiro Gyotoku.

REFERENCES

1. Cameron, E. and Campbell, A. The orthomolecular

treatment of cancer II. Clinical trial of high-dose ascorbic acid supplements in advanced human cancer. Chem-Biol. Interactions. 9:285-315, 1974.

2. Cameron, E. and Pauling, L. Supplemental ascorbate in the supportive treatment of cancer: Prolongation of survival times in terminal human cancer. Proc. Natl. Acad. Sci. 73:3685-3689, 1976.

3. Foster, M.A., Pocklington, T., Miller, J.D.B., and Mallard, J.R. A study of electron spin resonance spectra of whole blood from normal and tumor bearing patients. Br. J. Cancer. 28:340-348, 1973.

4. Kawasaki, H., Akagi, Y., Nishi, K., Kakuda, T., Kimoto, E., Morishige, F., and Khono, M. Kurume Med. J. 25:273, 1978.

5. Kawasaki, H., Morishige, F., Tanaka, H., and Kimoto, E. Influence of oral supplementation of ascorbate upon the induction of N-methyl-N'-nitro-N-nitro-soguanidine. Cancer Letters. 16:57-63, 1982.

6. Kimoto, E., Tanaka, H., Gyotoku, J., Morishige, F., and Pauling, L. Enhancement of antitumor activity of ascorbate against ehrlich ascites tumor cells by the copper: Glycylglycylhistidine complex. Cancer Res. 43:824-828, 1983.

7. Kirini, Y. and Kwan, Y. Chem. Pharm. Bull. 20:2651, 1972.

8. Lagercrantz, C. Acta Chem. Scand. 18:562, 1964.

9. Morishige, F. and Murata, A. Intern. Acad. Prevent. Med. 5:47, 1978.

10. Morishige, F., Ohtsu, N., Tanaka, H., Yamaguchi, T., and Kimoto, E. Changes in paramagnetic species of blood plasma following a mega-vitamin C intake. J. Nutri. Growth & Cancer. 1:11-19, 1983.

11. Pocklington, T. and Foster, M.A. Electron spin resonance of caeruloplasmin and iron transferrin in blood of patients with various malignant diseases. Br. J. Cancer. 36:369-374, 1977.

12. Sylven, B. and Bois-Svensson, I. On the chemical pathology of interstitial fluid I. Proteolytic activities in transplanted mouse tumors. Cancer Res. 25:458-468, 1965.

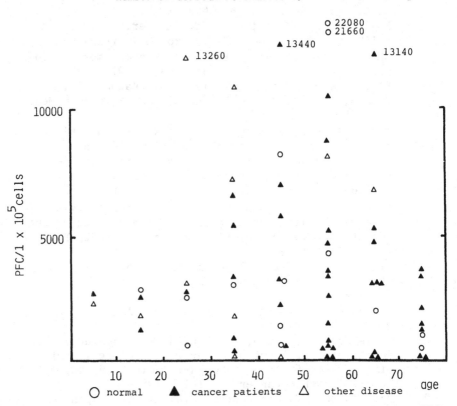

Chart 1. Many cancer patients do not necessarily show lower PFC (plaque forming cells). PFC tends to decrease with age.

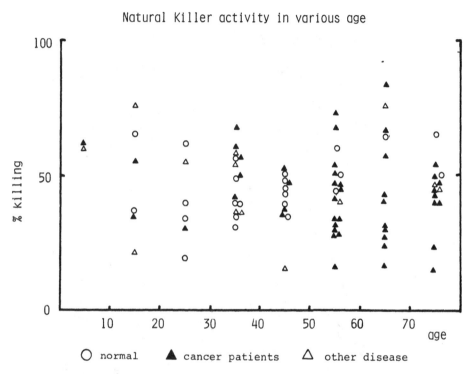

Chart 2. Cancer patients tend to show lower NK activity with age.

PWM stimulated PFC assay in Cancer patients

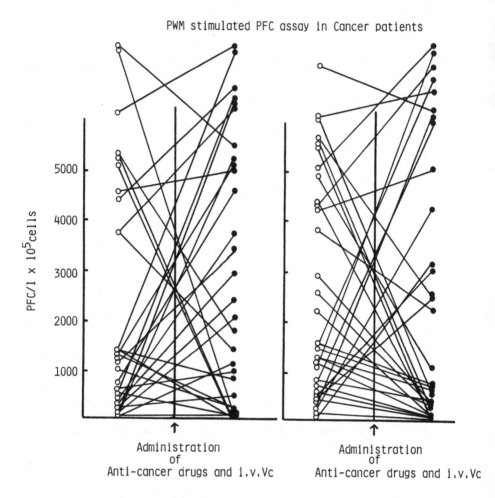

Chart 3. PWM stimulated PFC assay of cancer patients before and after administration of anticancer drugs plus i.v. infusion of vitamin C.

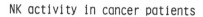

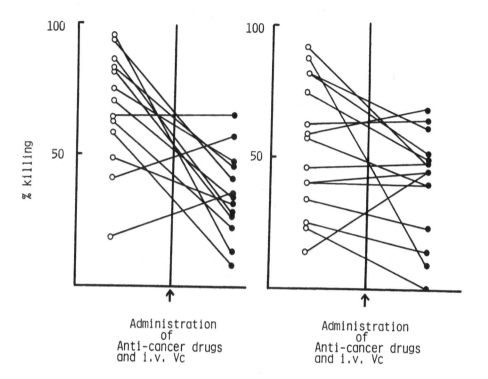

Chart 4. NK activity in cancer patients who received i.v. vitamin C infusion before and after anticancer drug administration.

Influence of Vc and IF in NK activity and PWM induced antibody production for Cancer Patients

A.K., 29, M. Osteo sarcoma

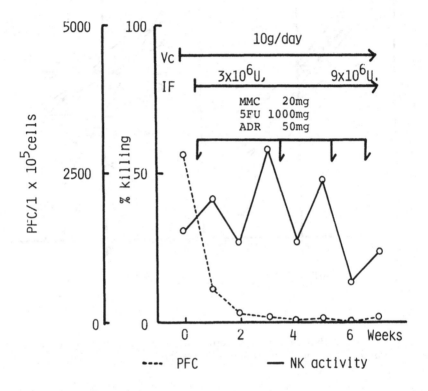

Chart 5. The change of both NK activity and PFC induced antibody production.

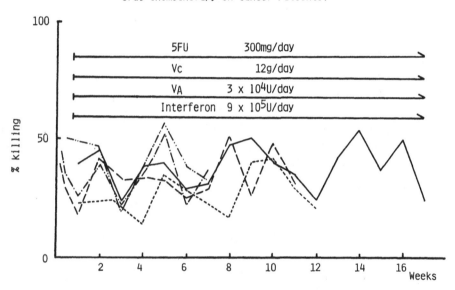

NK activity as a Result of Interferon injection in the course of oral Chemotherapy on Cancer Patients.

Chart 6. The NK activity did not take a down hill course despite chemotherapy.

Patients with Advanced Malignant Tumor

Diagnosis	Patients Participated	Patients aspirated BM	Patients infused BM
1. Gastric Cancer	51	66	43(34)
2. Pulmonary Cancer	32	40	24(13)
3. Mammary Cancer	18	26	17(13)
4. Hepatoma	16	22	9(6)
5. Osteo Sarcoma	8	15	11(5)
6. Malignant Lymphoma	8	12	6(4)
7. Pancreatic Cancer	7	11	3(2)
8. Ovarian Cancer	7	10	7(5)
9. Rectal Cancer	5	8	6(2)
10. Colon Cancer	5	6	6(5)
11. Esophageal Cancer	4	4	0(0)
12. Uterine Cancer	3	6	5(3)
13. Oral Malignant Tumor	3	5	5(3)
14. Cholecytic Cancer	3	3	1(1)
15. Thymoma	2	4	3(2)
16. Brain Cancer	2	4	2(1)
17. Intestinal Cancer	2	2	2(2)
18. Urinary Bladder Cancer	2	2	2(1)
19. Fatty Tissue Sarcoma	1	2	2(1)
20. Renal Cancer	1	2	2(1)
21. Thyroidal Tumor	1	2	1(1)
22. Maxillary Tumor	1	2	1(1)
23. Myeloma	1	2	0(0)
24. Vaginal Cancer	1	1	1(1)
25. Mediastinal Tumor	1	1	1(1)
26. Pharyngeal Cancer	1	1	1(0)
27. Melanoma	1	1	0(0)
28. Cervical Tumor	1	1	0(0)
29. Tongue Tumor	1	1	0(0)
30. Parotid Tumor	1	1	1(1)
Total	190	263	160(109)

Table 1.   As of now, 190 patients with advanced solid cancer have been subjected to treatment with mega-doses of ascorbate, 10g per day or more.

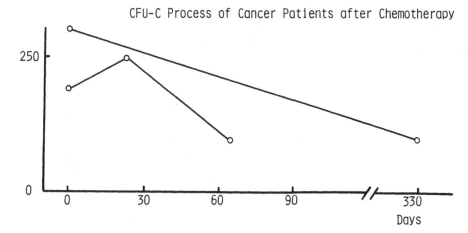

Chart 7. Bone marrow cells were separated by Ficoll-paque gradient. CFU-C, which represents the hematopoietic function, gradually decreased in cancer patients after chemotherapy.

Influence of Nuclear-C on NK activity, PWM induced antibody production, and Hemopoiesis in Chemotherapy for Cancer Patients

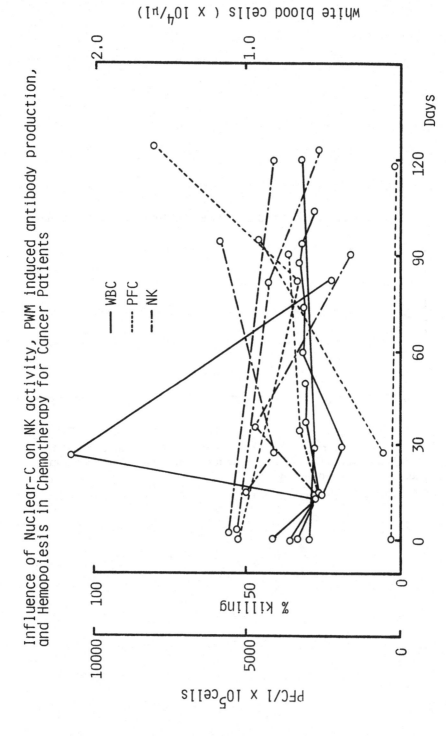

Chart 8.   Cancer patients who received Nuclear-C$_D$ did not often show the decrease of leucocytes, NK activity and PWM induced antibody production despite chemotherapy.

Blood Uric Acid Process of Cancer Patients received
Nuclear Acid with Intravenous Hyperalimentation

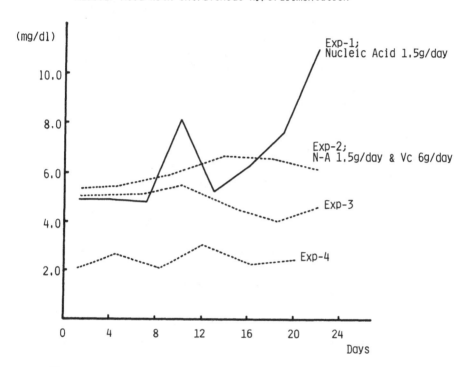

Chart 9. Patients who received nucleic acid alone (Exp-1) show high uric acid: on the other hand, the groups that received Nuclear-C_D (Exp-2, 3 and 4) are in a normal range.

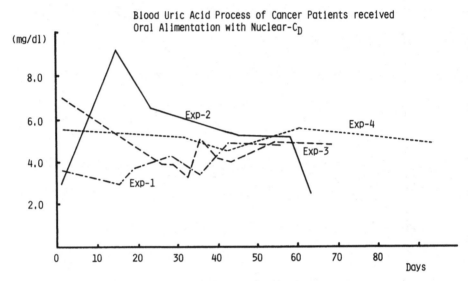

Chart 10. Cancer patients who received Nuclear-C_D do not show the increasing uric acid. It is suspected vitamin C inhibits the formaton of uric acid.

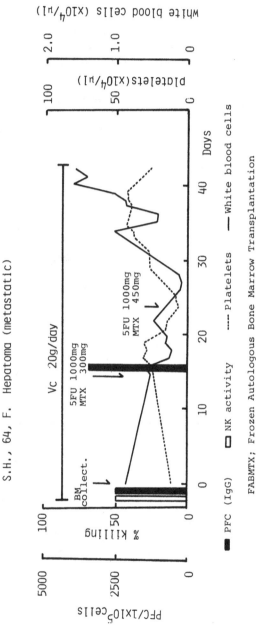

Chart 11. The effect of the i.v. injection of vitamin C. ɪns patient received 20g per day of vitamin C injection; bone marrow did not show myelosuppresion.

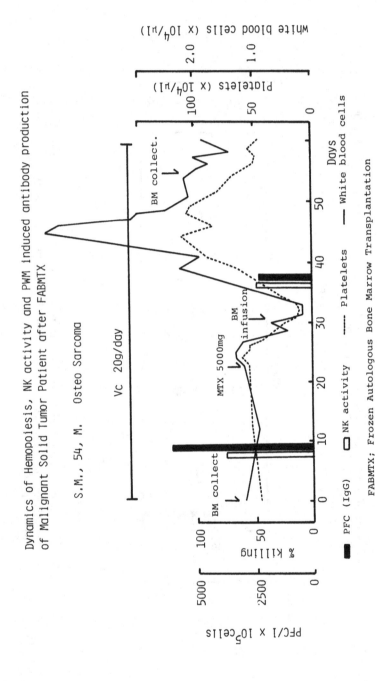

Dynamics of Hemopoiesis, NK activity and PWM induced antibody production of Malignant Solid Tumor Patient after FABMTX

S.M., 54, M.   Osteo Sarcoma

FABMTX; Frozen Autologous Bone Marrow Transplantation

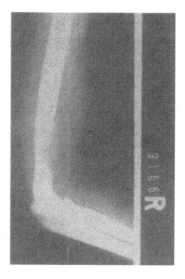

Fig. 1. X-ray film, made on December 11, 1980.

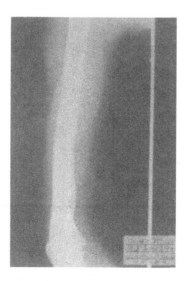

Fig. 2. X-ray film, made on April 7, 1981.

Advanced Malignant Tumors Treated with Cryosurgery & Ascorbate (10g/day)

Diagnosis	Patients	Cryosurgery
1. Gastric Cancer	9	11
2. Mammary Cancer	6	7
3. Pulmonary Cancer	5	7
4. Hepatoma	4	5
5. Cervical Cancer	4	7
6. Maxillary Tumor	3	7
7. Colon Cancer	3	3
8. Esophageal Cancer	2	4
9. Uterine Cancer	2	2
10. Mediastinal Cancer	2	2
11. Urinary Bladder Cancer	2	2
12. Ovarian Cancer	2	2
13. Malignant Melanoma	1	5
14. Parotid Tumor(Cancer)	1	2
15. Malignant Lymphoma	1	1
16. Pancreatic Cancer	1	1
17. Osteosarcoma	1	1
18. Cholecystic Cancer	1	1
19. Prostate Cancer	1	1
20. Osteocarcinoma	1	1
21. Pelvic Tumor(Cancer)	1	1
Total	53	73

Table 2. Advanced malignant tumors treated with cryosurgery and ascorbate, 10g per day.

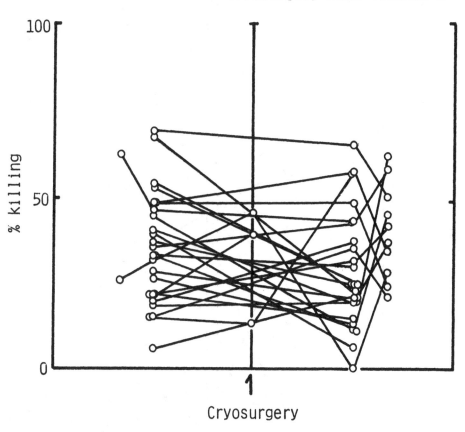

NK activities before & after
        Cryosurgery plus Vitamin C

hart 13.

Number of Secreting cells induced by PWM
before & after Cryosurgery plus Vc

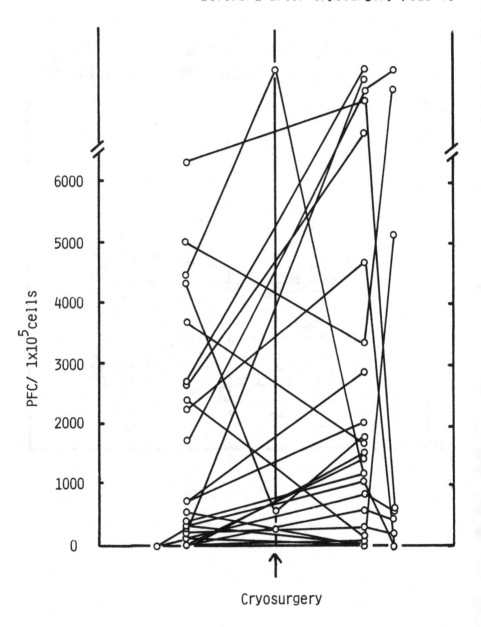

Chart 14.

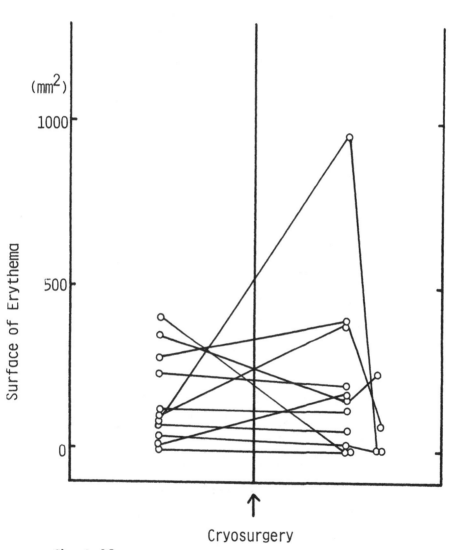

Tuberculin Skin Reaction before
& after Cryosurgery plus Vc

Chart 15.

Autopsy No.208 (TAH-35) Hata H. 49M

Gastric cancer with liver metastasis.
Histological diag.: well differentiated adenocarcinoma.

May, 18 '81   Diagnosis : Probe laparatomy

Jan. 30 '82   Admission

Apr. 5   UMD : 5FU 2000mg, MMC 30mg.

Jun. 10   UMD : 5FU 1000mg, MMC 10mg.

Jun. 17   UMD : 5FU 1000mg, MMC 10mg.

Jun. 22   Death

5 days ⌐ 12 days ⌐ 78 days ⌐ Vc 90 days

Chart 16. The patient's protocol in autopsy. There is one case that suffered from liver metastasis with gastric cancer.

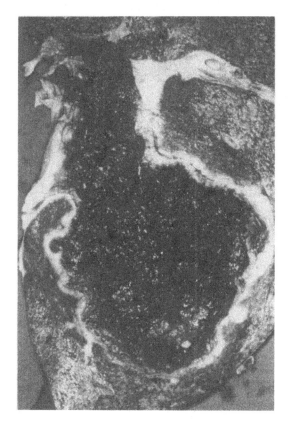

Fig. 3. Liver autopsy. A thick connective tissue formation surrounded the liver tumor which had had two mega-doses of vitamin C for 90 days.

VITAMIN B$_6$ STATUS AND ADMINISTRATION

DURING RADIATION THERAPY

Ladner, H.-A. and R.M.Salkeld

Ladner,H.-A., M.D., Professor, University of

Freiburg, W.-Germany, Dpt.of gynecol.Radiology

It has been demonstrated in man and experimental animals by biochemical investigations with vitamin A and C during both carcinogenesis and cancer therapy that there is a correlation between the vitamin status of the host and the tumor growth. Similar findings have also been observed in vitamin B$_1$ (RIVLIN 1975), B$_2$ (BASU 1976) and B$_6$ research.

VITAMIN B$_6$ AND CANCER

In animal experiments, metabolic function (e.g. enzyme activity) was altered in growing tumors in the presence of vitamin B$_6$ deficiency. It is also know that in some animals tumors growth was distinctly inhibited when dietary intake of pyridoxine was reduced (HA et al. 1984). This has also been observed in patients with advanced tumors (GAILANI et al. 1968). Consequently, antivitamin substances such as fluorouracil oder L-penicillamine have inhibited the growth of test tumors (TRYFIATES and COWORKERS 1974-1980, see review: TRYFIATES et al. 1981). This concern with the influence merely of vitamin B$_6$ deficiency on tumor growth has also been partly responsible for the fact that vitamin B$_6$ research in the field of oncology has been run on a very tight budget and that vitamin B$_6$ supplementation has been avoided during treatment of cancer. However, some of the more recent findings in the field of clinical oncology
- changes in tryptophan metabolism (similar to vitamin B$_6$ deficiency) in Hodgkin´s disease, bladder and breast

429

cancer (ALLEGRI et al. 1972, DE VITA et al. 1971, BELL
et al. 1975, BROWN et al. 1969, WOLF 1974).
- plasma pyridoxal-5-phosphate (PLP), the coenzyme form of
vitamin B_6, was reduced both in cases of local recurrences and systemic metastases of breast cancer patients
(POTERA et al. 1977) or in patients with advanced Hodg-
kin`s disease (DE VITA et al. 1971)
- suggestion that vitamin B_6 may correct the abnormalities of tryptophan metabolism and prevent recurrences of
bladder cancer (BAYARD and BLACKARD 1977) together with
some aspects of tumor and vitamin B_6 research show that we
should try a another approach to this problem. In the clinical analysis we have to mention some further relationships between vitamin B_6 metabolism and cancer. First, there
are interactions between estrogens and vitamin B_6 (ROSE
1978): PLP influences the DNA-binding activity of steroid
hormone receptors (WESTPHAL and BEATO 1981), especially in
breast and endometrium carcinoma, and receptor status is
one factor affecting the cure rate. The elevated urinary
excretions of tryptophan metabolites in patients with
breast cancer correlated with lower urinary steroid excretion (DAVIS et al. 1972). Secondly, vitamin B_6 status has
been demonstrated to influence immune responses (ROBSON
and SCHWARZ 1980).

VITAMIN B_6 AND IRRADIATION

In a few words we have to summarize the special situation
of vitamin B_6 metabolism after irradiation: it was observed that during radiation therapy for malignant tumor supplementation with vitamin B_6 markedly improved the general
condition of the patients and reduced the side effects of
radiation, such as nausea and vomiting. Subsequently the
work of LANGENDORFF and his collegues showed similar biochemical changes in experimental animals both in vitamin
B_6 deficiency syndrome and in acute radiation syndrome
(LANGENDORFF et al. 1960, STREFFER 1970). MELCHING 1963
and STREFFER 1970 as well as our group (LADNER) found in
the mouse, rat and dog a definite impairment of the activity of enzymes dependent on pyridoxal 5-phosphate (LANGEN-
DORFF et al. 1964) as well as a radioprotective effect of
individual B-vitamins, especially vitamin B_6, administered
immediately before total body irradiation in the lethal
range (LADNER and DÜSTERLHO 1964, LADNER and SCHWEIKERT

1964). During the last 10 years by means of new biochemical assay methods we have found at first in animals (LADNER et al. 1980) and later in patients with tumors (LADNER and VAN DE WEYER 1970) pronounced metabolic changes even during local irradiation, for example an increase in the urinary excretion of tryptophan metabolites (xanthurenic acid, kynurenine and kynurenic acid), and reduction of the activity of erythrocyte glutamic oxaloacetate transaminase (EGOT). It became apparent that, especially in man, there is a clear difference between tumor-induced and irradiation-induced metabolic changes. Furthermore, the changes in cases of certain tumors, e.g. the tryptophan metabolism, in carcinoma of the bladder (BROWN et al. 1969, WOLF 1975), breast (BELL et al. 1975) and in Hodgkin`s disease (DE VITA et al. 1971, ALLEGRI et al. 1972) were so marked that the investigation of the vitamin B status in large groups of cancer patients was indicated.

PATIENTS AND METHODS

Therefore we assessed the status of vitamin B_1, B_2 and B_6, and in certain subgroups also of vitamin A, C and E, in patients with gynecological cancers before and during the course of high-voltage radiation. Initially the EGOT-activation tests were carried out by the hospital laboratory and later by Hoffmann-La Roche in Basle. During the last 6 years the erythrocyte PLP concentrations were also measured. Shortage of room does not allow a detailed description of the groups of 5700 patients (Fig.1) or the analytical methods (Fig.2) (details see LADNER and HOLTZ 1979, VILLEUMIER et al. 1983).

Patients investigated   (1964 - 1984)
                                 n = 5700

(a)   gynecological cancer (carcinoma of cervix uteri, endometrium, ovary and breast)

(b)   gynecological cancer with special problems (diabetes mellitus, incipient uremia, etc.)

(c)   irradiation

(d)   cytostatic agents

(e)   irradiation with vitamin B_6 supplementation

Vitamin	Coenzyme	Erythrocyte enzyme	Activation test
B_1	thiamine pyrophosphate (TPP)	transketolase	ETK
B_2	flavine adenine dinucleotide (FAD)	glutathione reductase	EGR
B_6	pyridoxal 5-phosphate (PLP)	glutamate-oxalacetate transaminase	EGOT
B_6	pyridoxal 5-phosphate (PLP) (in Erythrocytes)	concentration: ng/ml (blood, hematocrit 40 %)	

In the evaluation of the findings, patients were excluded who had additional diseases which influenced the vitamin B_6, B_1 and B_2 status, such as diabetes (BEREZIN 1974) and uremia (SPANNUTH et al. 1978). In the light of the following results 1 + 2, we extended our investigations to the question of how far the observed vitamin B_6 deficiency could be reduced or prevented by pyridoxine supplementation. In patients treated with radiation for gynecological carcinomas, a dose of 40 mg pyridoxine daily was not always adequate to prevent the biochemical vitamin B_6 deficiency after radiation of up to 50 Gy. Daily administration of 300 mg pyridoxine was required to prevent impairment of the biochemical parameters of vitamin B_6 status (EGOT-activation and PLP). Since the effects, such as diarrhea, in irradiated patients could be only partly alleviated by daily oral doses of 300 mg pyridoxine, we investigated the influence of these doses on the survival rate in a large group of patients irradiated for gynecological tumors at various stages. During the last 20 years patients treated with local radiation were randomized to pyridoxine or no pyridoxine supplementation.

RESULTS

1. The extent of tumor-induced changes before the start of radiation therapy were dependent on the stage of the tumor; the more the carcinoma had progressed, and this applies to uterus, ovary and breast, the more pronounced was the impairment of the vitamin B_6, B_1 and B_2 activation tests.

2. Soon after the start of radiation – mostly after 10 days of radiation with a total dose in the target area of 20 Gy – the enzyme activities, especially those for vitamin B_6 and B_1, were definitely reduced (Fig.3), so that a biochemical deficiency of vitamin B_6 and B_1 was provoked, in particular in those patients with an already poor vitamin status before local radiation. Radiation-induced changes in the vitamin B_2 enzymes were less marked. After higher radiation doses in the target area or after widefield (abdominal) radiation, especially when the total radiation dose exceeded 40 Gy, the vitamin B_6, B_1 and even B_2 enzyme activities were even more impaired.

Gy (=100 rad)	Vitamin B_6 α-EGOT deficiency > 2,0	Vitamin B_6 Erythrocyte PLP deficiency < 3 ng/ml	Vitamin B_1 α-ETK deficiency > 1,25
0	22	31	25
1–15	24	74	43
16–40	49	82	43
41–60	43	83	53

Vitamin B_6 (α-EGOT and PLP) and vitamin B_1 (α-ETK) status before and during radiotherapy in 185 patients with gynecological carcinoma (frequency in %)

3. Similar reduction of the vitamin B_6 and B_1 enzyme activities were observed together with A. PFLEIDERER, Freiburg, in 120 patients with carcinoma of the ovary and breast after administration of cytostatic drugs, especially after cis-platinum.

4. The vitamin A, C and E status, as indicated by their plasma concentrations, was also impaired following local radiation, however not to the same degree as the vitamin B_6 and B_1-status.

5. If patients in stage II and III with similar radiation type and dosage are compared, the five years survival rate was about 10-15 % better in the groups which received pyridoxine than in the groups which did not. In 210 patients with endometrium carcinoma, stage II, the 5 years cure rate was 15 % better in the group with pyridoxine than in the group without pyridoxine.

Parallel to the changes in the vitamin B_6 status, several parameters of immune function were also impaired. Since in recent years vitamin B_6 has been reported (ROBSON and SCHWARTZ 1980) to play a role in immunocompetence, this aspect will also be investigated further. Nevertheless, on the basis of the present results, it can already be recommended that during high-voltage radiation therapy for cancer vitamin B_6 administration is of value.

CONCLUSIONS

We think it is important to show the difference between our aim and the approach of the other vitamin B_6 research in the field of oncology: Our problem in radiotherapy, especially intracavitary curietherapy and high-voltage therapy, was to find an adjuvant medication to improve tolerance to irradiation but which does not promote tumor growth. We believe that this problem may be solved to the extent that pyridoxine presumably protects only the healthy adjacent organs in patients with gynecological cancer against the effects of radiation. It should be stressed that in our study the pyridoxine was administred only during the period of irradiation and subsequent two weeks.

The biochemical deficiency of vitamin B_6, which we have
demonstrated both in experimental animals and in a large
group of patients with gynecological tumors, is a more
important effect of radiation than previously assumed.
This finding together with our observation about the positive influence of vitamin B_6 in 5700 irradiated patients
should provoke further investigations not only into the
effect of vitamin B_6 deficiency (for example on immunocompetence) during radiation therapy but also into the
effect of a deficiency of vitamin A, C and E.

REFERENCES

1 BASU,T.K.: Significance of vitamins in cancer.
   Oncology 33: 183-187 (1976)
2 BELL,E.D.; BULBROOK,R.D.; HAYWARD,J.L.; TONG,D.:
   Tryptophan metabolism and recurrence rates of patients
   with breast cancer after mastectomy. Acta vitamin.
   enzymol. 29: 104-107 (1975)
3 BEREZIN,M.: Vitamins and diabetes mellitus.
   Diabetologia 10: 380 (1974)
4 BROWN,R.R.; PRICE,J.M.; FRIEDELL,G.H.; BURNEY,S.W.:
   Tryptophan metabolism in patients with bladder cancer:
   Geographical differences. J.Nat.Cancer Inst. 43: 295-
   301 (1969)
5 BYAR,H.L.; BLACKARD,C.: Comparisons of placebo, pyridoxine, and topical thiotepa in preventing recurrence of
   stage I bladder cancer. Urology 10: 556-561 (1977)
6 DAVIS,H.L.; BROWN,R.R.; LEKLEM,J.; CARLSON,I.H.:
   Tryptophan metabolism in breast cancer. Correlation
   with urinary steroid excretion. Cancer 31: 1061-1064
   (1973)
7 GAILANI,S.D.; HOLLAND,J.F.; NUSSBAUM,A.; OLSON,K.B.:
   Clinical and biochemical studies of pyridoxine deficiency in patients with neoplastic diseases. Cancer 21:
   975-988 (1968)
8 HA,C.; KERKVLIET,N.I.; MILLER,L.T.: The effects of
   vitamin B_6 deficiency on host susceptibility to moloney
   sarcoma virus-induced tumor growth in mice. J.Nutr.114:
   938-945 (1984)

9 LADNER,H.-A.; SCHWEIKERT,C.H.: Zur Wirksamkeit resis-
   tenzsteigernder Substanzen bei Strahlenbelastung und
   Trauma. In: Melching,H.-J, et al. (eds.): Strahlenschutz in Forschung und Praxis 4: 299-302 (1964) Rom-
   bach, Freiburg

10 LADNER,H.-A.; VON DÜSTERLHO,R.: Zur Strahlenschutz-
   wirkung des Pyridoxal-5-phosphats. Naturwissenschaften
   51: 407 (1964)

11 LADNER,H.-A.; VAN DE WEYER,K.H.: Zur Erkennung strah-
   leninduzierter Vitamin B_6-Mangelzustände beim Menschen.
   Fortschr.Röntgenstr. 112: 382-388 (1970)

12 LADNER,H.-A.; HOLTZ,F.: Zum Verhalten einiger B-Vitamine nach Strahlen und/oder Zytostatikabehandlung
   gynäkologischer Karzinome. In: Wannenmacher,M.; Gau-
   werky,F.; Streffer,Ch. (eds.). Kombinierte Strahlen-
   und Chemotherapie. Urban u. Schwarzenberg, München-
   Wien-Baltimore 191-195 (1979)

13 LADNER;H.-A.; MITCHELL;J.S.; KING,E.A.; WEISSELBERG,R.:
   Das Verhalten einiger B-Vitamine beim Karzinompatien-
   ten während der Strahlentherapie. Strahlentherapie 156:
   856-860 (1980)

14 LANGENDORFF,H.; MELCHING,H.-J.; RÖSLER,H.: Untersu-
   chungen über einen biologischen Strahlenschutz.
   XXXVII.Mitteilung: Über den Anteil des Adenylsäure-
   systems und des Pyridoxal-5-phosphats am Strahlenschutz-
   effekt des Serotonins. Strahlentherapie 113: 603-609
   (1960)

15 LANGENDORFF,H.; SCHEUERBRANDT,G.; STREFFER,Ch.; MEL-
   CHING;H.-J.: Die Wirkung einer Ganzkörperbestrahlung
   von Mäusen auf die Aktivität der Dekarboxylase aroma-
   tischer Aminosäuren in Leber und Milz. Naturwissenschaften 51: 290-291 (1964)

16 MELCHING,H.-J.: Zur Frage einer Beeinflussung der Strah-
   lenempfindlichkeit bei Säugetieren. Strahlentherapie
   120: 34-73 (1963)

17 POTERA,C.; ROSE,D.P.; BROWN,R.R.: Vitamin B_6 deficiency
   in cancer patients. Am.J.Clin.Nutr. 30: 1677-1679 (1977)

18 RIVLIN,R.S.: Riboflavin and cancer. In: Rivlin,R.S.(ed)
   : Riboflavin, Plenum press, New York and London. 369-
   391 (1975)

19 ROBSON,L.C.; SCHWARZ,M.R.: The effects of vitamin B_6
   deficiency on the lymphoid system and immune responses.
   In: Tryfiates,G.B. (ed): Vitamin B_6 metabolism and role
   in growth. Food and Nutrition press, Westport 205-222
   (1980)

20 ROSE,D.P.: Oral contraceptives and vitamin B_6. In: Human vitamin B_6 requirements. National academy of sciences, Washington, 193-201 (1978)

21 STREFFER,Ch.: Zum Stoffwechsel der Aminosäuren und Proteine nach Bestrahlung von Säugetieren. In: Gerber, G.B.; Ladner,H.-A.; Rausch,L; Streffer,Ch (eds): Biochemisch nachweisbare Strahlenwirkungen und deren Beziehungen zur Strahlentherapie. G.Thieme, Stuttgart 51-63 (1970)

22 SPANNUTH,C.L.; MITCHEL,D.;STONE,W.J.; SCHENKER,S.; WAGNER;C.: Vitamin B_6 nutriture in patients with uremia and with liver diasease. In: Human vitamin B_6 requirements. National Academy of Sciences, Washington, 180-192 (1978)

23 TRYFIATES,G.P.; MORRIS,H.P.; SONIDIS,G.P.: Vitamin B_6 and cancer (Review). Anticancer Res. 1: 263-268 (1981)

24 DE VITA,V.T.; CHABNER,B.A.; LIVINGSTON,D.M.; OLIVERIO, V.T.: Anergy and tryptophan metabolism in Hodgkin's disease. Am.J.Clin.Nutr. 24: 835-840 (1971)

25 VUILLEUMIER,J.P.; KELLER,H.E., RETTTENMEIER,R; HUN-ZIKER,F.: Clinical chemical methods for the routine assessment of the vitamin status in human populations Part II: The water-soluble vitamin B_1, B_2 and B_6. Internat.J.Nutr.Res. 53: 359-370 (1983)

26 WESTPHAL,H.M., BEATO,M.: Influence of pyridoxal-5-phosphate on the DNA-binding activity of steroid hormone receptors and other DNA binding proteins. FEBS Letters 124: 189-192 (1981)

27 WOLF,H.: Studies on tryptophan metabolism in man. Scand.J.Clin.Lab.Invest. 33: Suppl. 136 (1974)

RETINOIDS AND VITAMIN E: MODULATORS OF IMMUNE FUNCTIONS

AND CANCER RESISTANCE

Ronald Ross Watson
Department of Family and Community Medicine
and Cancer Center, University of Arizona,
Tucson, Arizona 85724

For centuries man has recognized the association
between nutrition and health. One compelling hypothesis
that explains the increased morbidity and mortality is
that nutritional deficiencies impair responsiveness
(1,2). How different nutrient intakes alter career growth
and development has been more of a mystery. Nutritional
modulation of immune functions, either enhancement or
suppression, is a significant component in retarding
cancer development or growth. For example, nutritional
intakes reduced in animals enhance longevity by, in part,
changing development of immune responses and increasing
resistance to cancers (3,4,5). Moderately undernourished
Australian aborigine children had increased incidences of
bacterial infections and reduced incidence of tumors,
which suggests improved cellular immunity (6). It also
suggests that more needs to be known about the effects of
diet on various host defenses and the proper intakes for
optimum immune functions. Human nutrition in different
populations is most often both quantitatively and
qualitatively distinct. It may include deficiencies or
excesses in protein, calories, vitamins, and trace
minerals, usually in a large variety of permuted
combinations.

A major aim of clinical and experimental cancer
research is to develop agents or ways to increase the
tumor-directed immunological response of the host (7).
Clearly, vitamins have stimulating effects on some aspects

of cellular and humoral immune functions (8). While
immunoalteration by high dietary intakes of vitamins is
not the most prominent explanation for resistance to
cancer, it is an important side effect and may be a
significant component of resistance. Naturally occurring
and synthetic retinoids have been shown to prevent and/or
cure several chemically induced benign and malignant
animal tumors. There is also evidence that blood levels
of vitamin A and the ingestion of vegetables containing
large amounts of beta-carotene are inversely associated
with cancer risk. On the other hand, low levels of
dietary retinoids are associated with immunosuppression
(9) and perhaps explain part of the increased risk of
certain types of cancer in countries with chronic
undernutrition. In this paper Vitamin A and E will be
used as models to show an association between low or very
high intake and immune functions which affect cancer
resistance.

VITAMIN A DEFICIENCY AND IMMUNE FUNCTION

Is immunosuppression associated with low vitamin A
intake and can it be a significant contributing factor to
cancer development from dysplasia? The association
between hypovitaminosis A and microbial infections suggest
a major role due to suppressed host defenses in incidence
and severity of infections (10). Vayas and Chandra (9)
recently summarized the effects of hypovitaminosis A on
immune functions with most reports showing significant
immunosuppression. Most research was done with animal
models as relatively little is known about vitamin A
deficiency and immune functions in humans (9). A diet
deficient in vitamin A in rats reduced the size of the
thymus and spleen (11). The magnitude of change was much
greater in the vitamin A-deficient group than pair fed
controls. The cortical region of the thymus of vitamin
A-deficient animals was devoid of lymphocytes. Involution
of the thymus and bursa of Fabricius were observed in
vitamin A-deficient chicks (12). The associated presence
of protein-calorie malnutrition also confounds the picture
in vitamin A-deficient children. Thus, the reduction in
the number of T cells may well be due to concomitant
protein-calorie malnutrition in addition to vitamin A
deficiency (13). Surprisingly the level of serum thymic
factor is unaltered even with reduction in thymus size in

animals fed a low vitamin A diet (14). In vitamin A
deficiency, the differential count revealed a relative
increase in neutrophils and a decrease in lymphocyte
number. However, its effects on natural kill or
regulatory lymphocytes important in cancer resistance,
appears unstudied (9). The mitogenic response of splenic
lymphocytes of vitamin A–deficient rats is significantly
less than pair-fed animals (15). Vitamin A
supplementation for 3 days was shown to increase
circulating lymphocytes and to restore the mitogenic
response of splenic lymphocytes to normal levels (15).
Decreased nucleic acid synthesis may be due to defective
synthesis of membrane receptors. Marked changes in
membrane glycoproteins of lymphocytes (9) may contribute
to impaired cell-mediated immunity seen in vitamin A
deficiency. Alternatively, if changes in T cells in
vitamin A deficiency are accompanied by increased
suppressor T cells, then decreased mitogenic response
would also result. Vitamin A deficiency could
significantly reduce immune responses to cancer antigens
by loss of the adjuvant effects of vitamin A. It acts as
an adjuvant at nontoxic doses and enhances cell-mediated
and humoral immune responses (12). Injections of vitamin
A increased cellularity of regional lymph nodes (16). The
vitamin was also shown to stimulate antibody production to
bovine gamma globulin, which would otherwise have resulted
in immunological paralysis (17). The adjuvant property of
vitamin A was thought to be due to its membrane-labilizing
effect on lysosomes. Lysosomal membrane labilization can
induce lymphoid cell proliferation (18). Vitamin A
enhances cell-mediated immunity response when administered
simultaneously with the antigen challenge (9). Moreover,
injection of vitamin A at a site remote to that of antigen
was shown to be ineffective in enhancing cell-mediated
immunity (19).

THE ROLE OF HIGH INTAKES OF RETINOIDS ON IMMUNOALTERATION AND ANTICANCER RESISTANCE

Epidemiologic evidence suggests that natural retinoids
can cause a reduction of cancer risk in several types of
cancer. Some different postulated modes of action of high
vitamin A are: prevention of association of the
carcinogens or their active metabolites to the target
site, interference with the normal metabolic pathway of

certain carcinogens via inhibition of certain mixed
function oxidases, lysosomal labilization and subsequent
breakdown of premalignant cells, reversal of squamous cell
dysplasia, and immunosuppression (19). Routinely vitamin
A (retinol) has been shown to increase the T-cell
mitogenic response in lymphocytes (20). Retinoic acid
stimulation of cell-mediated immune reactions is indicated
by the enhancement of skin graft rejection in mice (21)
and induction of cytotoxic T-cells in mice fed high
intakes (22,23). However, stimulation of mitogenesis is
not universal for all retinoids and at all
concentrations. For example, retinol at high
concentrations inhibited human T-cell mitogenesis (24).
In mice effector activity of spleen cells against a
syngeneic tumor was specifically augmented by low doses of
retinoic acid, whereas high doses had a suppressive effect
(25). In addition, effector cell generation time was
shortened and subsequent persistence was extended by
retinoic acid (25). It was not clear in this study
whether retinoic acid acted on immunoregulatory hormone
production, directly affected T-cells, or perhaps, first
affected macrophages carrying antigens which then helped
activate effector T-cells. Cellular immune enhancement
with increased tumor resistance by retinoids in vivo
suggest that this property of retinoids is a major
responsible system for retinoids' ability to inhibit the
growth and developments of certain types of tumors (26).
For example, retinoid inhibition was only seen with tumors
which are strongly immunogenic or in immunocompetent mice
(26). Using adult thymectomized, lethally irradiated and
fetal liver reconstituted mice, it was found that
inhibition of tumor growth was not due to direct toxic
effects of retinoic acid (26), but rather appeared to be
the result of stimulation of thymus-dependent,
immune-mediated effectors able to suppress tumor growth.
However, there is much evidence that the direct effects of
retinoids on tumors in vivo is a major system of antitumor
activity (27). Clearly, there are limits to the benefits
to the immune system of high doses of retinoids. Some
very high doses caused depletion of spleen and thymus
lymphocytes while leaving bone marrow unaffected (28). In
vitro treatment of lymphocytes with retinol at a high
concentration suppressed immune functions. In a mouse
model, induction of cell-mediated cytotoxicity to
allogenic tumor cells is stimulated by low doses of

retinoic acid while high doses suppress cell-mediated
cytotoxicity induction (28). In humans, natural killer
cell activity was regulated by retinoic acid (29), which
suppressed tumor growth. Synthetic retinoids such as
13-cis retinoic acid are sometimes more effective in
prevention of experimentally induced cancers and less
toxic than vitamin A. The role of altered immune defenses
in the action of 13 cis retinoic acid is unclear due to
limited experimentation, particularly in humans (7). It
has recently been shown to inhibit in vitro human
T-lymphocyte mitogenesis (30). In humans with
unresectable bronchogenic cancer there are immune
potentiating effects of 13 cis retinoic acid. The authors
concluded that these effects are as important as any
direct ones on the tumor itself (20). Perhaps of greater
interest is recent animal experiments showing a 10-fold
increase in cell-mediated cytotoxicity by 13 cis retinoic
acid, after challenge with suboptimal immunogen inoculum
(31). At high dosages, cell-mediated cytotoxicity was
inhibited by some other retinoids while 13 cis retinoic
acid increased cell-mediated cytotoxicity (32). This
suggests that correlation of cellular immune functions,
cancer resistance, and dose of each retinoid needs to be
studied carefully at several doses in humans. The
helper/suppressor T-cell ratio tended to increase with
prolonged use of 13 cis retinoic acid (Watson, Alberts and
Jackson, unpublished data). Serum immunoglobulins were
significantly decreased due to prolonged use of this
retinoid. Changes in hormone production or release caused
by high intakes of vitamins may be part of the mechanics
on which alter immune functions. We have shown that high
dietary levels of vitamin E in mice decrease basal serum
glucocorticoid levels (33) as well as summarized a number
of studies confirming its role in changing immune function
(34). We recently found that high intakes of 13 cis
retinoic acid suppressed significantly corticosteroid
levels. Plasma cortisol levels decreased from 15.3 ug/dL
to 9.6 ug/dL (Watson--unpublished data). This might
explain in part some of the apparent changes seen in
regulatory T-cell markers or the lower serum
immunoglobulin levels. Altered cellular immunity
functions could play a major role in prevention of
carcinogenesis with hypovitaminosis A suppressing and
hypervitaminosis A sometimes enhancing cellular immunity
(7,9). Recently high vitamin A intake enhanced immune

functions suppressed by burns (35) and surgical trauma
(36). Hypervitaminosis A may be able to elevate
suppressed normal or immune functions in the cancer
patient for optimum functioning of host defenses to
pathogens and tumor cells. It appears critical to monitor
the cellular immune system when attempting to achieve
enhancement of tumor resistance with retinoid
supplementation. Enhancement or activation of macrophages
was caused by high retinol palmitate intakes in mice with
increased numbers of peritoneal exudate cells. Thus, the
strong possibility exists for assessment in humans of
optimum doses of several retinoids via observations of
their effects on key anticancer defenses. In summary
retinoids appear to be potent antipromoters for
carcinogenic agents (37). They may effectively inhibit
initial malignant cell growth directly and/or via a
modulation of cellular functions, including immune
defenses systems.

EFFECTS OF HIGH VITAMIN E INTAKE ON IMMUNE FUNCTIONS
AND DISEASE RESISTANCE

Most human or animal diets contain enough vitamin E to
prevent the generalized, recognized signs of deficiency.
However, the optimum amount for enhanced longevity, immune
responses, and resistance to disease or tumor growth is
less clear and is poorly defined (38). Several recent
studies suggest that it is necessary to understand the
effects of intake above that routinely found in what is
now considered a "reasonable and prudent" diet. For
example, following high vitamin E intake, carcinogenesis
was inhibited, patients were protected from adverse side
effects of radiation therapy, humoral immune responses to
antigen stimulation or resistance to bacterial infection
were enhanced (39,40), helper T-cell activity was altered,
and attainment of adult cellular immune functions (41) in
young mice was accelerated. Clearly absence of vitamin E
in the diet will eventually cause significant suppression
of disease resistance (42,43). However, to determine what
are optimal as well as toxic or suppressive levels for
disease or cancer resistance, not only must deficient
diets be used, but those with high intakes. A review of
all but the more recent literature showed that
supplementation of routine diets in animals improved the
humoral immune responses of mice, chickens, turkeys, and

guinea pigs (44). Why do these limited animal studies suggest that high intakes of vitamin E improve disease and possibly tumor resistance? We believe that enhanced disease resistance, and tumor resistance in mice based on our work (41,45,46), is due to altered cellular immune functions and secretory immune functions. For example, we found that there were increased amounts of secretory IgA in the intestinal secretions of young mice fed a high vitamin E diet (41,45,46). We also found elevated numbers of cytotoxic lymphocytes in young mice, which could be important in anticancer defenses and which perhaps result from more rapid maturation of T-cell functions (41,45,46). It appeared that vitamin E was accelerating maturation of only certain types of T cells. Under several conditions, high vitamin E increased the phytohemagglutinin/concanavalin A response ratio, suggesting that the vitamin has an effect on maturation of T cells (47). Hypothetically, stimulation of T-cell responses may be the result of an effect on Ia + T cells (47). Vitamin E did not function as a mitogen in nude (athymic) mice or enhance the lipopolysaccharide (LPS) response of spleen as it does in normal mice (47). These data suggest that vitamin E may act with thymic factors to produce a mature T-helper cell. Thus, vitamin E may act in part by selectively stimulating certain populations of T-cells and/or reducing hormonal control on these T-cell functions.

In the area of hormonal regulation, we have shown consistently in mice that high intakes of vitamin E reduce serum corticosteroids (41,45,46). They have been clearly shown to affect T-cell function and thymus gland development. This may be a partial explanation for enhanced immune functions via decreased regulation of the thymus and, directly, T cells. Vitamin E may directly affect the lymphocyte cell itself by altering prostaglandin synthesis (48). There is growing evidence that prostaglandins regulate immune responses and are clearly immunosuppressive at high levels. Vitamin E may directly affect the lymphocyte cell itself by alterine prostaglandin synthesis (48). There is growing evidence that prostaglandins regulate immune responses and are clearly immunosuppressive at high levels. Vitamin E is an effective inhibitor of prostaglandin synthetase. Vitamin E as an antitoxidant may prevent the oxidation of

arachidonic acid in the biosynthetic pathway leading to
prostaglandins. Chickens fed supplemental vitamin E at
six times the normal level had decreased levels of
prostaglandins E, E2 and F2a in immunopoietic organs
(bursa and spleen). Aspirin, a known prostaglandin
inhibitor, acted synergestically with vitamin E in
depressing endogenous prostaglandin levels and decreasing
mortality from Escherichia coli infection (48). Improved
defenses and antibody production may also be due to
increased T-cell helper function (49). These T cells may
be active in host defenses per se and play a critical role
in optimum B-cell production of IgG and IgA (49).

Although a number of investigations show either
enhancement or at least little effect of supplementary
vitamin E, recent reports suggest that high levels may be
inhibitory. In one of the only human studies of vitamin E
supplementation and immune response, Prasad (50) reported
suppression of bactericidal activity and mitogen-induced
lymphocyte transformation after 3 weeks of
supplementation. This does not agree with our unpublished
data from a long-term supplementation with higher levels
of vitamin E (Petro, Ismail, and Watson, unpublished work)
or with the animal work cited above. Of more relevance is
a very recent animal study showing that some levels of
vitamin E supplementation enhanced whereas very high
levels suppress immune functions. Vitamin E is generally
considered to be relatively nontoxic at high dosages. In
the study by Yasanga et al. (57), vitamin E was given
intravenously rather than by diet and high serum levels
were maintained. They found enhancement with injection of
5-20 IU/kg per day. The optimum level was not determined
from these two dosages. (In many of the human and animal
studies cited previously, the serum levels of
alpha-tocopherol were not measured, so that correlation
between dietary supplementation, altered immune function,
and serum levels of alpha-tocopherol is difficult.) In
unpublished work, Yasanaga et al. indicate that they have
data in mice confirming our preliminary study (67), which
showed some suppression of cancer growth in vivo by
supplementary vitamins in mice. It should also be
emphasized that, though most studies manipulate one
nutrient in an experiment, there can be significant
interations between several components in the diet.
Recently, Chen (52) found an increased vitamin E

requirement when rats were fed large amounts of vitamin C. She found that adverse effect of high supplementation of vitamin C on tissue antioxidant potential was overcome by increased vitamin E and that the vitamin E requirement was increased by vitamin C supplementation. Clearly, there is a need to define accurately the levels of vitamin E that produce the best host defenses in humans. Whether supplementation of normal diets with vitamin E is considered "overcoming a deficiency disease" or "producing optimum functions" is largely irrelevant. What is critical is defining and determining what is important for health in humans and animals, including cancer resistance.

ACKNOWLEDGMENTS

Research supported in part by grants from National Cancer Institute CA-27502, Wallace Genetics, Inc. and Phi Beta Psi Sorority.

REFERENCES

1. Watson R. R., and McMurray D. N. Effects of malnutrition on secretory and cellular immunity. CRC Crit. Rev. Food Sci. Nutr., 12:113-159, 1979.

2. Scrimshaw N. S., Taylor C. E., and Gordon J. E., Interactions of nutrition and infection. WHO Monogr. Ser., 57:3, 1968.

3. Weindruch R. H., Kristie A., Chevey K. E., and Walford R. L. Influence of controlled dietary restriction on immunological function and aging. Fed. Proc., 38:2007-2016, 1979.

4. Watson R. R., and Safranski D. Dietary restrictions and immune responses in the aged. CRC Handbook Immunol. Aging., 125-139 1981.

5. Fernandes G., Yanis E. J., and Good R. A. Suppression of adenocarcinoma by the immunological consequences of caloric restriction. Nature (London), 263:504-507, 1976.

6 Jose D. G., Shelton, M., and Tauro, G. P., et al Deficiency of immunological and phogocytic function in aboriginal children with protein-calorie malnutrition. Med. J. Aust., 2:699-705, 1975.

7. Watson R. R. Regulation of immunological resistance to cancer by beta carotene and retinoids. In: Watson

R. R., ed. Nutrition, Disease Resistance and Immune Function. New York: Marcel Dekker, 299–312, 1984.

8. Watson, R. R., ed. Nutrition, Disease Resistance and Immune Function. New York: Marcel Dekker, 299–312, 1984.

9. Vyas D. and Chandra R. K. Vitamin A and Immunocompetence. In: Watson R. R., ed. Nutrition, Disease Resistance and Immune Function. New York: Marcel Dekker, 325–356, 1984.

10. Chandra R. K., and Newberne P. M., eds. Nutrition, Immunity and Infection: Mechanisms of Interactions. New York: Plenum Press, 1977.

11. Krishnan S., Bhuyan U. N., Talwar G. P., and Ramalingaswami V. Effect of vitamin A and protein-calorie undernutrition on immune responses. Immunology, 27:383–392, 1974.

12. Bang B. G., Foard M. A., and Bang F. B. The effect of vitamin A deficiency and Newcastle disease on lymphoid cell system in chickens. Proc. Soc. Exp. Biol. Med., 143:1140–1146, 1973.

13. Bhaskaram C., and Reddy V. Cell-mediated immunity in iron and vitamin-deficient children. Br. Med. J., 3:522, 1975.

14. Chandra R. K., Heresi G., and Au B. Serum thymic factor activity in deficiencies of calories, zinc, vitamin acid pyridoxine. Clin. Exp. Immunol., 43:332–335, 1980.

15. Nauss K. M., Mark D. A., and Suskind R.M. The effect of vitamin A deficiency on the in vitro cellular immune response of rats. J. Nutr., 109:1815–1823, 1979.

16. Taub R. N., Krantz A. R., and Dresser D. W. The effect of localized injection of adjuvant material on the draining lymph node. I. Histology. Immunology, 18:171–186, 1970.

17. Dresser D. W. Adjuvanticity of vitamin A. Nature (Lond.), 217:527–529, 1968.

18. Allison A. C., and Mallucci L. Lysosomes in dividing cells with special reference to lymphocytes. Lancet, 2:1371–1373, 1964.

19. Kummet T., Moon T. E., and Meyskens F. L. Vitamin A: Evidence for its preventive role in human cancer. Nutr. Cancer, 5:96–106, 1983.

20. Micksche M., Cerni C., Kokron O., Titscher R., and Wrba H. Stimulation of immune response in lung cancer

patients by vitamin A therapy. Oncology, 34:234-238, 1977.

21. Floersheim G. L., and Bollog W. Accelerated rejection of homografts by vitamin A acid. Transplantation, 15:564-567, 1972.

22. Dennert G., and Laton R. Effects of retinoic acid on the immune system: Stimulation of T-killer cell induction. Eur. J. Immunol., 8:23-29, 1978.

23. Dennert G., Crowley C., Douba J., and Lotan R. Retinoic acid stimulation of the induction of mouse killer T-cells in allogenic and syngeneic systems. J. Natl. Cancer Instit., 62:89-94, 1979.

24. Skinnider L. F., and Geisbrecht K. Inhibition of phorbol myristate acetate and phytohemagglutinin stimulation of human lymphocytes by retinol. Cancer Res., 39:3332-3334, 1979.

25. Glaser M., Lotan R. Augmentation of specific tumor immunity against a syngeneic SV40-induced sarcoma in mice by retinoic acid. Cellular Immunol. 45:175-181, 1979.

26. Patek P. Q., Collins J. L., Yogeeswaran G., and Dennert G. Antitumor potential of retinoic acid: Stimulation of immune mediated effectors. Int. J. Cancer, 24:624-628, 1979.

27. Lotan R., and Nicholson G. L. Inhibitory effects of retinoic acid or retinylacetate on the growth of untransformed, transformed and tumor cells in vitro. J. Nat. Cancer Instit., 59:1717-1722, 1977.

28. Dennert G., and Lotan R. Effects of retinoic acid on the immune system: Stimulation of T killer cell induction. Eur. J. Immunol., 8:23-29, 1978.

29. Goldfarb R. H., and Herberman R. B. Natural killer cell reactivity: Regulatory interactions among phorbol ester, interferon, cholera toxin, and retinoic acid. Immunology, 45:2129-2135, 1981.

30. Moriguchi S., Jackson J. C., and Watson R.R. In vitro effects of retinoids on human lymphocyte functions. Human Tox., in press, 1985.

31. Lotan R., and Dennert G. Stimulatory effects of vitamin A analogs on induction of cell-mediated cytotoxicity in vivo. Cancer Res., 39:55-58, 1979.

32. Skinnider L. F., and Giesbrecht K. Inhibition of phorbol myristate acetate and phytohemagglutinin stimulation of human lymphocytes by 13-cis retinoic acid and ethyl etrinoate. Experientia, 37:1345, 1981.

33. Lim T. S., Putt N., Safranski D., Chung C., and Watson
    R. R. Effect of vitamin E on cell-mediated immune
    responses and serum corticosterone in young and
    maturing mice. Immunology, 44:289-295, 1981.
34. Watson R. R. Stress caused by dietary changes:
    Corticosteroid production, a partial explanation for
    immunosuppression in the malnourished. In:
    Malnutrition, Disease Resistance and Immune Function.
    New York: Mercel Dekker, 273-283, 1984.
35. Fusi S., Kupper T.S., Green D.R., and Ariyan S.
    Reversal of postburn immunosuppression by
    administration of vitamin A. Surgery, 96:330-335,
    1984.
36. Cohen B. E., Gill G., Cullen P. R., and Morris P. J.
    Reversal of postoperative immunosuppression in man by
    vitamin A. Surgery Gynec. Obstet., 149:658-662, 1979.
37. Meyskens F. L. Jr., Gilmartin E., Alberts D. S.,
    Levine N. S., Brooks R., Salmon S. E., and Surwit
    E. A. Activity of 13-cis retinoic acid against
    squamous epithelial premalignancies and malignancies.
    Cancer Treat. Rep., 66:1315-1319, 1982.
38. Van Vleet J. F. Current knowledge of selenium-vitamin
    E deficiency in domestic animals. J. Am. Vet. Med.
    Assoc., 176:321, 1980.
39. Heinzering R. H., Nockels C. F., Quarles C. L., and
    Tengerdy R. P. Protection of chicks against E. coli
    infection by dietary supplementation with vitamin E.
    Proc. Soc. Exp. Biol. Med., 146:279-283, 1974.
40. Tenegerdy R. P., Heinzerling, R. H., Brown G. L., and
    Mathias M. M. Enhancement of the humoral immune
    response by vitamin E. Int. Arch. Allergy Appl.
    Immunol., 44:221, 1973.
41. Lim T. S., Putt N., Safranski D., Chung C., and Watson
    R. R. Effect of vitamin E on cell-mediated immune
    responses and serum corticosterone in young and
    maturing mice. Immunology, 44:289-295, 1981.
42. Teige Jr. J., Nordstoga K., and Aursjo J. Influence
    of diet on experimental swine sysentery. 1. Effects
    of a vitamin E and selenium deficient diet
    supplemental with 6.8% cod liver oil. Acta Vet.
    Scand., 18:384-396, 1977.
43. Teige Jr. J., Saxegaard F., and Frooslie A. Influence
    of diet on experimental swine dysentery. 2. Effects
    of vitamin E and selenium deficient diet supplemented
    with 3% cod liver, vitamin E or selenium. Acta Vet.
    Scand., 19:133-146, 1978.

44. Nockels C. F. Protective effects of supplemental vitamin E against infection. Fed. Proc., 38:2134-2138, 1979.

45. Watson R. R., Chung C., and Petro T. M. Resistance to leukemia L-1210 and Listeria monocytogenes growth in mice fed a high vitamin E diet. In Vitamin E: Biochemical, Hematological and Clinical Aspects. New York Academy of Sciences, New York, 393:205-209, 1982.

46. Watson R. R., and Messiha N. Enhancement of IgA in intestinal secretions and antibody dependent cellular cytotoxicity in intestinal mucosal cells of mice fed a high vitamin E diet. (Submitted for publication)

47. Corwin L. M., and Schloss J. Influences of vitamin E on the mitogenic response of murine lymphoid cells. J. Nutr., 110:916-923, 1980.

48. Likeoff R. O., Guptill D. R., Lawrence L. M., McKay C. C., Mathias M. M., Nockels C. F., and Tenegerdy R. P. Vitamin E and aspirin depress prostaglandins in protection of chickens against Escherichia coli infection. Am. J. Clin. Nutr., 34:245-251, 1981.

49. Tanaka J., Fujiwara H., and Torisu M. Vitamin E and immune response. Enhancement of helper T cell activity by dietary supplementation of vitamin E in mice. Immunology, 38:727-734, 1979.

50. Prasad J.S. Effect of vitamin E supplementation on leukocyte function. Am. J. Clin. Nutr., 33:606-608, 1980.

51. Yasunaga T., Kato H., Ohgaki K., Inamoto T., and Hikasa Y. Effect of vitamin E as an immunopotentiation agent for mice at optimal dosage and its toxicity at high dosage. J. Nutr., 112:1075-1084, 1982.

52. Chen L. H. An increase in vitamin E requirement induced by high supplementation of vitamin C in rats. Am. J. Clin. Nutr., 34:1036-1041, 1981.

CLINICAL TRIALS AND IN VITRO STUDIES OF

13 CIS RETINOIC ACID IN THE

MYELODYSPLASTIC SYNDROME

Emmanuel C. Besa[1], Martin Hyzinski[2], Peter Nowell[3], Janet Abrahm[2]
Department of Medicine, Section of Hematology-Oncology of Medical College of Pennsylvania[1], Philadelphia Veterans Administration Medical Center[2], and Department of Pathology and Laboratory Medicine of the University of Pennsylvania School of Medicine [3], Philadelphia, Pennsylvania.

The myelodysplastic syndrome (MDS) occurs in a heterogenous group of patients with varying degrees of cytopenia and an associated morphologic change in their peripheral blood and bone marrow cells which indicate an abnormality in cellular maturation. This condition is also considered to be a pre-leukemic state because of the tendency to progress into acute myelogenous leukemia in approximately 40% of the patients. A significant number of these patients succumb to the complications of bone marrow failure such as infection and hemorrhage from the resulting cytopenia. Currently, there is no satisfactory specific therapy available for MDS.

Retinoic acids have been shown to induce differentiation in a human promyelocytic leukemia cell line (1), inhibit clonal growth of other human myeloid leukemic cells (2), and to enhance normal erythroid (3) and myeloid (4) progenitor cell responses to stimulating factors in vitro. A phase 1 clinical study using 13 cis retinoic acid (13

CRA) in MDS patients indicated some clinical benefit (5).

This report presents the results of our current clinical trial of 13-cis retinoic acid in MDS patients. In addition it includes our preliminary in vitro studies which were initiated to determine whether the marrow culture growth pattern could predict the patient's clinical response and whether we could elucidate the mechanism of action of 13 CRA therapy in the responding patients.

Patients and Methods

Twenty four patients with MDS using the French-American-British (FAB) criteria and classification (6) were entered into a 13 CRA at 100 mg/m^2 with the resultant classification distribution: 1 patient with refractory anemia (RA), 10 patients with refractory anemia with excess blast (RAEB), 1 patient with refractory anemia with excess blast in transformation (RAEBIT), 9 patients with idiopathic acquired sideroblastic anemia (IASA), and 2 patients with chronic myelo-monocytic leukemia (CMML). One patient had malignant myelofibrosis following adjuvant chemotherapy with cyclophosphamide, 5 fluoro-uracil and methotrexate for breast cancer. The initial 12 patients received 13 CRA and the rest were randomized in a double-blind fashion against a placebo for 6 months. Three patients received corticosteroids concomitantly with 13 CRA in the initial studies and were excluded in the randomized study. Parallel studies with hydrocortisone and dexamethasone in the in vitro studies were done because of these patients.

Marrow Culture:
Marrow was obtained from normal donors (7) and patients enrolled in the clinical trial of 13 cis retinoic acid therapy (8) with their informed consent. Ficoll-Paque inter-face cells from the marrow aspirates were

placed into duplicate or triplicate semisolid agar cultures as previously described (8) and into quadruplicate methylcellulose cultures prepared using a modification of the method of Worton (7) and Iscove (9). Medium conditioned by normal human peripheral blood leukocytes exposed to 1% v/v PHA according to the method of Aye (10) served as the source of Granulocyte-Monocyte colony stimulating factor. The medium was shown to be most active undiluted. Hydrocortisone sodium succinate ($5 \times 10-5$ to $10-6M$), dexamethasone ($10-7$ to $10-5M$) and 13 cis retinoic acid ($10-9$ to $5 \times 10-6M$) were included in the stimulating material alone and in combination in some dishes. Drug concentrations are those achieved in vivo by oral administration (11-14). At the end of 10-14 days incubation, the agar cultures were fixed, transferred to glass slides and histochemically stained for chloroacetate and alpha napthyl acetate esterases as previously described (8). Colonies were considered granulocytic if more than 90% of the cells in the colony contained chloroacetate esterase, monocytic if more than 90% of the colony cells contained alpha napthyl acetate esterase and mixed if neither enzyme predominated by 90%.

Chromosome Studies
a) Marrow aspirates
Bone marrow specimens were processed on the day of aspiration and after 24 hours in culture and stained by the Trypsin-Giemsa banding method as described (15). For each study, a total of 18-38 chromosome counts were done with a least 3 karyotype analyses. Periodically, studies were repeated to determine the effects of therapy on the karyotype abnormality.

Table I - <u>Clinical Characteristics of the</u>
<u>24 Patients with MDS on the 13 CRA Trial</u>

	Non-Randomized	Randomized
Median Age: (range)	63 (44-78)	65 (57-88)
Sex:(male/female)	9/3	7/5
FAB Classification		
RA		1
RAEB	6	4
RAEBIT		1
IASA	5	4
CMML		2
Others	1	
"de Novo"	9	12
Post Chemotherapy	3	0
Treatment:		
13 CRA	12	6
Placebo	0	6
Chromosomes		
Normal	2	6
Abnormal	9	5
Unsuccessful	1	1
Hematologic Problems		
Anemia Alone	2	4
Bicytopenia	3	4
Pancytopenia	7	3
High WBC	–	1

b) In Vitro Culture

On day 8 or 9 of culture, individual plucked colonies or the entire culture dish were washed free of methylcellulose in Hank's Balanced Salt solution (GIBCO), placed into hypotonic solution and further processed by standard methods for chromosome analysis (16).

Statistical Methods

Student T-test for paired samples was used.

Results

The clinical characteristics of the 24 MDS patients are summarized in Table I. The initial non-randomized patients were more severely affected with pancytopenia (62 vs 25%), and more patients had abnormal karyotypes detected in their bone marrow cells (75 vs 42%) compared to the randomized patients. Three patients in the initial group were previously exposed to cytotoxic chemotherapeutic agents.

Clinical Outcome in the Clinical Trial of 13 CRA in MDS:

There were 2 early deaths occurring in the severely affected non-randomized group and only 3 of the 12 patients completed 6 months of therapy. Three of the patients in the randomized study who received a placebo dropped out because of non-specific symptoms which the patient attributed to the drug in 2 and the other because of progression of RAEBIT into acute leukemia within the first 3 weeks of therapy. The hematologic response and clinical outcome of the MDS patients in the two trials are summarized in table 2.

A complete response to 13 CRA in a patient with RAEB occurred after 6 months of therapy with disappearance of the morphologic cellular abnormalities in the peripheral blood and bone marrow in the initial study (17). A gradual decrease in the percentage of marrow cells bearing an abnormal karyotype occurred finally resulting in a cytogenetic remission. The patient had a hematologic and cytogenetic relapse 6 months after 13 CRA was discontinued and was again treated with the same dose of 13 CRA and the patient is again clinically stable

Table 2 - Hematologic Response and Clinical Outcome of 13 CRA in MDS

	Non Randomized	Randomized Placebo	13 CRA
Duration of Therapy:			
$\leq$ 1 mo.	2	3	0
$\leq$ 6 mo.	7	1	2
$>$ 6 mo.	3	2	4
Hematologic Response:			
Complete response	1	0	1
Partial response	1	0	2
Increased neutrophils	7		1
Increased platelets	1		1
Clinical Outcome:			
Clinically Well	1	0	1
Stable Disease	2	1	4
Progression of Disease	7	2	1
Early Death	2	2	0
Causes of Death:			
Total No.	11/12	3/6	1/6
Sepsis	4	1	1
Hemorrhage	3	1	0
Transformation to Leukemia	5	1	0

with improvement of the bone marrow cellularity. Another patient went into complete
remission on the 8th month of 13 CRA after
continuation of treatment when she entered a
partial remission at 6th week.

Three patients had partial responses
which lasted from 2 to 5 months. One patient
died from sepsis and hemorrhage after recurrence of severe pancytopenia. The other 2
patients however returned to stable but
transfusion dependent state.

Half of the patients (3/6) who received
the placebo had died within the first 6 months
of the study and only 1 remains in stable
condition while only 1 of 6 patients who
received 13 CRA progressed and died.

Side Effects of 13 CRA in MDS patients:

All patients that received 13 CRA had
dryness and hyperkeratosis of the skin of
varying severity and cheilosis. The other
symptoms such as conjunctivitis (30%), nasal
mucositis (20%) and vaginitis (10%) of
moderate severity improved after a decrease in
13 CRA dosage. Gradual return to full doses
were tolerated well. Elevation of the fasting
cholesterol and triglycerides were observed in
a third of the patients on 13 CRA. Two
patients complained of headaches, fever and
diarrhea during the first week of therapy in
the placebo group and these patients requested
to be removed from the study.

In Vitro studies:

Response of normal marrow to incubation
with Hydrocortisone, dexamethasone or 13 Cis

Retinoic Acid:

Figure 1 illustrates the effect of incubation with various concentrations of hydrocortisone and dexamethasone on the type of colony that develops in marrow cultures from normal donors. While the total number of colonies is unchanged, both drugs induce a mild inhibition of monocyte colony development (p=.006). When retinoic acid was added to the cultures, there was total inhibition of monocyte colonies in all conditions studied except $10-6M$ hydrocortisone (data not shown).

Figure 1 also illustrates the effect of retinoic acid concentration on the type of colony grown from normal donor marrows. As can be seen, in the range of retinoic acid con-centrations usually achieved by oral administration on the schedule used in the clinical trial, the percentage of colonies that are monocytic is significantly decreased (p<.01). The total number of colonies was not significantly changed in this set of experiments, though the number of clusters not containing either type of esterase was increased at retinoic acid concentrations of > $10-6M$ (data not shown).

Response of marrow from patients with myelodysplastic syndrome to incubation with hydrocortisone, dexamethasone or 13 cis retinoic acid:
Table 3 details the in vitro marrow growth patterns and the clinical response of the 7 MDS patients studied to date. Five patients were studied prior to study entry, one (AC) was studied while in clinical remission receiving 13 cis retinoic acid and one (JL) was studied on multiple occasions. Marrows from three of the five patients sampled prior

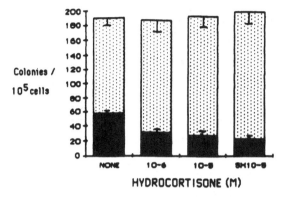

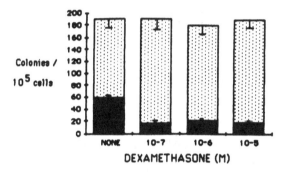

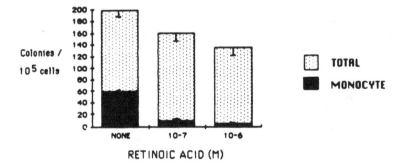

Figure 1. The effects of various concentrations of hydrocortisone (upper panel), dexamethasone (middle panel) and
retinoic acid (lower panel) on the total and monocytic
colony growth from normal marrows. Numbers are means of
duplicate studies from 8 normal donors.

Table 3 - MDS Patients Clinical Response
and Marrow Culture Results

Patient	Diagnosis†	Clinical Response	Marrow Growth*
VZ	RAEB	Worse	None
JG	AISA	Unchanged	None
MH	AISA	Worse	None
MC	CMML	Partial Remission	29 Colonies
AC	RAEB	Clinical Remission	24 Colonies
JL	RAEB	Unchanged	60 Colonies
LC	AISA	Died of Leukemia	39 Colonies

Mean Colony Number: Normals 190+/-24
                      Patients 38+/-8

---

* Greatest number of colonies that could be proven under any of the culture conditions.
† RAEB = refractory anemia excess blasts; AISA = acquired idiopathic sideroblastic anemia; CMML = chronic myelomonocytic leukemia.

---

to study entry failed to grow in vitro. All of these patients had abnormal chromosomes and responded clinically to the drug.

Marrows from the other four grew significantly fewer colonies than did the 7 normal donor marrows grown at the same time (mean colony number 38 +/-8 for the patients, 190 +/-24 for the normals). The colony type (ie granulocyte, monocyte or mixed) of the patients, including the two patients receiving retinoic acid at the time they were studied,

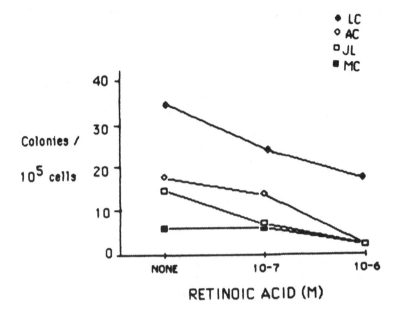

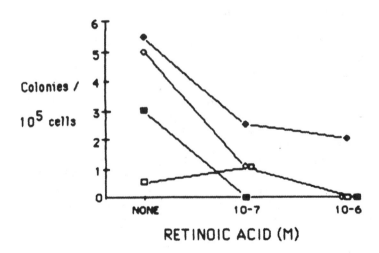

Figure 2. The effects of retinoic acid at concentrations achievable by oral administration on the total number (upper panel) and monocytic colony number (lower panel) in marrow from 4 MDS patients. Initials refer to individual donors. Points represent average of triplicate samples.

did not differ significantly from that of the normal donors.

One patient (MC) demonstrated a 2 fold increase in granulocyte colonies in the presence of either hydrocortisone or dexamethasone, and a 4 fold increase when 10-7M retinoic acid was also included (data not shown). This patient has achieved a partial response to 13 CRA but the patient was not treated with corticosteroids and the predictive value of this observation is not known. None of the patients was "steroid responsive" by the Bagby criteria (18,19).

However, as shown in Figure 2, all patient marrows were more sensitive to low doses of 13 cis retinoic acid than were normals. Also shown in Fig. 2, 10-7M RA halved or eliminated monocyte colony growth in patients, and 10-6M inhibited all GM-CFU growth in 3 of the 4. The marrow of patient JL contained an abnormal clone marked by the chromosomal rearrangement [t(2;11)]. He had had a complete clinical remission while receiving 13 cis retinoic acid and then had been taken off the drug. In vitro studies during remission were indistinguishable from those of other patients. When he developed a clinical relapse and was restarted on 13 cis retinoic acid, this clone became apparent in 100% of his marrow metaphases. In vitro studieswere repeated at this time. The patient's marrow cells were washed free of serum andany drugs the serum contained prior to being placed in agar culture. When the marrow cells were stimulated by colony stimulating factor, 100% of the colonies growing were monocytoid (ie they stained for alpha napthyl acetate esterase) and chromosome studies of the cultures indicated the presence

of the [t(2;11) translocation in vitro.
Furtherthe clone was not inhibited by the
inclusion either of hydrocortisone or dexamethasone. 13 cis retinoic acid, added in
vitro in concentrations he was receiving in
vivo, however, completely inhibited clonal
growth. Clinically, the patient achieved a
stabilization on the drug with a decrease in
marrow hypercellularity and percent of
myeloblasts.

Discussion

        Our clinical trials confirm the initial
observation that certain patients with MDS
could benefit from treatment with 13 CRA. The
achievement of a complete response without
marrow hypoplasia and a cytogenetic remission
in one patient is certainly a unique observation in the treatment of MDS. A significant
clinical response usually does not occur
within the first two months so that severely
affected patients or MDS patients on the verge
of transformation may not benefit from this
therapy. Relapse of the condition after
discontinuation of 13 CRA may indicate the
need for some form of maintenance therapy. The
disappearance of an abnormal chromosome is
useful in determining the completeness of the
response.

        We have found, as have others who have
studied much larger numbers of patients (22)
that the marrow of about half the patients
with myelodysplastic syndrome fails to grow in
standard in vitro agar or methylcellulose
cultures. We too have found the number of
colonies is less for the patients than the
normals. With the smaller number of patients
we have studied to date, we cannot yet suggest
that the lack of in vitro growth in patients

with abnormal chromosomes is a bad prognostic
feature, since it has not been noted by others
(22), but we will continue to monitor this as
the number of patients studied increases.

     None of the other marrow culture studies
of patients with myelodysplastic syndrome
have analyzed colony type. We found the type
of colony growth and the pattern of response
to retinoic acid to be similar in patients and
controls, though patients' abnormal marrow
cells were more sensitive to the toxic effects
of the retinoic acid.

     Thus with the small number of patients
studied to date, no assessment can be made as
to whether in vitro growth patterns of marrows
of patients with myelodysplastic syndrome will
predict clinical response to 13 cis retinoic
acid.   Studies of 12 other patients are
currently in progress and we hope to continue
to increase our experience in this area.

     Studies of patient JL who relapsed and
then achieved a new clinical stability when
the drug was restarted suggest a possible
mechanism of action for the drug. In vitro
studies showed that proliferation of his
abnormal monocytoid clone was completely
inhibited by concentrations of retinoic acid
he was receiving in vivo. It may be that
abnormal clones of cells that produce monocyte
colonies may have the same sensitivity to
retinoic acid as can be demonstrated in
monocyte colony progenitor cells in normal
marrows. Studies of other patients with
similar clinical courses and clonal chromosomal markers will be required to further
evaluate this hypothesis.

REFERENCES

1. Breitman TR, Collins SJ, Keene BR. Terminal differentiation of human promyelocytic cells in primary culture in response to retinoic acid. Blood 57:1000-1004, 1981.
2. Douer D, Koeffler P. Inhibition of the clonal growth of human myeloid leukemia cells. J Clin Invest 69: 277-283, 1982.
3. Douer D, Koeffler HP. Retinoic acid enhances growth of human early erythroid progenitor cells in vitro. J Clin Invest 69: 1039, 1982.
4. Douer D, Koeffler HP. Retinoic acid enhances colony-stimulating factor induced clinical growth of normal human myeloid progenitor cells in vitro. Exp Cell Res 138: 193-198, 1982.
5. Gold EJ, Mertelsmann RH, Itri LM, Gee T, Arlin Z, Kempin S, Clarkson B, Moore MAS. Phase-1 clinical trial of 13 cis retinoic acid in myelo-dysplastic syndrome. Cancer Treatment Reports 67: 981-986, 1983.
6. Bennett JM, Catovski D, Daniel MT, Flandrin G, Galton DAG, Gralnick HR, Salton C. The French-American-British (FAB) Cooperative Group: Proposals for the classification of the myelodysplastic syndromes. Brit J Haematol 51: 189-199, 1982.
7. Worton RG, McCullough EA, Till JE. Physical separation of hematopoietic stem cells forming colonies in culture. J Cell Physiol 74: 171-182, 1969.
8. Abrahm JL, Smiley R. Modification of normal human myelopoiesis by 12-0-tetradecanoyl-phorbol-13-acetate (TPA). Blood 58: 1119-1126, 1981.
9. Iscove NN, Sieber F, Winterhalter KH. Erythroid colony formation in cultures of mouse and human bone marrow. Analysis of the requirement for erythropoietin by gel filtration and affinity

chromatography on Agarose-Conconavalin A. J Cell
Physiol 83: 309-320, 1973.

10.Aye MT, Niho Y, Till JE, McCulloch EA.
Studies of leukemic cell populations in culture.
Blood 44: 205-219, 1974.

11.Claman HN.   Corticosteroids and lymphoid
cells. New Eng J Med 287: 388-397, 1972.

12.Duggan DE, Yeh KC, Matalia N, Ditzier CA,
McMahon FG. Bioavailability of oral dexamethasone. Clin Pharm and Therapeutics 18:
205-209, 1975.

13.Brophy TR O'R, McCafferty J, Tyrer JH,
Eadie MJ. Bioavailability of oral dexamethasone
during high dose steroid therapy in neuro-
logical patients.   Eur J Clin Pharmacol 24:
103-108, 1983.

14.Kerr IG, Lippman ME, Jenkins J, Myers CE.
Pharmacology of 13 cis retinoic acid in humans.
Cancer Research 42:2069-2073, 1982.

15.Seabright M. A rapid banding technique for
human chromosomes. Lancet 2: 971-972, 1971.

16.Dube ID, Eaves CJ, Kalousek DK, Eaves AC.
A method for obtaining high quality chromosome
preparations from single hemopoietic colonies
on a routine basis. Cancer Genetics and Cyto-
genetics 4: 157-168, 1981.

17.Besa EC, Granick JL, Itri L, Nowell PC.
Complete hematologic and cytogenetic remission
in a patient with dysmyelopoietic syndrome
treated with 13 cis retinoic acid. Blood 62:
199a, 1983.

18.Bagby GC.   Mechanisms of glucocortico-
steroid activity in patients with the
preleukemic syndrome (Hemopoietic dysplasia).
Leuk Res 4: 571-580, 1980.

19.Bagby GC.   Glucocorticoid therapy in the
preleukemic syndrome (Hemopoietic dysplasia).
Ann Intern Med 92: 55-58, 1980.

20.Koeppler H, Robinson WA. 13 cis retinoic
acid enhances granulocyte-monocyte colony
formation in vitro by normal human bone

marrow. Blood 58 (suppl. 1): 112a, 1981.
21.Asmar S, Beranek M, Herzig, G. Retinoic
    acid stimulates growth and affects differ-
    entiation of normal human myeloid precursors.
    Clin Res 31: 308A, 1983.
22.Bailey-Wood R, May S, Jacobs A. The effect
    of retinoids on CFU-GM from normal subjects
    and patients with myelodysplastic syndrome.
    Br J Hematol 59: 15-20, 1985.
23.Abrahm JL, Colucci A. 13 cis retinoic acid and
    dimethylsulfoxide inhibit monocyte differentiation
    of normal human colony forming units-culture.
    Blood 58 (Suppl. 1): 104a, 1981.

EXPERIENCE WITH RETINOIDS AS PREVENTION AND TREATMENT FOR HUMAN CANCERS

Frank L. Meyskens, Jr., M.D.

Arizona Cancer Center

Tucson, Arizona

INTRODUCTION

In laboratory studies retinoids have potent effects as inhibitors of carcinogenesis at the promotion phase and are stimulators of differentiation and maturation and growth inhibitors of established tumor cells in vitro (9,14). Additionally, epidemiological data in general supports the contention that vitamin A is a natural inhibitor (anti-promoter) of many human cancers (6,7). Early data suggested that vitamin A was necessary for normal epithelial cell maturation and limited studies over a decade ago suggested that retinoic acid was growth inhibitory to human skin cancers (2). These observations have prompted us to study retinoids in the prevention and treatment of human cancer and the results from these studies are summarized here.

PREVENTION

We have suggested that prevention of human cancers can be divided into three distinct phases: primary, secondary and tertiary (10). Primary prevention seeks to obviate contact with the proximate carcinogen - such as cessation of smoking or use of sunscreens. Secondary prevention has as its goal the supplementation of an antipromoter in individuals already exposed to the carcinogen. Examples would include correction of vitamin or multinutrient deficiencies in individuals at high risk for cancer or supplementation with natural or synthetic antipromoters.

We have sponsored two trials of secondary chemoprevention of skin cancer and these are diagrammatically
summarized in Table 1. Both studies are directed by Drs.
Moon and Levine and use different populations of patients
at risk for skin cancer. The first group must have had 8
or greater prior actinic keratoses and is at relatively
low risk for a subsequent actinic keratoses (10%/year) or
basal/squamous cell skin carcinoma (2-3%/year). Participants will be carefully stratified and randomized to placebo
or retinol (25,000 I.U. qd) and over 2,300 participants
will be required to assure meaningful results in a real
time frame. The second group of participants is at a
later phase of cutaneous carcinogenesis, requiring a prior
history of 8 resected squamous/basal cell carcinomas prior
to entry into study. These patients have a high risk of
subsequent cutaneous cancer, occurring at a rate of 60-100%/
year. Participants will be carefully stratified and randomized to placebo, retinol (25,000 I.U. qd), or 13 cis-
retinoic acid (0.10mg/kg po qd). Only 300 patients will
need to be accrued to be able to show significance between
the three groups.

Tertiary prevention has as its goal reversal of an
established preneoplastic focus such as leukoplakia or
cervical dysplasia. We have done extensive phase I and II
studies of the effects of vitamin A acid (β-trans retinoic
acid) delivered locally to the preneoplastic cervix (13,
15). The results from these studies are summarized in
Table 2. Our pre-phase I studies showed that a cervical
cap was a more effective delivery device than a diaphragm
and that a cream base was the most easily of the various
carrying vehicles delivered. Using a molded cervical cap
a formal phase I investigation was conducted and based on
side effects a concentration of 0.32% retinoic acid was
determined as the dose for phase II studies. In the phase
II trials a 50% response rate was seen in the 18 evaluable
patients treated. Based on these encouraging results, a
phase III study in patients with moderate and severe
dysplasia is planned. Three hundred patients will be
randomized between placebo cream and retinoic acid and
followed for several years thereafter.

TREATMENT

We have tested the activity of oral systemic 13 cis-
retinoic acid on tumor response in over 240 patients with

cancer who were not receiving concomitant therapy. These
results are summarized in Table 3 and detailed elsewhere
(1,3,4,5,8,11). No activity was seen in patients with
cancers of the breast, bladder, cervix, colon, stomach,
soft tissue, bone, pancreas or lymph glands. Minor activity was seen in 1 of 2 patients with esophageal cancer, 2
mixed responses in 22 patients with non-small cell lung
cancer, and one partial response in a patient with ovarian
cancer. In 16 patients with various myelodysplastic syndromes, three exhibited minor improvements in hematopoesis,
a result also reported by others.

Substantial activity was seen against patients with
advanced head and neck cancer, and melanoma. Partial
responses of subcutaneous and skin sites were seen in 3
patients with head and neck cancers. In 20 patients with
metastatic melanoma skin/subcutaneous responses were seen
in 3 patients and in one case pulmonary nodules responded
also. We have also seen disappearance of β-HCG in 2 of 5
women with persistent choriocarcinoma.

Highly significant responses were seen in three conditions: dysplastic nevi, laryngeal papillomatosis and
mycosis fungoides. These responses are detailed elsewhere,
but in brief summary dysplastic nevi were treated by local
application of retinoic acid in 3 patients and in all cases
complete responses were seen (8). We have also treated 6
patients with severe refractory laryngeal papillomatosis
with oral 13 cis-retinoic acid. Three sustained complete
responses were obtained, with 2 patients off therapy for
greater than one year (1). Others have also demonstrated
the responsiveness of this entity to retinoids. The most
striking responses have been in patients with the cutaneous
T-cell lymphoma mycosis fungoides (4). Of 18 evaluable
patients, 9 substantial partial responses were seen with a
median duration of responses of six months. In one case
the response lasted for over 30 months.

FUTURE STUDIES

Maturation of results from the two current secondary
prevention of skin cancer trials will be required before
combination studies are entertained. The results from the
randomized phase III trials will also be eagerly awaited.
A major consideration is whether a prevention trial in
patients with dysplastic nevus syndrome is presently

warranted. Since the data is presently limited to 3
patients treated by local application of retinoic acid, a
formal phase II trial using oral systemic 13 cis-retinoic
acid will be conducted in 14 patients with severe dysplastic nevus syndrome.

Based on our results and those of others, large randomized trials of placebo versus oral 13 cis-retinoic acid
are being conducted in patients with laryngeal papillomatosis, surgically cured high risk head and neck cancer,
and stage I cutaneous malignant melanoma. The effects of
retinol in both stage I and II cutaneous melanoma are also
being studied in randomized trials.

Another potential avenue of exploration is combining
13 cis-retinoic acid with other biological modifiers, such
as interferon, or with cytotoxic drugs.

Acknowledgement. I thank various colleagues for participating in these studies (particularly D. Alberts, R. Dorr,
D. Earnest, N. Levine, T. Moon, R. Watson, B. Greenberg,
S. Jones, J. Kessler, T. Miller and S. Salmon) and also
Karla Ramos for typing the manuscript. Supported in part
by the National Cancer Institute (CA 27502, CM-NO 17500)
and Hoffman LaRoche, Inc. (Nutley, N.J.).

LITERATURE CITED

1.   Alberts, D.S., Coulthard, S.W., Meyskens, F.L., Jr.
      Regression of aggressive laryngeal papillomatosis with
      13-cis-retinoic acid (Accutane[R]). Arch. Otolog., in
      press, 1985.
2.   Bollag, W., Ott, F. Vitamin A acid in benign and
      malignant epithelial tumors of the skin. Acta Dermat.,
      74:163-166, 1975.
3.   Greenberg, B.R., Durie, B.G.M., CoBarnett, T., and
      Meyskens, F.L., Jr. Phase II study of 13-cis-retinoic
      acid (Isotretinoin) in myelodysplastic disorders.
      Cancer Treat. Rep., submitted, 1984.
4.   Kessler, J.F., Levine, N., Meyskens, F.L., Jr., Lynch,
      P.J., and Jones, S.E. Treatment of cutaneous T-cell
      lymphoma (mycosis fungoides) with 13-cis-retinoic
      acid. The Lancet, pp. 1345-1348, June 18, 1983.
5.   Kessler, J.F., Meyskens, F.L., Jr. Clinical results
      with retinoids as preventive and therapeutic anti-

cancer agents. In: Prasad, K.N. (ed) <u>Vitamins and Cancer</u>, (Karger, Basel), in press, 1985.

6. Kummet, T. and Meyskens, F.L., Jr. Vitamin A: a potential inhibitor of human cancer. Sem. Oncol., 10:281-289, 1983.

7. Kummet, T., Moon, T.E., and Meyskens, F.L., Jr. Vitamin A: evidence for its preventive role in human cancer. Nutrition and Cancer, 5:96-106, 1983.

8. Levine, N., Edwards, L., and Meyskens, F.L., Jr. Topical retinoic acid therapy for multiple dysplastic nevi. In preparation.

9. Lotan, R. Effects of vitamin A and its analogs (retinoids) on normal and neoplastic cells. Biochem. Biophy. Acta, 605:33-91, 1980.

10. Meyskens, F.L., Jr. Prevention and treatment of cancer with vitamin A and the retinoids. In: Prasad, K.N. (ed) <u>Vitamins, Nutrition and Cancer</u>, (Karger, Basel), pp. 266-273, 1984.

11. Meyskens, F.L., Jr., Gilmartin, E., Alberts, D.S., Levine, N.S., Brooks, R., Salmon, S.E., and Surwit, E.A. Activity of Isotretinoin against squamous cell cancers and preneoplastic lesions. Cancer Treat. Rep., 66:1315-1319, 1982.

12. Meyskens, F.L., Jr., Goodman, G.E., and Alberts, D.S. 13-cis-retinoic acid: pharmacology, toxicology and clinical applications for the prevention and treatment of human cancer. Critical Reviews in Hematology/ Oncology, in press, 1985.

13. Meyskens, F.L., Jr., Graham, V., Chvapil, M., Dorr, R.T., Alberts, D.S., and Surwit, E.A. A phase I trial of β-all-trans-retinoic acid for mild or moderate intraepithelial cervical neoplasia delivered via a collagen sponge and cervical cap. J. Natl. Cancer Inst., 71:921-925, 1983.

14. Sporn, M.B., Dunlap, N.M., Newton, D.L., and Smith, J.M. Prevention of chemical carcinogenesis by vitamin A and its synthetic analogs. Fed. Proc., 35:1332-1338, 1976.

15. Surwit, E.A., Graham, V., Droegemueller, W., Chvapil, M., Dorr, R.T., Davis, J.R., and Meyskens, F.L., Jr. Evaluation of topically applied trans-retinoic acid

in the treatment of cervical intraepithelial lesions.
Am. J. Obst. Gyn., 143:821-823, 1982.

TABLE 1

SECONDARY CHEMOPREVENTION OF HUMAN SKIN CANCER

EARLY CARCINOGENESIS

DISEASE - ACTINIC KERATOSIS

NUMBER   2300 PARTICIPANTS
              22 DERMATOLOGISTS

SCHEMA

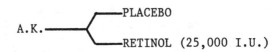

LATE CARCINOGENESIS

DISEASE - AT LEAST 8 PRIOR BASAL OR SQUAMOUS CELL
                    CARCINOMA OF SKIN

NUMBER   300 PARTICIPANTS
              22 DERMATOLOGISTS

SCHEMA

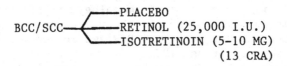

TABLE 2

TERTIARY CHEMOPREVENTION OF CERVICAL

DYSPLASIA WITH LOCAL β-ALL TRANS RETINOIC ACID

<u>PHASE I TRIAL(S)</u>
- CERVICAL CAP BEST DELIVERY DEVICE
- CONCENTRATION 0.372%

<u>PHASE II TRIAL</u>
- 50% COMPLETE RESPONSE

TABLE 3

TRIALS WITH SYSTEMIC ORAL ISOTRETINOIN

(13 CIS-RETINOIC ACID) IN ADVANCED CANCERS

NO ACTIVITY

DISEASE	NUMBER OF EVALUABLE PATIENTS
BREAST	11
BLADDER	5
CERVIX	5
COLON	17
GASTRIC	2
SARCOMA	10
PANCREATIC	4
LYMPHOMA	4

MINOR ACTIVITY		NUMBER OF RESPONSES
ESOPHAGEAL	2	1 MINOR
LUNG (NON-SC)	22	2 MIXED
OVARIAN	15	1 PR
MYELODYSPLASTIC SYNDROME	16	3 PR

SUBSTANTIAL ACTIVITY

HEAD/NECK	19	3 PR
MELANOMA	20	2 PR, 1 MR
CHORIOCARCINOMA (FEMALE, MINIMAL DISEASE)	5	2 CR

HOME RUNS

DYSPLASTIC NEVUS SYNDROME	3	3 CR
LARYNGEAL PAPILLOMATOSIS	6	3 CR
MYCOSIS FUNGOIDES	18	9 PR, 2 MINOR

INDEX